Teen Health Series
Diet Information for Teens
Drug Information for Teens
Mental Health Information
  for Teens
Sexual Health Information
  for Teens

Pain
SOURCEBOOK

Second Edition

Health Reference Series

Second Edition

Pain
SOURCEBOOK

*Basic Consumer Health Information about
Specific Forms of Acute and Chronic Pain,
Including Muscle and Skeletal Pain, Nerve Pain,
Cancer Pain, and Disorders Characterized
by Pain, Such as Fibromyalgia, Shingles,
Angina, Arthritis, and Headaches*

*Along with Information about Pain Medications
and Management Techniques, Complementary and
Alternative Pain Relief Options, Tips for People
Living with Chronic Pain, a Glossary, and a
Directory of Sources for Further Information*

Edited by
Karen Bellenir

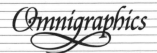

615 Griswold Street • Detroit, MI 48226

Bibliographic Note

Because this page cannot legibly accommodate all the copyright notices, the Bibliographic Note portion of the Preface constitutes an extension of the copyright notice.

Edited by Karen Bellenir

Health Reference Series

Karen Bellenir, *Managing Editor*
David A. Cooke, MD, *Medical Consultant*
Elizabeth Barbour, *Permissions Associate*
Dawn Matthews, *Verification Assistant*
Carol Munson, *Permissions Assistant*
Laura Pleva, *Index Editor*
EdIndex, Services for Publishers, *Indexers*

* * *

Omnigraphics, Inc.

Matthew P. Barbour, *Senior Vice President*
Kay Gill, *Vice President — Directories*
Kevin Hayes, *Operations Manager*
David P. Bianco, *Marketing Consultant*

* * *

Peter E. Ruffner, *President and Publisher*

Frederick G. Ruffner, Jr., *Chairman*

Copyright © 2002 Omnigraphics, Inc.

ISBN 0-7808-0612-3

Library of Congress Cataloging-in-Publication Data

Pain sourcebook : basic consumer health information about specific forms of acute and chronic pain, including muscle and skeletal pain, nerve pain, cancer pain, and disorders characterized by pain, such as fibromyalgia, shingles, angina, arthritis, and headaches; along with information about pain medications and management techniques, complementary and alternative pain relief options, tips for people living with chronic pain, a glossary, and a directory of sources for further information / edited by Karen Bellenir.-- 2nd ed.
    p. cm.-- (Health reference series; 104)
  ISBN 0-7808-0612-3 (lib.bdg.: alk. paper)
  1. Pain--Popular works. I. Bellenir, Karen. II. Series.

RB127 .P346 2002
616'.0472--dc21

                                     20020266221

Table of Contents

Part III: Pain Management

Part IV: Living with Pain

Part V: Pain Research

Part VI: Additional Help and Information

Preface

About This Book

The problem of pain is virtually universal. Almost everyone experiences it at one time or another. It is also a costly malady. For example:

- Every year in the United States, low-back pain accounts for 93 million lost work days and costs more than $5 billion in healthcare.

- An estimated 40 million Americans suffer chronic headaches. This includes migraine sufferers who lose 65 million workdays each year.

- Arthritis affects 20 million Americans and costs an estimated $4 billion each year in lost income, productivity, and healthcare.

People with pain problems often feel isolated and sometimes hopeless, but many who suffer can be helped. Treatment options for pain relief have become more varied over the past several decades as researchers have discovered more about how the brain functions and how pain-relievers work. Additionally, alternative therapies, including acupuncture, biofeedback, and hypnosis have joined the pain relief arsenal.

Pain Sourcebook, Second Edition, updates the first edition, which was published in 1998. It provides basic consumer health information on the nature and mechanism of pain and gives attention to common complaints associated with pain. It offers practical help for living with pain and reports on research initiatives into the causes and treatment of pain. A glossary of pain-related terms, a directory of resources, and other helps to guide pain patients seeking relief are also included.

How to Use This Book

This book is divided into parts and chapters. Parts focus on broad areas of interest. Chapters are devoted to single topics within a part.

Part I: Pain summarizes what is currently known about pain. It describes theories about the origins of pain, the differences in pain perception between men and women, and the varying experiences of pain in infants, children, and the elderly.

Part II: Types of Pain and Disorders Characterized by Pain provides details about some of the most common diseases and disorders that underlie chronic and acute pain. These include arthritis, back pain, cancer pain, carpal tunnel syndrome, fibromyalgia, headache, kidney stones, phantom pain, shingles, and many others.

Part III: Pain Management offers facts about various strategies used to manage pain. It describes frequently used medications, examines the question of addiction to narcotic pain relievers, and provides facts about some newer pharmaceutical products. Frequently used non-drug alternatives and adjuncts, including acupuncture, biofeedback, hypnosis, and massage, are also described.

Part IV: Living with Pain explains strategies used for coping with chronic pain and offers information about concerns related to pain patients' daily lives, including potential adverse effects of pain medications, alcohol-medication interactions, depression, and emotional well being.

Part V: Pain Research gives updates on some important areas of current pain investigation, including research into new product development, determining drug effectiveness, complementary and alternative medicine, and brain functioning.

Part VI: Additional Help and Information includes a glossary of pain-related terms, a description of the different types of pain treatment facilities, a directory of resources, and a list of books, magazine and journal articles, and websites for additional reading.

Bibliographic Note

This volume contains documents and excerpts from publications issued by the following U.S. government agencies: Center for Drug Evaluation and Research (CDER); National Center for Complementary and Alternative Medicine (NCCAM); National Center for Research Resources (NCRR); National Heart, Lung, and Blood Institute (NHLBI); National Institute for Occupational Safety and Health (NIOSH); National Institute of Arthritis and Musculoskeletal and Skin Disease (NIAMS); National Institute of Dental and Craniofacial Research (NIDR); National Institute of Diabetes and Digestive and Kidney Diseases (NIDDK); National Institute of Neurological Disorders and Stroke (NINDS); National Institute on Alcohol Abuse and Alcoholism (NIAAA); National Institute on Deafness and Other Communication Disorders (NIDCD); National Institute on Drug Abuse (NIDA); National Institutes of Health (NIH); and the U.S. Food and Drug Administration (FDA).

In addition, this volume contains copyrighted documents from the following organizations and individuals: About.com; American Academy of Orthopedic Surgeons; American Academy of Pain Management; American Academy of Pain Medicine; American Association of Endodontists; American Association of Neurological Surgeons; American College of Physicians/American Society of Internal Medicine; American Pain Foundation; American Pain Society; American Society of Anesthesiologists; Bedard, Marcia, PhD; Berg, David (PainOnline); Continuum Health Partners, Inc.; Inlet Medical, Inc.; International Association for the Study of Pain; International Pelvic Pain Society; Janssen Pharmaceutica; Lippincott Williams and Wilkins; Mid Atlantic Society for Biofeedback and Behavioral Medicine; National Vulvodynia Association; New York State Department of Health; North American Chronic Pain Association of Canada; San Francisco Medical Society; School of Medicine at Washington University Medical Center; University of California Davis Medical Center; University of Iowa College of Nursing; Wanlass, Richard, Ph.D.; and Werner, Kristine R., Ph.D.

Full citation information is provided on the first page of each chapter. Every effort has been made to secure all necessary rights to reprint the copyrighted material. If any omissions have been made, please contact Omnigraphics to make corrections for future editions.

Acknowledgements

In addition to the organizations, agencies, and individuals listed above, special thanks go to many others who worked behind the scenes to help bring this book to fruition. They include permissions associate Liz Barbour, verification assistant Dawn Matthews, document engineer Bruce Bellenir, indexer Edward J. Prucha, and operations manager Kevin Hayes.

Note from the Editor

This book is part of Omnigraphics' *Health Reference Series*. The *Series* provides basic consumer health information about a broad range of medical concerns. The information is intended to help facilitate communication between people and their health care providers. It is not intended to serve as a tool for diagnosing illness, in prescribing treatments, or as a substitute for the physician/patient relationship. The editorial staff and Omnigraphics' encourage all persons concerned about medical symptoms or the possibility of disease to seek professional care from an appropriate health care provider.

Our Advisory Board

The *Health Reference Series* is reviewed by an Advisory Board comprised of librarians from public, academic, and medical libraries. We would like to thank the following board members for providing guidance to the development of this series:

Dr. Lynda Baker, Associate Professor of Library and Information Science, Wayne State University, Detroit, MI

Nancy Bulgarelli, William Beaumont Hospital Library, Royal Oak, MI

Karen Imarisio, Bloomfield Township Public Library, Bloomfield Township, MI

Karen Morgan, Mardigian Library, University of Michigan-Dearborn, Dearborn, MI

Rosemary Orlando, St. Clair Shores Public Library, St. Clair Shores, MI

Medical Consultant

Medical consultation services are provided to the *Health Reference Series* editors by David A. Cooke, MD. Dr. Cooke is a graduate of Brandeis University, and he received his M.D. degree from the University of Michigan. He completed residency training at the University of Wisconsin Hospital and Clinics. He is board-certified in Internal Medicine. Dr. Cooke currently works as part of the University of Michigan Health System and practices in Brighton, MI. In his free time, he enjoys writing, science fiction, and spending time with his family.

Health Reference Series *Update Policy*

The inaugural book in the *Health Reference Series* was the first edition of *Cancer Sourcebook* published in 1989. Since then, the *Series* has been enthusiastically received by librarians and in the medical community. In order to maintain the standard of providing high-quality health information for the layperson the editorial staff at Omnigraphics felt it was necessary to implement a policy of updating volumes when warranted.

Medical researchers have been making tremendous strides, and it is the purpose of the *Health Reference Series* to stay current with the most recent advances. Each decision to update a volume will be made on an individual basis. Some of the considerations will include how much new information is available and the feedback we receive from people who use the books. If there is a topic you would like to see added to the update list, or an area of medical concern you feel has not been adequately addressed, please write to:

Editor
Health Reference Series
Omnigraphics, Inc.
615 Griswold Street
Detroit, MI 48226

The commitment to providing on-going coverage of important medical developments has also led to some format changes in the *Health Reference Series*. Each new volume on a topic is individually titled and called a "First Edition." Subsequent updates will carry sequential edition numbers. To help avoid confusion and to provide maximum flexibility in our ability to respond to informational needs, the practice of consecutively numbering each volume has been discontinued.

Part One

Pain

Chapter 1

Pain: Theories, Treatments, and Hope

Introduction

What was the worst pain you can remember? Was it the time you scratched the cornea of your eye? Was it a kidney stone? Childbirth? Rare is the person who has not experienced some beyond-belief episode of pain and misery. Mercifully, relief finally came. Your eye healed, the stone was passed, the baby born. In each of those cases pain flared up in response to a known cause. With treatment, or with the body's healing powers alone, you got better and the pain went away. Doctors call that kind of pain acute pain. It is a normal sensation triggered in the nervous system to alert you to possible injury and the need to take care of yourself.

Chronic pain is different. Chronic pain persists. Fiendishly, uselessly, pain signals keep firing in the nervous system for weeks, months, even years. There may have been an initial mishap—a sprained back, a serious infection—from which you've long since recovered. There may be an ongoing cause of pain—arthritis, cancer, ear infection. But some people suffer chronic pain in the absence of any past injury or evidence of body damage. Whatever the cause, chronic pain is real, unremitting, and demoralizing—the kind of pain New England poet Emily Dickinson had in mind when she wrote:

"Chronic Pain—Hope Through Research," National Institute of Neurological Disorders and Stroke (NINDS), NIH Pub. No. 98-2406, reviewed July 2001.

3

Pain—has an Element of Blank—
It cannot recollect
When it begun—or if there were
A time when it was not

Pain's "Terrible Triad"

Pain of such proportions overwhelms all other symptoms and becomes the problem. People so afflicted often cannot work. Their appetite falls off. Physical activity of any kind is exhausting and may aggravate the pain. Soon the person becomes the victim of a vicious circle in which total preoccupation with pain leads to irritability and depression. The sufferer can't sleep at night and the next day's weariness compounds the problem—leading to more irritability, depression, and pain. Specialists call that unhappy state the "terrible triad" of suffering, sleeplessness, and sadness, a calamity that is as hard on the family as it is on the victim. The urge to do something—anything—to stop the pain makes some patients drug dependent and drives others to undergo repeated operations or resort to questionable practitioners who promise quick and permanent "cures."

Many chronic pain conditions affect older adults. Arthritis, cancer, angina—the chest-binding, breath-catching spasms of pain associated with coronary artery disease—commonly take their greatest toll among the middle-aged and elderly. Trigeminal neuralgia (tic douloureux) is a recurrent, stabbing facial pain that is rare among young adults. But ask anyone living in a community for retired persons if there are any trigeminal neuralgia sufferers around and you are sure to hear of cases. So the fact that Americans are living longer contributes to a widespread and growing concern about pain.

Neuroscientists share that concern. At a time when people are living longer and painful conditions abound, the scientists who study the brain have made landmark discoveries that are leading to a better understanding of pain and more effective treatments.

In the forefront of pain research are scientists supported by the National Institute of Neurological Disorders and Stroke (NINDS), a component of the National Institutes of Health (NIH). Other institutes at NIH that support pain research include the National Institute of Dental Research (NIDR), the National Cancer Institute (NCI), the National Institute of Nursing Research (NINR), the National Institute on Drug Abuse (NIDA), and the National Institute of Mental Health (NIMH).

Theories of Pain

In the past several decades, important discoveries about pain-suppressing chemicals came about because scientists were curious about how morphine and other opium-derived painkillers, or analgesics, work. For some time neuroscientists had known that chemicals were important in conducting nerve signals (small bursts of electric current) from cell to cell. In order for the signal from one cell to reach the next in line, the first cell secretes a chemical, called a "neurotransmitter," from the tip of a long fiber that extends from the cell body. The transmitter molecules cross the gap separating the two cells and attach to special receptor sites on the neighboring cell surface. Some neurotransmitters excite the second cell—allowing it to generate an electrical signal. Others inhibit the second cell—preventing it from generating a signal.

When investigators injected morphine into experimental animals, they found that the morphine molecules fit snugly into receptors on certain brain and spinal cord neurons. Why, the scientists wondered, should the human brain—the product of millions of years of evolution—come equipped with receptors for a man-made drug? Perhaps there were naturally occurring brain chemicals that behaved exactly like morphine.

Numerous studies around the world led to the discovery of not just one pain-suppressing chemical in the brain, but a whole family of such proteins. The smaller members of the family were named enkephalins (meaning "in the head"). In time, the larger proteins were isolated and called endorphins, meaning the "morphine within." The term endorphins is now often used to describe the group as a whole.

The discovery of the endorphins lent weight to an overarching theory of pain: endorphins released from brain nerve cells might inhibit spinal cord pain cells through pathways descending from the brain to the spinal cord. Laboratory experiments subsequently confirmed that painful stimulation led to the release of endorphins from nerve cells. Some of these chemicals then turned up in cerebrospinal fluid, the liquid that circulates in the spinal cord and brain. Laced with endorphins, the fluid could bring a soothing balm to quiet nerve cells.

A New Look at Pain Treatments

Further evidence that endorphins figure importantly in pain control came from studies of some of the oldest and newest pain treatments.

5

These studies involved the use of a drug called naloxone that prevents endorphins and morphine from working. Injections of naloxone resulted in a return of pain which had been relieved by morphine and certain other treatments. But, interestingly, some pain treatments are not affected by naloxone: their success in controlling pain apparently does not depend on endorphins. Thus nature has provided us with more than one means of achieving pain relief.

Acupuncture. Probably no therapy for pain has stirred more controversy in recent years than acupuncture, the 2,000-year-old Chinese technique of inserting fine needles under the skin at selected points in the body. The needles are manipulated by the practitioner to produce pain relief which some individuals report lasts for hours, or even days. Does acupuncture really work? Opinion is divided. Many specialists agree that patients report benefit when the needles are placed near the site of the pain, not at the body points indicated on traditional Chinese acupuncture charts. The case for acupuncture has been made by investigators who argue that local needling of the skin excites endorphin systems of pain control. Wiring the needles to stimulate nerve endings electrically (electroacupuncture) also activates endorphin systems, they believe. Further, some experiments have shown that there are higher levels of endorphins in cerebrospinal fluid following acupuncture.

Those same investigators note that naloxone injections can block pain relief produced by acupuncture. Others have not been able to repeat those findings. Skeptics also cite long-term studies of chronic pain patients that showed no lasting benefit from acupuncture treatments. Current opinion is that more controlled trials are needed to define which pain conditions might be helped by acupuncture and which patients are most likely to benefit.

Local electrical stimulation. Applying brief pulses of electricity to nerve endings under the skin, a procedure called transcutaneous electrical nerve stimulation (TENS), yields excellent pain relief in some chronic pain patients. The stimulation works best when applied to the skin near where the pain is felt and where other sensibilities like touch or pressure have not been damaged. Both the frequency and voltage of the electrical stimulation are important in obtaining pain relief.

Brain stimulation. Another electrical method for controlling pain, especially the widespread and severe pain of advanced cancer, is through surgically implanted electrodes in the brain. The patient determines when and how much stimulation is needed by operating an external transmitter that beams electronic signals to a receiver under the skin that is connected to the electrodes. Stimulation-produced analgesia is a costly procedure that involves the risk of brain surgery. However, patients who have used this technique report that their pain "seems to melt away." The pain relief is also remarkably specific: the other senses remain intact, and there is no mental confusion or cloudiness as with opiate drugs.

Placebo effects. For years doctors have known that a harmless sugar pill or an injection of salt water can make many patients feel better—even after major surgery. The placebo effect, as it is called, has been thought to be due to suggestion, distraction, the patient's optimism that something is being done, or the desire to please the doctor (placebo means "I will please" in Latin).

Later experiments suggested that the placebo effect may be neurochemical, and that people who respond to a placebo for pain relief—a remarkably consistent 35 percent in any experiment using placebos—are able to tap into their brains' endorphin systems. To evaluate it, investigators designed an ingenious experiment. They asked adults scheduled for wisdom teeth removal to volunteer in a pain experiment. Following surgery, some patients were given morphine, some naloxone, and some a placebo. As expected, about a third of those given the placebo reported pain relief. The investigators then gave these people naloxone. All reported a return of pain.

How people who benefit from placebos gain access to pain control systems in the brain is not known. Scientists cannot even predict whether someone who responds to a placebo in one situation will respond in another. Some investigators suspect that stress may be a factor. Patients who are very anxious or under stress are more likely to react to a placebo for pain than those who are more calm, cool, and collected. But dental surgery itself may be sufficiently stressful to trigger the release of endorphins—with or without the effects of placebo. For that reason, many specialists believe further studies are indicated to analyze the placebo effect.

As research continues to reveal the role of endorphins in the brain, neuroscientists have been able to draw more detailed brain maps of the areas and pathways important in pain perception and control and have found other members of the endorphin family. At the same time, clinical investigators have tested chronic pain patients and found that they often have lower-than-normal levels of endorphins in their spinal

7

fluid. If we could just boost their stores with man-made endorphins, perhaps the problems of chronic pain patients could be solved.

Not so easy. Some endorphins are quickly broken down after release from nerve cells. Other endorphins are longer lasting, but there are problems in manufacturing the compounds in quantity and getting them into the right places in the brain or spinal cord. In a few promising studies, clinical investigators have injected an endorphin called beta-endorphin under the membranes surrounding the spinal cord. Patients reported excellent pain relief lasting for many hours. Morphine compounds injected in the same area are similarly effective in producing long-lasting pain relief.

But spinal cord injections or other techniques designed to raise the level of endorphins circulating in the brain require surgery and hospitalization. And even if less drastic means of getting endorphins into the nervous system could be found, they are probably not the ideal answer to chronic pain. Endorphins are also involved in other nervous system activities such as controlling blood flow. Increasing the amount of endorphins might have undesirable effects on these other body activities. Endorphins also appear to share with morphine a potential for addiction or tolerance.

Meanwhile, chemists are synthesizing new analgesics and discovering painkilling virtues in drugs not normally prescribed for pain. Much of the drug research is aimed at developing nonnarcotic painkillers. The motivation for the research is not only to avoid introducing potentially addictive drugs on the market, but is based on the observation that narcotic drugs are simply not effective in treating a variety of chronic pain conditions. Developments in nondrug treatments are also progressing, ranging from new surgical techniques to therapies like exercise, hypnosis, and biofeedback.

New and Old Drugs for Pain

When you complain of headache or low back pain and the doctor says take two aspirins every 4 hours and stay in bed, you may think your pain is being dismissed lightly. Not at all. Aspirin, one of the most universally used medications is an excellent painkiller. Scientists still cannot explain all the ways aspirin works, but they do know that it interferes with pain signals where they usually originate, at the nerve endings outside the brain and spinal cord: peripheral nerves. Aspirin also inhibits the production of chemicals called prostaglandins that are manufactured in the blood to promote blood clotting and wound healing. Unfortunately, prostaglandins, released from cells at the site

8

of injury, are pain-causing substances. They actually sensitize nerve endings, making them—and you—feel more pain. Along with increasing the blood supply to the area, these chemicals contribute to inflammation—the pain, heat, redness, and swelling of tissue damage.

Some investigators now think that the continued release of pain-causing substances in chronic pain conditions may lead to long-term nervous system changes in some patients, making them hypersensitive to pain. People suffering such hyperalgesia can cry out in pain at the gentlest touch, or even when a soft breeze blows over the affected area. In addition to the prostaglandins, blister fluid and certain insect and snake venoms also contain pain-causing substances. Presumably these chemicals alert you to the need for care—a fine reaction in an emergency, but not in chronic pain.

There are several prescription drugs that usually can provide stronger pain relief than aspirin. These include the opiate-related compounds codeine, propoxyphene, morphine, and meperidine. All these drugs have some potential for abuse, and may have unpleasant and even harmful side effects. In combination with other medications or alcohol, some can be dangerous. Used wisely, however, they are important recruits in the chemical fight against pain.

In the search for effective analgesics, physicians have discovered pain-relieving benefits from drugs not normally prescribed for pain. Certain antidepressants are used to treat several particularly severe pain conditions, notably the riveting pain of facial neuralgias like trigeminal neuralgia and the excruciating pain that can follow an attack of shingles.

Interestingly, pain patients who benefit from antidepressants report pain relief before any uplift in mood. Pain specialists think that the antidepressant works because it increases the supply of a naturally produced neurotransmitter, serotonin. (Doctors have long associated decreased amounts of serotonin with severe depression.) But now scientists have evidence that cells using serotonin are also an integral part of a pain-controlling pathway that starts with endorphin-rich nerve cells high up in the brain and ends with inhibition of pain-conducting nerve cells lower in the brain or spinal cord.

Antiepileptic drugs have also been used successfully in treating trigeminal neuralgia. The rationale for the use of antiepileptic drugs (principally carbamazepine) is based on the theory that a healthy nervous system depends on a proper balance of incoming and outgoing nerve signals. Trigeminal neuralgia and other facial pains or neuralgias are thought to result from damage to facial nerves. That means that the normal flow of messages to and from the brain is disturbed.

9

The nervous system may react by becoming hypersensitive: it may create its own powerful discharge of nerve signals, as though screaming to the outside world "Why aren't you contacting me?" Antiepileptic drugs—used to quiet the excessive brain discharges associated with epileptic seizures—quiet the distress signals and in that way may relieve pain.

Nondrug Treatments

Treatment for pain can include counseling, relaxation training, meditation, hypnosis, biofeedback, or behavior modification. The philosophy common to all of these approaches is the belief that patients can do something on their own to manage their pain. That something may mean changing attitudes, feelings, or behaviors associated with pain.

Psychotherapy. Some patients may benefit from individual or group counseling. Trained professionals can help the chronic pain sufferer learn valuable coping skills. They also provide the patient with much needed support—both psychological and emotional—for dealing with pain.

Relaxation and meditation therapies. These methods enable people to relax tense muscles, reduce anxiety, and alter mental states. Both physical and mental tension can make pain worse, and in conditions such as headache or back pain, tension may be at the root of the problem. Meditation, which aims at producing a state of relaxed but alert awareness, is sometimes combined with therapies that encourage people to think of pain as something remote and apart from them. The methods promote a sense of detachment so that the patient thinks of the pain as confined to a particular body part over which he or she has control. The approach may be particularly helpful when pain is associated with fear, as in cancer.

Hypnosis. No longer considered magic, hypnosis is a technique in which an individual's susceptibility to suggestion is heightened. Normal volunteers who prove to be excellent subjects for hypnosis often report a marked reduction or obliteration of experimentally induced pain, such as that produced by a mild electric shock. The hypnotic state does not lower the volunteer's heart rate, respiration, or other autonomic responses. These physical reactions show the expected increases normally associated with painful stimulation.

The role of hypnosis in treating chronic pain patients is uncertain. Some studies have shown that 15 to 20 percent of hypnotizable patients with moderate to severe pain can achieve total relief with hypnosis. Other studies report that hypnosis reduces anxiety and depression. By lowering the burden of emotional suffering, pain may become more bearable.

Biofeedback. Some individuals can learn voluntary control over certain body activities if they are provided with information about how the system is working—how fast their heart is beating, how tense their head or neck muscles are, how cold their hands are. The information is usually supplied through visual or auditory cues that code the body activity in some obvious way—a louder sound meaning an increase in muscle tension, for example. How people use this biofeedback to learn control is not understood, but some practitioners of the art report that imagery helps: they may think of a warm tropical beach, for example, when they want to raise the temperature of their hands. Biofeedback may be a logical approach in pain conditions that involve tense muscles, like tension headache or low back pain. But results are mixed.

Behavior modification. This psychological technique (sometimes called operant conditioning) is aimed at changing habits, behaviors, and attitudes that can develop in chronic pain patients. Some patients become dependent, anxious, and homebound—if not bedridden. For some, too, chronic pain may be a welcome friend, relieving them of the boredom of a dull job or the burden of family responsibilities. These psychological rewards—sometimes combined with financial gains from compensation payments or insurance—work against improvements in the patient's condition, and can encourage increased drug dependency, repeated surgery, and multiple doctor and clinic visits.

There is no question that the patient feels pain. The hope of behavior modification is that pain relief can be obtained from a program aimed at changing the individual's lifestyle. The program begins with a complete assessment of the painful condition and a thorough explanation of how the program works. It is essential to enlist the full cooperation of both the patient and family members. The treatment is aimed at reducing pain medication and increasing mobility and independence through a graduated program of exercise, diet, and other activities. The patient is rewarded for positive efforts with praise and attention. Rewards are withheld when the patient retreats into negative attitudes or demanding and dependent behavior.

How effective are any of these treatment methods? Are some superior to others? Who is most likely to benefit? Do the benefits last? The answers are not yet in hand. Patient selection and patient cooperation

11

are all-important. Analysis of individuals who have improved dramatically with one or another of these approaches is helping to pinpoint what factors are likely to lead to successful treatment.

Surgery to Relieve Pain

Surgery is often considered the court of last resort for pain: when all else fails, cut the nerve endings. Surgery can bring about instant, almost magical release from pain. But surgery may also destroy other sensations as well, or, inadvertently, become the source of new pain. Further, relief is not necessarily permanent. After 6 months or a year, pain may return.

For all those reasons, the decision for surgery must always involve a careful weighing of the patient's condition and the outlook for the future. If surgery can mean the difference between a pain-wracked existence ending in death, versus a pain-free time in which to compose one's life and see friends and family, then surgery is clearly a humane and compassionate choice.

There are a variety of operations to relieve pain. The most common is cordotomy: severing the nerve fibers on one or both sides of the spinal cord that travel the express routes to the brain. Cordotomy affects the sense of temperature as well as pain, since the fibers travel together in the express route.

Besides cordotomy, surgery within the brain or spinal cord to relieve pain includes severing connections at major junctions in pain pathways, such as at the places where pain fibers cross from one side of the cord to the other, or destroying parts of important relay stations in the brain like the thalamus, an egg-shaped cluster of nerve cells near the center of the brain. In addition, surgeons sometimes can relieve pain by destroying nerve fibers or their parent cell bodies outside the brain or spinal cord. A case in point is the destruction of sympathetic nerves (a part of the autonomic nervous system) to relieve the severe pain that sometimes follows a penetrating wound from a sharp instrument or bullet.

When pain affects the upper extremities, or is widespread, the surgeon has fewer options and surgery may not be as effective. Still, skilled neurosurgeons have achieved excellent results with upper spinal cord or brain surgery to treat severe intractable pain. These procedures may employ chemicals or use heat or freezing treatments to destroy tissue, as well as the more traditional use of the scalpel.

Some surgeons have reported success with a brain operation called cingulotomy to relieve intractable pain in patients with severe psychiatric problems. The nerve fibers destroyed are part of a pathway important in emotions and motivation. The surgery appears to eliminate the discomfort and suffering the patient feels, but does not interfere with other mental faculties such as thinking and memory.

Prior to operating, physicians can often test the effectiveness of surgery by using anesthetic drugs to block nerves temporarily. In some chronic pain conditions—like the pain from a penetrating wound—these temporary blocks can in themselves be beneficial, promoting repair of nerve damage.

How do these current treatments apply to the more common chronic pain conditions? What follows is a brief survey of major pain disorders and the treatments most in use today.

The Major Pains

Headache. Tension headache, involving continued contractions of head and neck muscles, is one of the most common forms of headache. The other common variety is the vascular headache, involving changes in the pressure of blood vessels serving the head. Migraine headaches are of the vascular type, associated with throbbing pain on one side of the head. Genetic factors play a role in determining who will have migraines, but many other factors are important as well. A major difficulty in treating migraine headache is that changes occur throughout the course of the headache. Blood vessels may first constrict and then dilate. Changing levels of neurotransmitters have also been noted. While a number of drugs can relieve migraine pain, their usefulness often depends on when they are taken. Some are only effective if taken at the onset. Several drugs for the prevention of migraine have been developed in recent years, including serotonin agonists which mimic the action of this key brain chemical. Prompt administration of these drugs is important.

Drugs are also the most common treatment for tension headache, although attempts to use biofeedback to control muscle tension have had some success. Physical methods such as heat or cold applications often provide additional, if only temporary, relief.

Low back pain. The combination of pain-killers and modest amounts of a muscle relaxant are usually prescribed for the first-time low back pain patient. At the initial examination, the physician will also note if the patient is overweight or works under conditions (such as driving a truck or sitting at a desk for long hours) that offer little opportunity for exercise. Some authorities believe that low back pain is particularly prevalent in Western society because of the combination of overweight, bad posture (made worse if there is added weight up front), and infrequent exercise.

Although bed rest may be necessary for severe back problems, exercise is now considered to be an important addition to treatment and can help speed recovery for many patients with low back pain. Exercise helps reduce stress on the lower back by increasing flexibility and strength. To avoid injury, however, carefully follow the exercise routine prescribed by your doctor. In some cases, a full neurological examination may be necessary, including tests to determine if there may be a ruptured disc or other source of pressure on the cord or nerve roots.

Sometimes x-rays will show a disc problem that can be helped by surgery. Milder analgesics (aspirin, acetaminophen, or stronger non-narcotic medications) and electrical stimulation—using TENS or implanted brain electrodes—can be very effective for low back pain. What is not effective is long-term use of muscle-relaxant tranquilizers. Many specialists are convinced that chronic use of these drugs is detrimental to the back pain patient, adding to depression and increasing pain. Massage and manipulative therapy are used by some clinicians but, except for individual patient reports, their usefulness is still undocumented.

Cancer pain. The pain of cancer can result from the pressure of a growing tumor or the infiltration of tumor cells into other organs. Or the pain can come about as the result of radiation or chemotherapy. These treatments can cause fluid accumulation and swelling (edema), irritate or destroy healthy tissue causing pain and inflammation, and possibly sensitize nerve endings. Ideally, the treatment for cancer pain is to remove the cancerous tissue. When that is not possible, pain can be treated by any or all of the currently available therapies: electrical stimulation, psychological methods, surgery, and strong painkillers.

Arthritis pain. Arthritis is a general descriptive term meaning a disorder of the joints. The two most common forms are osteoarthritis that typically affects the fingers and may spread to important weight-bearing joints in the spine or hips, and rheumatoid arthritis, an inflammatory joint disease associated with swelling, congestion, and thickening of the soft tissue around joints. Current treatments for arthritis include aspirin, acetaminophen, and nonsteroidal anti-inflammatory drugs like indomethacin and ibuprofen. Steroid drugs—important anti-inflammatory agents modeled after the body's own chemicals produced in the adrenal glands—were introduced and hailed as lifesavers in the 1950's. But the long-term use of steroids has serious consequences, among them the lowering of resistance to infection, hemorrhaging, and facial puffiness—producing the so-called moonface.

TENS and acupuncture have been tried with mixed results. In cases where tissue has been destroyed, surgery to replace a diseased joint with an artificial part has been very successful. The total hip replacement operation is an example.

Arthritis is best treated early, say the experts. A modest program of drugs combined with exercise can do much to restore full function and forestall long-term degenerative changes. Exercise in warm water is especially good since the water is both relaxing and provides buoyancy that makes exercises easier to perform. Physical treatments with warm or cold compresses are helpful sources of temporary pain relief.

Neurogenic pain. The most difficult pains to treat are those that result from damage to the peripheral nerves or to the central nervous system itself. Mentioned earlier in this chapter as examples of extraordinarily searing pain were trigeminal neuralgia and shingles, along with several drugs that can help in these conditions. In addition, trigeminal neuralgia sufferers can benefit from surgery to destroy the nerve cells that supply pain-sensation fibers to the face. An advantage to using a treatment called "thermocoagulation"—which uses heat supplied by an electrical current to destroy nerve cells—is that pain fibers are more sensitive to the treatment resulting in less destruction of other sensations (such as touch and temperature).

Sometimes specialists treating trigeminal neuralgia find that certain blood vessels in the brain lie near the group of nerve cells supplying sensory fibers to the face, exerting pressure that causes pain. The surgical insertion of a small sponge between the blood vessels and the nerve cells can relieve the pressure and eliminate pain.

Among other notoriously painful neurogenic disorders is pain from an amputated or paralyzed limb—so called "phantom" pain—that affects a significant number of amputees and paraplegia patients. Various combinations of antidepressants and weak narcotics like propoxyphene are sometimes effective. Surgery, too, is occasionally successful. Many experts now think that the electrical stimulating techniques hold the greatest promise for relieving these pains.

Psychogenic pain. Some cases of pain are not due to past disease or injury, nor is there any detectable sign of damage inside or outside the nervous system. Such pain may benefit from any of the psychological pain therapies listed earlier. It is also possible that some new methods used to diagnose pain may be useful. One method gaining in popularity is thermography, which measures the temperature of surface tissue as a reflection of blood flow. A color-coded "thermogram" of a person with a headache or other painful condition often shows an altered blood supply to the painful area, appearing as a darker or lighter shade than the surrounding areas or the corresponding part on the other side of the body. Thus an abnormal thermogram in a patient who complains of pain in the absence of any other evidence may provide a valuable clue that can lead to a diagnosis and treatment.

Where to Go for Help

People with chronic pain have usually seen a family doctor and several other specialists as well. Eventually they are referred to neurologists, orthopedists, or neurosurgeons. The patient/doctor relationship is extremely important in dealing with chronic pain. Both patients and family members should seek out knowledgeable specialists who neither dismiss nor indulge the patient, physicians who understand full well how pain has come to dominate the patient's life and the lives of everyone else in the family.

Contrary to what many people think, pain patients are not malingerers or hypochondriacs. They are men and women of all ages, education, and social background, suffering a wide variety of painful conditions.

People with pain problems may feel isolated, helpless, or hopeless. But many of those who suffer with a pain problem can be helped if they—and their families—understand all the causes of pain, and the many and varied steps that can now be taken to undo what chronic pain has done. As a result of the strides neuroscience has made in tracking down pain in the brain—and in the mind—we can expect more and better treatments in the years to come. The days when patients were told "I'm sorry, but you'll have to learn to live with the pain" will be gone forever.

Chapter 2

What We Know about Pain

Pain! This very important English word is uttered through pursed lips and with an expulsion of air causing the speaker to pause a moment before proceeding with the next word or phrase. Pain has been experienced to some degree by everyone, regardless of age, status or economic level. The word can evoke fear. Experience with pain can leave lasting emotional and physical impressions. It can alter and destroy lives.

Advances in medical research and the discovery of analgesic drugs has given us some answers to questions about the origins and persistence of pain. Recent advances have led to new depths of understanding and control. We now know, for instance, that pain is not merely a passive symptom of disease. Acute pain can be a warning symptom. Persistent pain is now thought to be an aggressive disease in itself, producing changes in the brain that underlie the pathology of what we term chronic pain.

A major success story is the effect this new knowledge has had on the treatment of acute and chronic pain. However, many problems remain unsolved, and there are many mysteries of chronic pain that remain unexplained and misdiagnosed.

Pain is a product of the nervous system, the most difficult component of the human body to understand. The complexity and subtlety of the

"What We Know about Pain," an undated document produced by the National Institute of Dental Research (NIDR). Some of this information is focused on dental pain, but the discussion is still relevant to understanding pain in general.

17

nervous system can be compared to futuristic electronic circuitry—yet even the most advanced computer is primitive by comparison.

The nervous system consists of a peripheral web of nerve cells of varying diameter. A single nerve cell may be as small as 4 one-thousandths of a millimeter thick. These nerves extend throughout the body—to toes, fingers, teeth, tongue and scalp as well as to the central organs of heart, liver, lung and gut.

The nerves endlessly gather information, transmitting it to the mainframe, the central nervous system, which consists of the brain and spinal cord. The central nervous system interprets the information from the nerves and coordinates the body's response. The brain then integrates higher functions involving memory, comparison and decision making.

As early as 400 B.C., Hippocrates realized that the brain (not the heart) was the organizational center of the body, the seat of intelligence. Other Greek anatomists in the third and fourth centuries B.C. recognized that the nerves traveling from the skin to the spinal cord were sensory in nature, while those nerves going to the muscles effected motor response.

A nerve is a single cell consisting of a nucleus and various subcellular inclusions or organelles with the same microstructures as every other cell of the body. But the nerve cell is differentiated from other cells by having a tuft of short rootlike projections called dendrites at one end of the cell body and a long, thin projection from the other end called an axon.

Although the cell may be only 4 one-thousandths mm in diameter, it can be astonishingly long. In an average-sized human being, for example, the nerve from the base of the spine to the tip of the toe is 3 feet long. The tip of the axon may subdivide 150 times and attach to 150 separate muscle fibers.

Most axons, however, do not end in a block of muscle and may be as short as an inch in length. These nerve cells are only a single link in a chain of nerve cells, each axon making near contact with the dendrite of the next nerve cell. The tip of the axon secretes a chemical substance known as a neurotransmitter, which aids in transmitting the nerve impulse from one cell over the gap or synapse to the next cell.

Each synapse offers a certain amount of resistance to the passage of the nerve message. This resistance gradually loses strength the farther it travels from the point of origin. Because individual nerve cells usually exist together in great numbers forming a nerve cord, a transmitting nerve cell may receive information from more than one cell type above it in the chain.

18

The nerve impulse is subjected to many different and, at times, opposing influences that provide a greater sensitivity and control of the nerve impulse in humans. Nerve impulses can travel in only one direction from axon to dendrite. Information is transported away from the central nervous system by motor neurons, which trigger motor activity or movement. Sensory neurons originating in the peripheral sense organs send their messages from axon to dendrite and back to the central nervous system. The two types of nerve cells exist together in the 31 pairs of spinal nerves. In English, the terms nerve and nerve cord are used interchangeably.

The human face, the cranio-oral-dental complex, is the facade for the central nervous system. Dentistry deals most often with sensations in the 12 pairs of cranial nerves.

These nerves originate at the base of the brain where the brain stem juts out and proceeds down the vertebral column forming the spine. In the area around the first few centimeters of this brain stem, and passing out of the cranium through special foramen in the bone, are the cranial nerves, which serve the sensory and motor needs of the head, neck, chest and abdomen.

The sensory and motor cells travel in separate cords in these specialized tracts. The 12 nerves are known by name and Roman numeral: (I) olfactory, (II) optic, (III) oculomotor, (IV) trochlear, (V) trigeminal, (VI) abducens, (VII) facial, (VIII) acoustic, (IX) glossopharyngeal, (X) vagus, (XI) spinal accessory and (XII) hypoglossal.

The trigeminal nerve has three major divisions: the maxillary, mandibular and ophthalmic nerves, providing sensory innervation over the facial and oral area and motor innervation to the muscles of mastication.

The facial nerve has motor fibers in the face and scalp and sensory fibers from the taste buds. The spinal accessory nerve controls head and neck movement, and the hypoglossal nerve leads to the tongue. There is considerable overlap and individualized innervation of the areas of the craniofacial, oral and dental tissues.

Stimulus vs. Perception

The relationship between pain and injury or disability has led to the assumption that pain must be proportional to the severity of the injury. In many instances, however, this relationship fails to hold up. About 65 percent of soldiers who are severely wounded and 20 percent of civilians who undergo major surgery report feeling little or no pain for hours or days after injury or incision. In contrast, about 70

19

percent of people who suffer from chronic, low-back pain do not show any readily detectable injury. Clearly, the link between pain stimulus and pain perception is highly variable. Injury may occur without pain, and pain without apparent injury.

Perception of pain is a multi-step process, originating at the site of insult with the stimulation of specific nerve fibers known as nociceptors. Some nociceptors react to several kinds of painful stimulation. Others are more selective. Certain nociceptors will react to a pinprick, for example, but ignore painful heat.

After these nerve fibers or nociceptors are stimulated, the damaged cells release chemical mediators of pain and inflammation. These mediators include potassium ions, bradykinin, prostaglandins, serotonin and histamine.

The resulting sensitization of the peripheral nerve endings produces an exaggerated and prolonged sensitivity to later stimuli (peripheral hyperalgesia). Analgesic drugs such as aspirin and ibuprofen block some of these chemical mediators and decrease sensitization of nociceptors at the periphery.

The pain stimulus is then sent through the peripheral nervous system to the central nervous system, or CNS, where the pain message is processed at several levels. Touching a hot stove causes the pain signal to be routed immediately from the pain site to the dorsal horn of the spinal cord. Here it synapses with a second neuron, which picks up the signal, passes it to the other side of the spinal cord and up the spinothalamic tract to the thalamus. A message is then sent back down the spinal column to nerve cells that signal muscles to contract. That streamlined pathway is used for perception of sharp or acute pain and can be automatic as in a reflex.

An alternative pathway exists in which the neuron at the site of injury enters the dorsal horn of the spinal cord, transfers its message to the other side of the spinal cord, and then through a series of interconnected neurons, which transmit and modulate the pain message. The message travels up the spinal cord to the brain stem, the thalamus, and is finally perceived at the cerebral cortex. This slower ascending pathway allows perception of duller, more persistent pain.

Pain transmission also alerts another major division of the CNS—the autonomic nervous system. This system regulates involuntary processes such as breathing, blood flow, pulse rate, digestion and elimination, adjusting these activities to changing body needs. The autonomic nervous system also signals the release of hormones like epinephrine (adrenalin).

In 1965, Ronald Melzack, a Canadian scientist, and Patrick Wall, a British scientist, suggested a new gate theory of pain and speculated that pain-suppressing pathways must exist. Their idea was that when pain signals first reach the nervous system, they excite activity in a group of small neurons that form a kind of pain pool.

When the total activity of these neurons reaches a certain minimal level, a hypothetical gate opens to allow the pain signals to be sent to higher brain centers. However, nearby neurons in contact with the pain cells could suppress the cells so that the gate stayed closed. The gate-closing cells include large neurons that are stimulated by nonpainful touching or pressing of the skin. The gate also could be closed from above by brain cells activating a descending pathway to block pain.

This theory stimulated research to find the conjectured pathways and required mechanisms. For some time, neuroscientists knew that chemicals were important in conducting nerve signals (small bursts of electrical current) from cell to cell. Since serotonin was first identified as an inhibitory neurotransmitter in the early 1970s, scientists have discovered other neurotransmitters that inhibit pain. These include the opioid peptides, beta-endorphin and met-enkephalin.

All of the most potent pain-relieving drugs, called opioids, have the same effect as opium, with similar chemical characteristics and structure. Morphine is the purest, most active alkyloid of opium. The opioid receptors are found near synapses in the dorsal horn of the spinal cord. But these and other neurotransmitters have been traced to receptor sites throughout the body, including pathways in the face, and are believed to be involved in a pain-control network. These opioids serve as ligands or signals that bind with specificity and tenacity to their opioid receptors. In this way, they induce a signal transduction pathway in the responding neuronal cell.

Acute vs. Chronic Pain

Pain is generally divided into two main types: acute and chronic. Acute pain is often short-lived. It has a specific cause and purpose, and generally produces no persistent psychological reactions. Acute pain can occur during tooth extraction, tooth and soft tissue injury, and with infection and inflammation. It can be modulated and removed by treating its cause and through combined strategies using analgesics to treat the pain and antibiotics to treat the infection.

Chronic pain is distinctly different and more complex. Chronic pain has no time limit, often has no apparent cause and serves no apparent biological purpose. Chronic pain can trigger multiple psychological problems that confound both patient and health care provider, leading to feelings of helplessness and hopelessness.

The urge to do something—anything!—to stop pain makes some patients drug-dependent. It drives others into repeated operations and submits many to the mercies of anyone promising a cure. Chronic pain may be the most costly health problem in the United States. Estimated annual costs—including direct medical expenses, lost income, lost productivity, compensation payments and legal fees—are close to $50 billion. Some of the most common causes of chronic pain include:

Low-back pain. About 15 percent of U.S. adults have persistent low-back pain at some time in their lives. Five million Americans are partially disabled by back problems and another two million are so severely disabled that they cannot work. Low-back pain accounts for 93 million lost workdays and costs more than $5 billion in health care each year.

Headache. At least 40 million Americans suffer chronic, recurring headaches. They spend $4 billion a year on medications. Migraine sufferers alone lose 65 million workdays each year.

Recurrent facial pain. An estimated 7.5 million people—about 4 percent of the U.S. population aged 18 years or older—report pain in the face or jaw joint. Of these, 5.2 million are women, accounting for about 5.5 percent of the U.S. female population; 2.2 million are men, about 2.6 percent of the U.S. male population. The estimated nonsurgical direct costs for treating recurrent facial pain amount to about $874 million each year. The annual direct cost of treating patients with temporomandibular disorders—excluding surgery and medications—is at least another $1 billion.

Cancer pain. Most cancer patients in the intermediate or advanced stages of the disease suffer moderate-to-severe pain. More than 800,000 new cases of cancer are diagnosed each year in the United States, and some 430,000 people die.

Arthritis pain. The great crippler affects 20 million Americans and costs more than $4 billion each year in lost income, productivity and health care. Osteoarthritis may be significant in the etiology and pathogenesis of TMD [temporomandibular joint disorder].

Other pain disorders cost society many billions of dollars. These disorders include the neuralgias and neuropathies (diabetic and post-herpetic) that affect nerves throughout the body; pain triggered by damage to the central nervous system (the brain and spinal cord); and pain having no readily apparent cause.

Many chronic pain conditions affect mainly older adults. These include arthritis, cancer and angina. Tic douloureux (trigeminal neuralgia) is a recurrent, stabbing facial pain that is rare among young adults but becomes more common with increasing age.

Today, 32 million Americans are 65 years of age and older. By the year 2010, about one in five Americans will be 65 or older. These facts make chronic facial pain a remarkably significant area for our concern and clinical attention. Our challenge is how to best manage chronic facial pain.

Managing Pain

For those with responsibilities in oral health care, pain often creates a difficult situation. It is easy to be tricked by the source of the pain stimulus. The dentist wishes to help a patient with severe pain in a particular tooth, or group of teeth, or in the TMJ [temporomandibular joint] region, but can find nothing apparently abnormal.

The pain persists. Something must be done. In a few cases, all available techniques are tried to no avail. It is difficult to explain to a patient that the pain may be due to injury or disease not at the site where it is perceived, but rather at some other site. The problem may not be dental in origin but referred pain. The possibility of referred pain caused by some other condition—trigeminal neuralgia, for example, or diabetic neuropathy—is not easy to diagnose and can be presented as an apparent dental problem. It is the diagnosis that must be considered.

Pain management has long been important in dental practice, where there is heavy emphasis on pain prevention and control. Dentists routinely block trigeminal nerve pathways during painful procedures by administering a local anesthetic, which inhibits transmission of nociceptive information to the CNS. However, the analgesic should last long enough for the peak of inflammatory mediators to pass.

There are many procedures advertised for pain control. Most have their advocates, some detractors and many skeptics. When effective, these procedures can transform the life of a person plagued by chronic pain. But before complicated pain treatments are attempted, a variety of simpler treatments should be tried.

The value of rest, for instance, is often underestimated. Wearing a cervical collar or a lumbar support may reduce the head or back muscle spasms that contribute to the pain. Heat treatment can help by dilating blood vessels in the affected area, removing local pain-causing substances and possibly closing the pain gate or just causing relaxation and comfort. More attention should be given to the psychosocial, behavioral and functional aspects of chronic pain. If these methods do not help, other treatments may help:

Acupuncture. Although the Chinese have used this technique for 2,000 years, it remains controversial. The technique involves inserting fine needles under the skin at selected points and agitating them. The acupuncture mechanism is not well-established, although it is believed that the procedure excites an endorphin method of pain control. Some experiments have shown high levels of endorphin in the cerebrospinal fluid after acupuncture.

Local electrical stimulation. Applying brief pulses of electricity to nerve endings under the skin in the affected area—a procedure called transcutaneous electrical nerve stimulation, or TENS—reportedly gives excellent pain relief to some chronic pain sufferers. Frequency and voltage are important in achieving the sense of tingling and warmth that provides relief. Relief is believed to result from the stimulation of large-fiber activity that can close the pain gate. The TENS device can be small enough to be worn on a belt and used when necessary.

Brain and spinal cord stimulation. Surgically implanting electrodes in areas of the brain rich in opiate receptors has been done mainly in patients with widespread and severe cancer. Electrodes have also been placed onto the dorsal columns of the spinal cord, where they are believed to stimulate the large fibers involved in pain modulation. The patient operates the transmitter when relief is needed.

Placebo effect. Experiments suggest that the placebo effect may be neurochemical. Those who respond to a placebo for pain relief—a remarkably consistent 35 percent in any experiment using placebos—are believed to be able to tap into their brain's endorphin system, naturally inhibiting pain transmission.

Surgery. Surgical pain relief may involve cutting a nerve that supplies the painful area. This usually involves some sensory loss and possibly some motor loss.

Psychological treatment. Such treatments range from psycho-analysis and other forms of psychotherapy to relaxation training, meditation, hypnosis, biofeedback and behavioral modification. Underlying these approaches is the belief that patients can do something to control their own pain. Understanding how unconscious forces and past events contribute to their fears and pain is helpful for some people in providing relief. Changing behaviors, attitudes and feelings about pain may aid other chronic pain sufferers.

Analgesics. The use of analgesics or pain-killing drugs is a $30 billion-a-year business in the United States. These medications are effective in treating acute pain and often work in treating chronic pain as well. In 1750, the Rev. Edward Stone of Chipping Norton, England, isolated from a willow tree the first of a group of analgesic drugs derived from salicylic acid (from the Latin "salix," which means "willow"). The acetylated salicylic acid, having fewer side effects than Rev. Stone's original, is better known as aspirin. It has become the most popular, effective, universally used reliever of pain.

Scientists cannot explain as yet all the ways aspirin works, but it is known to interfere with the transmission of pain signals in the peripheral nociceptive nerve endings. Aspirin also inhibits the production of chemicals manufactured in the blood and released in injured tissue. These include prostaglandins, which contribute to inflammation at the injury site and result in pain.

Aspirin and other drugs used in treating inflammations (examples: phenylbutazone and indomethacin) were shown by John Vane in 1971 to inhibit the action of the enzyme that converts arachidonic acid to prostaglandins. Arachidonic acid metabolites acting in the brain also produce fever, explaining the effectiveness of aspirin in reducing fever.

Synthesis

One of the earliest forms of analgesic was the drug opium, popular even before the times of the ancient Greeks. Opioid receptors are found in the dorsal horn of the spinal cord near the neuron synapse region, where they effect the production of pain sensation.

Opiate-related compounds include codeine, propoxyphene (Darvon), morphine, heroin (diacetyl morphine) and meperidine (Demerol). All provide stronger pain relief than aspirin and some other nonsteroidal analgesics. The opioids, however, have some well-known potential for abuse and may have unpleasant and harmful side effects.

Because these drugs do not have an efficacy ceiling like that of the nonsteroidal analgesics, the dosage can be increased. Doing so also increases the side effects, including respiratory depression. In combination with other medications or alcohol, some of the opiates can be very dangerous. Used wisely, opiates are important agents in the chemical fight against pain.

Our challenge is to discover nonopiate drugs that have the same specificity and efficacy for managing chronic and severe craniofacial-oral-dental pain.

Local analgesics or nerve blocks may be effective for temporary pain relief when the pain is restricted to a well-defined area. Lidocaine (lignocaine) is often used to treat trigger spots where injections are made into painful areas of muscle.

Certain anti-depressants as well as anti-epileptic drugs also are used to treat severe pain conditions, including shingles and facial neuralgias. The anti-depressants are believed to increase the production of serotonin. Cells using serotonin are an integral part of a pain-controlling pathway that inhibits pain-conducting neurons in the brain or spinal cord.

The use of anti-epileptic drugs centers on the premise that the nervous system depends on a proper balance of incoming and outgoing nerve signals. In damaged facial nerve cells, the normal flow of messages to the brain is disturbed and becomes hyperactive. Excessive nerve discharges may occur. The anti-epileptic drugs may reduce the excessive frequency of discharges.

In a nation with an aging population, there is an increasing challenge to reduce chronic and debilitating diseases. Pain is a disease, not just a symptom. It results in pathology within the nervous system, which can affect all the systems of the body. Chronic pain can have enormous cost, for the individual patient and society as a whole.

The dental profession has always been proactive in pain prevention, management and research, beginning with early studies of tooth decay and tooth extraction. Although enormous progress has been made in understanding the molecular and cellular neurobiology and the neuroscience of pain, our knowledge of this elusive and complicated system is still fragmentary. Pain remains one of our most challenging and important problems in research and health care.

Chapter 3

Chronic Nonmalignant Pain

A growing amount of media attention has been given to the unspeakable suffering of millions of Americans with incurable conditions causing severe chronic pain. In addition to articles in the popular press and segments on network television, the Internet is an increasingly rich source of information on this topic. Yet the agonizing pain of millions of chronic pain patients remains untreated. This is largely because the nation's War on Drugs has created a climate of fear among patients and health professionals alike—fear of using strong opioid medications which are often the only way to relieve severe pain when all other treatments have failed.

This information is intended to debunk some of the myths that fuel this unreasonable fear, and is being sent to legislators, patients, and health professionals throughout the nation. It will also enable members of the press to have quick access to credible facts about chronic pain. Although this text shows the devastating effects on physical and mental health when severe pain goes untreated, as well as the profound impact on the economy, there is no way to measure the "bankruptcies of the heart" that invariably accompany this condition. Yet the steady erosion of the quality of life for millions of pain patients and their families—as they struggle with divorce, poverty, homelessness, despair, and often suicide—is the real tragedy here.

By Marcia E. Bedard, Ph.D., Professor of Women's Studies, California State University, Fresno, July 15, 1997. © 1997 Marcia Bedard; reprinted with permission. Text available from the North American Chronic Pain Association of Canada.

CNP, pain that lasts six months or more and does not respond well to conventional medical treatment, affects more people than any other type of pain. Thirty-four million Americans suffer from chronic pain, and most are significantly disabled by it, sometimes permanently.[1, 2, 15]

The economic impact of CNP is staggering. Back pain, migraines, and arthritis alone account for medical costs of $40 billion annually, and pain is the cause of 25% of all sick days taken yearly. The annual total cost of pain from all causes is estimated to be more than $100 billion.[2, 4, 15]

Despite the magnitude of suffering, CNP remains grossly under-treated in most patients. The reasons for this are: the low priority of pain relief in our health care system; lack of knowledge among both health professionals and consumers about pain management; exaggerated fears of opioid side effects and addiction; and health professionals' fear of medical board and DEA scrutiny, even when controlled substances are used appropriately for pain relief.[2, 13, 14, 15]

Contrary to common fears, numerous studies have shown addiction is extremely rare in pain patients taking opioid drugs, even in patients with histories of drug abuse and/or addiction. CNP patients will develop a physical dependence on opioid drugs, but this is not the same thing as addiction, which is an aberrant psychological state.[2, 3, 4, 5, 6, 7, 8, 9, 10, 11, 13, 14]

Unrelieved pain has many negative health consequences including, but not limited to: increased stress, metabolic rate, blood clotting and water retention; delayed healing; hormonal imbalances; impaired immune system and gastrointestinal functioning; decreased mobility; problems with appetite and sleep, and needless suffering. CNP also causes many psychological problems, such as feelings of low self-esteem, powerlessness, hopelessness, and depression.[12, 15, 16, 18, 19]

Undertreatment of CNP often results in suicide. In a recent survey, 50% of CNP patients had inadequate pain relief and had considered suicide to escape the unrelenting agony of their pain. Unrelieved pain also leads to requests for physician-assisted suicide, another indicator of pain's harsh impact on the quality of life of many patients and their families.[7, 8, 13, 14, 15, 16]

Discrimination against CNP patients is pervasive in the American health care system. Women, racial/ethnic minorities, children, the elderly, worker's compensation patients, and previously disabled patients (e.g., those with cerebral palsy, or who are deaf, blind, amputees, survivors of childhood polio, etc.) are at great risk for undertreatment of their pain, even though patients belonging to one or more of these groups are the vast majority of all CNP patients.[2, 13, 17]

CNP patients with severe, unrelenting pain from permanent structural damage to the neurologic or musculo-skeletal systems are often subjected to expensive and unnecessary surgeries and other painful invasive procedures. Arachnoiditis and reflex sympathetic dystrophy are the most common causes of severe CNP. Other common causes include: post-trauma, adhesions, systemic lupus, headaches, degenerative arthritis, fibromyalgia, and neuropathies.[8, 15, 18, 19]

Sources

1. American Chronic Pain Association. "Coping with Chronic Pain." 1995.

2. Brownlee, Shannon, and Joannie M. Schrof. "The Quality of Mercy." *U.S. News and World Report*, March 17, 1997: 55-57, 60-62, 65, 67.

3. Pasero, Christine L., R.N., B.S.N., and Margo McCaffery, R.N., M.S., F.A.A.N. "Pain Control." *American Journal of Nursing*. Vol. 97, No. 6., June, 1997: 20-21.

4. American Academy of Pain Medicine and American Pain Society. "The Use of Opioids for the Treatment of Chronic Pain." *Clinical Journal of Pain*, Vol. 13, March, 1997: 6-8.

5. Medina J.L., M.D., and S. Diamond, M.D. "Drug Dependency in Patients with Chronic Headache." *Headache*, 1977, Vol. 17: 12-14.

6. Porter J., M.D. and H. Jick, M.D. "Addiction Rare in Patients Treated with Narcotics." *New England Journal of Medicine* 1980, Vol. 302: 123.

7. Hitchcock, Laura S., Ph.D., et al. "The Experience of Chronic Nonmalignant Pain." *Journal of Pain and Symptom Management*, Vol. 9, No. 5, July 1994: 312-318.

8. Tennant, Forest, M.D., Dr. P.H., and Harvey Rose, M.D. "Guidelines for Opioid Treatment of Stage III Intractable Pain." California Task Force on Opioid Treatment of Stage III Intractable Pain. January 1, 1997. Research Center for Dependency Disorders and Chronic Pain Community Health Projects Medical Group, West Covina, CA

9. Zenz, Michael M.D., et al. "Long-Term Oral Opioid Therapy in Patients With Chronic Nonmalignant Pain," *Journal of Pain and Symptom Management*, Vol. 7, No. 2, February 1992: 69-77.

10. Friedman, David P., Ph.D. "Perspectives on the Medical Use of Drugs of Abuse." *Journal of Pain and Symptom Management*, Vol. 5, No. 1 (Suppl.) February 1990: S2-S5.

11. Portenoy, Russell K., M.D. "Chronic Opioid Therapy in Non-malignant Pain." *Journal of Pain and Symptom Management*, Vol. 5, No. 1 (Suppl) February 1990: S46-S62.

12. Dellasega and Keiser. "Pharmacologic Approaches to Chronic Pain in the Adult." *Nurse Practitioner*. Vol. 22, No. 5, May 1997: 20-25.

13. Medical Board of California. "Prescribing for Pain Management." May 6, 1996.

14. California Board of Pharmacy. "Health Notes: Pain Management." 1996.

15. Canine, Craig. "Pain, Profit, and Sweet Relief." *Worth*. March, 1997: 79-82, 151-157.

16. Liebeskind, J.C. "Pain Can Kill." *Pain*, Vol. 44, No. 1, January 1991: 3-4.

17. Morse, T.B. "America's War on the Disabled." Albuquerque, NM: 60's Press.

18. National Institute of Arthritis and Musculoskeletal and Skin Diseases. "Scientific Workshop Summary: The Neuroscience and Endocrinology of Fibromyalgia." July 1996. Bethesda, MD.

19. Davis, Nadyne, et al. (eds.). "Third Annual Fibromyalgia Research Conference." February 1994. Inland Northwest Fibromyalgia Association. Spokane, WA 99206

— by Marcia E. Bedard, Ph.D., Professor of Women's Studies, California State University, Fresno, CA 93740-0078

Special thanks to Barbara Acello, MSEd, RN, Ann LeBlanc, and Rachael McKenna for research assistance, as well as CNP patients on the internet who sent me so many excellent suggestions for additions.

Chapter 4

How Is Nerve Pain Different from Physical Pain?

Pain is an experience common to everyone. And because everyone has experienced physical pain on some level, most people think they have a reasonable understanding of what pain is like for everyone else. However, when we're dealing with pain caused by nerve injury, such as Central Pain Syndrome or peripheral neuropathy, the normal concept of pain is thrown out the window. The sensations experienced in nerve pain are unlike anything else, ranging from the odd, "buzzing" sensation doctors call paresthesia that you might feel from a minor case of peripheral nerve damage, to the devastating complex, bizarre burning called dysesthesia that results from more severe nerve injury. The one thing common in neuropathic (nerve) pain is that there are no words sufficient to describe how these types of pain feel, because the sensations are so different from anything experienced by a person without nerve damage.

In order to understand the processes involved in pain we need to discuss nerve fibers and how they behave during pain. A nerve is a collection of many nerve cells, which are also called neurons. These nerve cells can be fibers up to a yard long, or they can be very short, such as some of the modifying neurons (interneurons) in the spinal

---

This chapter includes text excerpted from "How Pain Nerve Cells Act When *They* Are in Pain," produced by PainOnline with medical advice from consultant Kenneth McHenry, MD. © 2001 David Berg, reprinted with permission. The full text, which includes a more complete discussion of the biochemical processes involved in nerve pain, is available online at http://www.painonline.org.

cord. Sometimes the vocabulary used in medical literature can be a little vague and "nerve" can mean either one nerve cell or many.

Chemical Batteries in the Nervous System

The molecules that carry pain signals do not function unless they have a power source available. For the sake of simplicity we'll refer to that power as a battery. That battery comes in the form as a high-energy phosphate bond, which carries a negative charge. These batteries activate various chemicals in the body.

Molecules in the body are usually inert (nonreactive) unless something, usually a kinase, phosphorylates them (attaches a high-energy phosphate bond). The negative high-energy phosphate bond is taken from its supply carrier adenosine (a kind of delivery boy) and placed on the molecule that needs to be energized. The catalysts that accomplish this battery attachment are called kinases. Research by Ru-Rong Ji and Clifford Woolf indicates that mitogen-activated protein kinase (MAPK) is the master switch in Central Pain Syndrome. MAPK initiates a process that begins to place high-energy phosphate bonds, or batteries, on all kinds of pain neurotransmitters, making pain nerves fire out of control.

This action is taking place in the spinal cord, where first order neurons from the body are relaying signal to the second order neurons within the cord, which then travel to the thalamus (or perhaps the submedius, if they serve emotional messaging). This process of overblown excitation is probably recreated in the thalamus in its turn, but little is known about it.

In this chapter, "upstream" means closer to the brain, and "upregulate" means excite or make more excitable. Pain neurons leading from the skin-level are called first order neurons. Neurons are referred to by higher numbers as they get closer to the brain. For example, marginal cells in the spinal cord are one type of second order neuron.

It is more difficult to study neurons in the brain than elsewhere in the body, so science has been more successful in discovering treatments for injury to peripheral nerves. Opioids, like morphine, act to quiet the pain signal in the cord, but Central Pain originates upstream of the opioid point of action in the cord, so they don't stop Central Pain. Most people feel opioids act by sedating the patient, but do not actually stop the pain. Sometimes anticonvulsants are used as an alternative way to quiet the central nervous system and make Central Pain a little easier to bear, but there is no current treatment that is truly satisfactory.

The features of Central Pain and peripheral neuropathy can be difficult to distinguish and assign their specific point of origin. Some believe that in at least some instances the effects and actions of Central Pain and peripheral neuropathy are inescapably intertwined.

The Pain Path

At the nerve endings in the skin, the chronic pain process is ignited by persistent production of excess inflammatory chemicals, like prostaglandins, which cause an acid pH. The irritated first order neuron sends its signal toward the cord along a long extension, called the axon, which goes clear to the dorsal region (back) of the cord. It enters the cord just beyond where the neuron cell body is located. The pain signal crosses to the other side of the cord, while being influenced by connections with nearby neurons, and then connects via a synapse (or gap which is bridged by chemicals) to a second order neuron. Signals in the second order neuron rise to the thalamus, which is behind the eyes and optic nerves. The thalamus then forwards the pain signal through fibers that reach to the cortex, which results in conscious pain.

At the end of the first order axon, a long arm of the cell reaches to the skin surface. If you were to travel along this axon from the skin to the cord, you would meet the cell body to which the axon connects just outside the cord. On the other side of the cell body would be a little more axon, which is the part connecting to the next neuron. Inside the cord, the message is influenced by connections of the axon to other nerve cells, including some regulating neurons coming down from the brain. At the near end of each axon, is a small gap between it and the second order neuron, which is upstream (closer to the brain). The signal does not go across the gap directly, but by chemicals that are released into the gap, which then recreate a signal on the other side of the gap. The gap is called a synapse, or synaptic junction.

Making things more complicated, the cell body has the option of either forwarding the axon's signal into the cord or ignoring the signal. This decision by the cell body is determined by little fibers connecting to other cell bodies. The average cell body has thousands of these connections, about half are excitatory and about half are inhibitory of signal. So whether or not the near axon (end which enters the cord) actually carries pain signal is influenced by the connections that have already hit the cell body, which then decides the frequency of firing it will send to the near axon. Little globs or vesicles of excitatory chemicals are released from the near axon into the synaptic junction.

The action of the kinases you hear so much about, such as the ones that turn on NMDA (N-methyl D-aspartate; a big bad chemical of pain) occurs on the other side of the gap beyond the first order axon.

The genes in the second order neuron are influenced by the firing that reaches them to write (called transcription) for more pain-causing proteins from these genes, or in other words to make more messenger RNA, which results in the manufacture (called translation) of pain-causing proteins.

When the kinases attach batteries to the pain-causing proteins, the proteins are no longer silent. Very potent chemicals like NMDA initiate a powerful pain signal. The amino acid glutamate that enters the gap causes quick, short pain, while "Substance P" (which is composed of 11 amino acid residues) released from a vesicle acts in the second order neuron to cause persistent pain.

You remember that we said there are interneurons (in the zone crossing the cord) that act on the connection between first and second order neurons. These interneurons are mainly control devices coming down from the brain. Signals that come down from the brain are called efferent, while the signals carrying information to the brain are called afferent. We like efferent signals because they inhibit, but we don't like afferent signals, because they excite our pain.

It is worth mentioning that the axons of first order A-beta fibers are thick, insulated and rapidly tell about a very small area of skin, while C-fibers are thin, slow, have no insulation and tell about a much larger area of skin. If C-fibers get seriously and chronically irritated they can influence A-beta fibers entering the cord to send out signals to the normally quiet A-beta neighbors, so the whole neighborhood of A-betas is "buzzing" with pain. This is called "windup."

How Pain Works

A capacitor is a device to store electrical charge and the cell membrane is a capacitor. It can store about one microfarad (a tiny unit of electrical capacity) per square centimeter. This ability to store the electrical charge slows down conductance considerably in small nerve fibers like C fibers, so they are not suitable to warn about sudden pain, but operate for persistent pain.

Our pain system is configured to connect to our muscles to make them move away from pain. However, we don't want to go around twitching with every insignificant bump, so a place was provided where integration of sensory inputs could occur. That place is called a synapse. It is a physical break, which is crossed by chemicals, which are themselves under control from higher brain centers. The chemical message across the synaptic junction travels at a mere 2mm per minute. Fortunately the gap is only about one-millionth of an inch, so even at slow speed the signal requires only about 0.6 milliseconds to cross. This delay of the synapse allows interneurons time to excite or inhibit the system and upregulate or downregulate the reactivity in sensory and muscle fibers. If there were no input at the synapse, every signal might cause a muscle twitch.

What is the function of the brain in all of this? It's mainly to inhibit, or slow things down. We know the brain is primarily inhibitory, because if you remove the brain from a lab animal you still get nerve transmission from the cord and nerves, and it is faster without the brain. The time for signal to pass from toe to the cord is about 8 milliseconds, and the time added to allow for all the synaptic junctions is about 9 milliseconds, depending on size and insulation of the nerve fiber.

The speedy pain fibers, the A-betas, are covered with myelin, and are as big as 0.022 mm. People with multiple sclerosis have lost some of this myelin, which can cause pain signals to occur in nearby neurons. Normally only the nerve ending can generate an action potential, but in axons with damaged myelin, uninjured neighbor neurons can begin to fire automatically. This is called "crossed afterdischarge" by its discoverer, Marshall Devor. It provides clues to how a damaged axon might set off a huge pain process, building up an amplifying circuit of nerve fibers reacting to excitatory chemicals that are released into an area through injury.

"Adaptation" means that responses can reach saturation. For example, if you turn the hot water up a bit on a cold day and step into a hot bath, it might feel too hot at first but in a short time, it feels okay. This means the receptor signal is falling back. You have reached saturation and the nerve doesn't want to fire much anymore. If overproduced exciter chemicals drive the nerve ending receptor to fire at continuing high frequency, adaptation might never occur. Some touch receptors related to pain are never completely quiet, so adaptation would tend to be steady state and prominent in them, but if something removed the chemical means of adaptation, the nerves would refuse to be quiet at all. It is not hard to imagine how Central Pain patients might feel burning from touch, pressure, cramps, and tightness, if adaptation were abolished.

The brain hears a lot of noise from sensory fibers all the time. It's astounding it can "hear" these very small voltage differences and know what constitutes a real signal and is not just the "noise" of neuron voltage drifting up and down, right at the significant firing threshold. The state of readiness in sensory nerves, which drift over the firing threshold periodically, add up to a tremendous amount of noise that the brain must inhibit or ignore. Remember, in sensation most of the work of the brain is to inhibit or suppress signals. That is so you can think about only one thing at a time. The brain integrates all the many signals reaching the thalamus. Only when characteristics of a pain signal show a clear deviation from normal (one theory is that the brain has a template or pattern of normality against which to compare all sensory messages coming in) will the brain consciously generate a pain perception.

Pattern matching, or template comparison would be a highly sophisticated operation and susceptible to dysfunction. The chemical brew that churns up in synaptic junctions after nerve injury might be too much for the brain to inhibit; thus causing Central Pain. It is a paradox that incompletely injured nerves in sensory systems increase their signal powerfully, while nerves going to muscles simply carry less current when injured. Still, this makes sense when looking at the alerting function of pain systems.

In a normal pain system, "noise" is ignored by the brain, but how well the brain ignores "noise" in nerve injury is unknown. It is also unknown why adaptation fails to stop the burning pain of nerve injury. Perhaps adaptation does diminish it, but what persists is still so powerful that the burning continues.

A highly potent generation of pain signals could, over time, burn out the inhibitory control (dampening) neurons in the dorsal cord and in the thalamus, so that relatively light signals could make a major impact. This would be like pouring salt into a wound, or in this case, like pouring excitatory proteins into a system which has already been made vulnerable to them by injury. The end point of that injury may simply be to reset the regulatory genes in pain neurons so that they produce too much kinase, which attaches batteries to every excitatory protein, without waiting properly for the control signal from the brain, to do so. The downregulating center may have been burned out, like pointing a camera element directly at the sun can burn a hole in the shutter, the "bursting" pain signals may then pour on through the system.

Functional MRI shows metabolism (function) going on in the brain. Images of pain centers in the brain when nerve injury has occurred are inconsistent, even in the same individual. These imaging studies show anything from excessive metabolism, to normal metabolism, to shutdown in those areas of the brain. Perhaps the brain is damaged and is failing to regulate in its normal sense, giving in to adaptation, and then periodically tries unsuccessfully to bring things under control. Of course, "normal" brain metabolism in a system designed to actively inhibit, is highly abnormal if the brain ought to be powered up and doing its job of inhibiting pain signals. In Central Pain, pain centers appear confused, overwhelmed, and haphazard.

The Nerve Pain of Central Pain Syndrome

One of the questions from Central Pain patients is why they feel the pain so intensely. Often, patients will describe a type of nerve proximity feature to their pain, such as the direct feeling one gets when a dentist touches a filling with a metal instrument. It is a complex sensation that some describe as metallic, others as cold, but it is a common feature of Central Pain. The metallic/cold component of Central Pain suggests the brain is picking up on some very good conduction in the pain pathway.

Normal stimulation of pain nerves results in a rise in output of signal, but it may not correlate directly with the increase in stimulation. In fact, there are three ways the action potential may respond. These three are step, ramp, and oscillatory.

- **Step:** In a pure step arrangement, if the stimulus goes up a certain amount, the response goes up a certain amount, only to fade over time from saturation due to adaptation.

- **Ramp:** The ramp response is more even (linear) with continual increases, rather than discontinuous jumps in the nerve output.

- **Oscillatory:** Oscillatory output in sensory nerves would occur when walking, as weight shifts back and forth from one dysesthetic foot to the other. If this system failed completely, you wouldn't be able to walk because you couldn't sense when your foot hit bottom. CP patients often have a gait disturbance due to atopesthesia (not able to recognize of the location of a sensation) and loss of sensation so they cannot accurately tell when one foot has hit bottom.

The brain has a drive for survival. Your brain has an interest in sensation continuing, even if it is painful, because there are functions that require some sensation. The brain does not like to be shut out entirely from its environment, so it apparently recruits pain for information if it has to. It may even be withholding inhibition of which it is capable in order to maintain contact with the outside world.

Unfortunately, most pain fibers can't be tested for their output characteristics because the output occurs so close to the cell body that the results are unreliable, especially with thermal receptors. In Central Pain, nerves continue the sensation of burning after touch stimulus stops. In fact, the continual or spontaneous burning never stops, but evoked or elicited burning does. This suggests there are pain outputs operating at two different levels, each with its own characteristics.

Summary

Now is a good time to review what happens in Central Pain.

1. At the skin there is irritation

2. In the cord there is amplification

3. In the brain there is feature extraction and interpretation (integration)

Unfortunately, doctors can confuse these three steps. That is why pain clinics may grow frustrated when something shown to work in peripheral nerve injury does nothing to help a Central Pain patient. The clinician may be giving a drug that avoids irritation, or even amplification, but it may have no effect on the integration of signals in the thalamus, which causes the brain to mistake the signal's character and generate a pain message quickly. As stated, if integration fails in an injured neuron, the signal would be less clear and perhaps the sensation would also be harder to recognize.

Chapter 5

Gender and Pain

Male and Female Brains Process Pain Differently

Whether you are male or female influences how much pain you have, what type of pain it is, and how treatment affects you. Male and female brains process pain differently.

Women report pain more often than men do, said, Karen Berkley, Ph.D. (McKenzie Professor of Neuroscience at Florida State University, Tallahassee, Florida) and in more body regions. They also have more severe and more persistent pain. When women and men are given the same pain stimuli in laboratory studies—gradually increasing heat, for instance—women say "ouch!" before men do. Women discriminate better between types of pain.

Age and sex differences exist in the prevalence of many chronic pain conditions, according to Linda LeResche, Sc.D., research professor of oral medicine, at the University of Washington School of Dentistry, Seattle, Washington. Studying age/sex patterns, she said, may help identify causes of some pain conditions. Migraine headache, as one example, affects mainly women in their childbearing years, decreasing with age. This pattern suggests hormones may play a role

Excerpted from "Gender and Pain Conference," National Institutes of Health (NIH), April 1998. In 1996, the NIH established its Pain Research Consortium with representatives from all NIH divisions. Members of this group, plus other NIH centers and offices, sponsored the April 1998 conference on gender and pain. The full text of these reports is available online at http://www1.od.nih.gov/painresearch/genderandpain.

in migraines. That is less likely to be true, she said, for a pain problem that continues to rise with age, such as joint pain.

Despite their greater pain burden, women handle pain better than men do. Women use more coping strategies, honed perhaps by their more frequent encounters with pain, in menstruation and in labor and childbirth. Women prepare better for pain, Berkley asserted. They plan tactics to handle it. Men more often say, "I'll deal with it when I have to."

Even young boys and girls often differ in how they perceive and cope with pain. Many cultures around the world permit girls to be emotional, but discourage boys from showing pain. These attitudes then are carried into adulthood.

Some Medications Ease Pain Better in Women

Studies of dental pain in men and women offer scientists an opportunity to assess gender influences on the pain experience. Christine Miaskowski, R.N., Ph.D., professor of nursing at the University of California, San Francisco, California (UCSF), described how extraction of third molars, sometimes called wisdom teeth, affects men and women differently.

In a series of studies conducted at UCSF's schools of dentistry and nursing, the same oral surgeon performed standardized surgery. Miaskowski and her colleagues then evaluated the effectiveness of several pain-relieving medications on post-surgical pain. They found that certain medications at most doses eased pain in women better and longer than they did in men. The medications, all available only by prescription, belong to a family of pain-relieving medications known as kappa opioids. They include pentazocine, nalbuphine, and butorphanol. Further research is in progress, Miaskowski said, to discover why men and women respond differently. The researchers also plan to explore the impact of the menstrual cycle on pain sensitivity and medication effectiveness in women.

In another dental study, Jocelyne Feine, D.D.S., H.D.R., associate professor, Faculty of Dentistry, McGill University, Montreal, Quebec, Canada, followed 27 women and 21 men for 10 days after surgery to implant a replacement tooth. The women described the surgery as significantly more painful than the men did, Feine said, although both sexes rated the pain on a pain scale as similarly intense. In both sexes, pain fell by 50% within two days. In the 10 days following the surgery, women tolerated low levels of pain much better than did the men. As time passed, the men were more disturbed than the women by persisting discomfort.

Sexes Affected Differently by Common Diseases Associated with Pain

Osteoarthritis

Osteoarthritis (OA), the "wear and tear" disorder of the joints, affects 40% of middle aged adults and up to 70% of older adults. Some forms of OA are more common in women than men. OA of the knee, for example, is twice as common in women as in men. By contrast, OA of the hips affects men and women equally.

Pain is the most common symptom of OA. The extent of joint damage does not necessarily predict the amount of pain persons with OA feel, according to Francis J. Keefe, Ph.D., professor of health psychology at Ohio University, Athens, Ohio. One person with moderate OA, he said, may report little pain and be quite active, even able to play golf or tennis. Another may report severe pain and sometimes use a wheelchair.

Keefe and his colleagues asked 41 women and 30 men with OA to keep daily pain diaries. The women reported 40% more OA pain and more severe pain. But they coped more actively with it. They spoke more about their pain with others, looked for distractions, sought spiritual support, and asked for help. Women's energetic coping efforts, he said, paid off: the day after experiencing severe OA pain, they were less likely to report negative moods than men were.

Heart Disease

Before age 50, women have more chest pain but less heart disease than men do. Women over age 50 have more silent heart disease than men do.

Women in their premenopausal years experience chest pain more often than men. But they are far less likely than men to have underlying heart disease, said Noel Bairey-Merz, M.D., medical director of the Preventative and Rehabilitative Cardiac Center at Cedars-Sinai Medical Center, Los Angeles, California. Postmenopausal women, she said, are more likely than men to have silent heart disease.

Half of the young women with chest pain so severe that their doctors send them to a cardiac catheterization laboratory for further study, she said, prove to have normal arteries in the heart. That is true for only 17% of men with similar symptoms.

Preliminary findings suggest that female hormones may play a contributory role. Both premenopausal women with high estrogen

41

levels and postmenopausal women using estrogen replacement therapy, Bairey-Merz said, had more frequent and more severe chest pain that was not caused by heart disease.

In another study, David Sheps, M.D., professor and chair of cardiology at the James H. Quillen College of Medicine at East Tennessee State University in Johnson City, Tennessee, and his colleagues, explored differing perceptions of chest pain, or angina, in men and women with heart disease. Some 170 men and 26 women participated in the study. They were matched for age, disease severity, and other factors. All participants kept symptom diaries for 48 hours. They then completed separate day-long tests of mental and physical stress. On the mental stress day, they took a battery of psychological exams. Among them was a public speaking challenge: participants had to give a talk about a hassling life experience. The physical stress day included an upright bicycle exercise test and similar exertion. On both days, participants wore devices to monitor heart activity, had blood drawn, and had x-ray studies of heart functioning.

Women reported chest pain more often in daily life and on the mental stress day, but no more often after exercise stress. The researchers identified several factors that might account for this discrepancy. The women scored higher than the men did on psychological measures, such as "harm avoidance." They had lower levels of beta endorphins, brain chemicals related to feelings of well being. When challenged with a heat stimulus, they reported feeling pain sooner than the men did. These findings, Sheps and his colleagues say, suggest that men and women attend to and view certain symptoms differently.

Migraine Headaches

About one in 5 women and one in 17 men in the U.S. report experiencing migraine headaches, according to Rami Burstein, Ph.D., assistant professor of anesthesia and neurobiology at Beth Israel Deaconess Medical Center and Harvard Medical School, Boston, Massachusetts. Before puberty, Burstein said, migraines are more common in boys than girls.

Migraines cause dull pain, typically worse on one side of the head. Some people become extremely sensitive to light and experience nausea. Migraines usually last from 2 to 6 hours.

In women, migraines often occur at the time of ovulation, near menstruation, and in pregnancy. This fact has prompted attention to hormonal factors. One theory is that shifts in hormone levels may be a trigger: birth control pills make migraines worse in some women, better in others. During pregnancy, some women's migraines disappear, but other women get them for the first time. Migraines usually appear before age 35, but some women develop them only after menopause. In both women and men, other triggers include lack of sleep, hunger, stress, red wine, bright light, and heat.

Chronic Reproductive Organ Pain

Medications used for many common pain syndromes benefit men with chronic pain of the reproductive organs, but rarely help women with chronic pelvic pain, according to Ursula Wesselmann, M.D., Ph.D., assistant professor of neurology at the Johns Hopkins University School of Medicine, Baltimore, Maryland. She and her colleagues at the Hopkins pain clinic compared 39 women with chronic, non-cancerous, pelvic pain and 25 men with chronic, non-cancerous, testicular pain. Each patient received one of four different types of medication known to relieve other pain syndromes. The medications included antidepressants, anticonvulsants, membrane stabilizing agents, and opioids. A larger percentage of men than women improved in each case. With antidepressants, the most frequently used medication, for instance, nine of 11 men improved. Only four of 28 women did so.

Both women and men with these disorders, Wesselmann said, experience deep pain that often is hard to localize. Such pain often triggers changes in blood pressure, nausea, and sweating, making people feel quite ill. Both men and women, she said, often find the pain embarrassing and hard to talk about, even with a physician. As a result, some delay seeking help or don't assertively pursue the help they need.

Pelvic pain in women that lasts at least 6 months at the same location generally is thought to have a gynecological source, Wesselmann said, although physicians sometimes are not able to pinpoint it. A disorder such as endometriosis, an inflammation of the lining of the uterus, causes some women a great deal of pain, even when little disease is present. Yet some women with extensive disease have no pain.

Many of the women Wesselmann studied had undergone numerous surgical procedures, including hysterectomies, pelvic exploration, and treatment for endometriosis, before coming to the pain clinic still seeking relief. Studies of large groups of women, she noted, suggest that women have a 5% risk of having pelvic pain in their lifetime. The risk rises to 20% in women with pelvic inflammatory disease.

Chronic testicular pain is most common in men in their late 30s. This pain is defined as pain in one or both testes that lasts at least 3 months. In one in 3 men, there is no obvious cause. In the others, bicycle accidents, vasectomies, infections, tumors, and other medical disorders are identified as the trigger.

The men in the Hopkins study had undergone fewer surgical procedures on average than the women. Male urologists may be more reluctant to remove reproductive organs in male patients, Wesselmann suggested, than male gynecologists to remove reproductive organs in women.

Chronic reproductive organ pain interfered more with daily activities in women than it did in men. Women reported that the pain caused them to lose time from work and to be less productive. This was true regardless of whether or not they also were depressed. Only depressed men reported similar interference with daily life. Of the two types of chronic reproductive organ pain, Wesselmann said, women's pain is the more complex. There is an urgent need, she said, to better understand its causes and improve its treatment.

Fibromyalgia

Nine times more women than men have fibromyalgia (FM), a disorder causing widespread pain and fatigue, according to Laurence A. Bradley, Ph.D., professor of medicine at the University of Alabama, Birmingham, Alabama. Persons with FM report exquisite sensitivity to pressure stimulation both at specific locations, referred to as tender points, and at other sites on the body.

The lack of an obvious definitive cause for the disorder, the preponderance of women, and the long-held belief that women are more prone than men to "hysterical" disorders have served, Bradley said, to stigmatize persons with FM and to retard research. His research and that of other contemporary investigators suggest that FM has a biological basis.

Bradley and his colleagues studied pain perception, functional brain activity, and psychosocial factors, in three groups of women. They included:

- 66 women being treated in a medical clinic for FM. These women met the standard classification measures for FM: they had widespread pain lasting at least 3 months at 11 or more of the 18 standard tender points. None had other rheumatic illnesses, chronic fatigue syndrome, or a history of neck or back surgery.

44

- 40 women in the community who fit the same guidelines for FM, recruited via newspaper advertisements. None of these women had sought help for pain in the last 10 years.

- 40 healthy women.

The researchers found that regardless of whether or not the women had sought health care, those with FM perceived a pressure stimulus as painful at lower intensity levels than healthy women did. Women with FM also distinguished different types of sensations better than healthy women. Their cerebrospinal fluid contained significantly higher levels of substance P, a chemical messenger of pain. Studies using a device known as a single photon emission computerized tomographic (SPECT) scanner, showed differing activity in areas critical for pain perception in women with FM than in healthy women.

Temporomandibular Disorder

Seven times more women than men have Temporomandibular Disorder (TMD), a group of conditions involving pain and dysfunction of the temporomandibular joint in the jaw and surrounding muscles, according to William Maixner, D.D.S., Ph.D., co-director of the oral and maxillofacial pain program at the University of North Carolina, Chapel Hill, North Carolina. TMD is surprisingly common, he said, affecting an estimated one in four young adult women.

Persons with TMD, he and his colleagues found, are more sensitive to several types of painful stimuli than persons without the disorder. A heat stimulus applied to skin on the arm or the face, for example, caused more pain in persons with TMD than in healthy persons. When a heat stimulus was applied in a pulsating fashion to the hand, persons with TMD reached their maximum level of pain tolerance much faster than persons without TMD.

TMD may lower quality of life by disturbing both sleep and mood, Maixner said. It even may be an early stage of fibromyalgia (FM), he suggested. Some 75% of persons with fibromyalgia—again, mostly women—also report TMD symptoms. The progression from TMD to FM, he said, may be linked to the degree of disruption in a person's pain regulatory systems.

Postmastectomy Pain

Most women recover uneventfully from surgery for cancer of the breast, but some develop chronic pain starting days to weeks after their surgery. About one in 20 to one in five experience long-lasting pain, according to different studies. The pain typically affects the underarm, underside of the upper arm, and/or the chest wall, and sometimes, the shoulder. Women usually say this pain involves shock-like sensations overlying more continuous aching and burning. They describe it as "shooting," "stabbing," "piercing," and even "excruciating." Since movement such as reaching or lifting often makes the pain worse, women commonly protect the affected arm. This habit frequently produces shoulder stiffness and further pain. Women may have trouble sleeping, dressing, and performing household chores. Chronic postmastectomy pain, unfortunately, often does not lessen with time.

Researchers are studying both causes and treatments for this pain syndrome, including medications, physical therapy to restore function, and behavioral strategies to aid in coping with the pain. Some studies link the pain to surgical injury to a particular nerve in the underarm area. Researchers are exploring whether it is possible to spare this nerve without contributing to the further spread or recurrence of the cancer.

A study conducted in Finland found that chronic pain was more likely in women who remembered more postoperative pain. The researchers interviewed women with breast cancer 3 times in the year following their surgery. Those with chronic pain remembered having severe pain after the surgery, and their memory for it grew even stronger over time. By the end of the year, anxiety and depression returned to normal levels in women who had no chronic pain. It persisted, however, in those whose pain continued.

Researchers at the University of California, San Francisco, School of Nursing, studied 95 women who had breast cancer surgery. Nineteen reported postmastectomy pain. These women, the researchers found, often received inadequate pain relief. Some physicians, they suggested, may be unfamiliar with the postmastectomy pain syndrome and its potential treatment. Existing medications, including tricyclic antidepressants, topical anesthetics, and anticonvulsants, all requiring prescriptions, they said, may ease this type of pain.

Cancer Pain

Having a severe, chronic pain condition may have a greater influence on the individual's experience of pain than does their sex, according to Dennis Turk, Ph.D., John and Emma Bonica Professor of Anesthesiology and Pain, at the University of Washington School of

Medicine, Seattle, Washington. Turk and Akiko Okifuji, Ph.D., research assistant professor of anesthesiology, studied 91 men and 52 women who sought treatment at a cancer center for chronic cancer pain. The group included persons with both localized cancer and cancer that had spread, or metastasized. The patients were comparable in age, education, and other measures, although they were not matched by type of cancer or stage.

The researchers found no significant male/female differences among the patients in pain severity, emotional distress, adaptation, or limitations in activities of daily life. The results were comparable to those seen in an earlier study of 428 consecutive patients, approximately equal numbers of men and women, at a pain treatment center.

The majority of pain patients, Turk said, regardless of diagnosis, fall into three categories:

- *Dysfunctional.* These persons have high pain and emotional distress, and believe they have little control over their circumstances.

- *Interpersonally distressed.* These persons have moderate pain and emotional distress, but perceive they receive little support.

- *Adaptive copers.* These persons have low emotional distress and a "take-charge" attitude.

Proportionally fewer cancer patients were classified as dysfunctional than noncancer patients, Turk said. Fewer persons whose cancer had spread were interpersonally distressed than those in the other two groups. "There are very few patients with metastatic cancer and chronic pain," he observed, "who do not feel they get considerable support from others." Turk said he found no statistically significant differences between men and women with all types of chronic pain with regard to pain severity, adaptation, or effect of pain on their lives. Differences within each sex, he said, proved greater than those between the sexes. "How people perceive and interpret their particular situation," he said, "may be more important than whether they are male or female."

Chapter 6

Pain in Infants

Although physicians and nurses believe babies can feel as much pain as adults, they say that infants are not getting the pain relief they feel they need during circumcision and other medical procedures. Researchers at Washington University School of Medicine in St. Louis reported these findings in the October 1997 issue of *Pediatrics* after surveying 374 caregivers in premature and neonatal nurseries in St. Louis hospitals.

"Caregivers reported very large discrepancies between how pain is managed and how they believe pain should be managed. These caregivers reported a very low use of pain-relieving drugs and comfort measures, regardless of the painfulness of the procedure," said Fran L. Porter, Ph.D., assistant professor of pediatrics and lead author of the study, which was funded by the National Institute of Child Health and Human Development.

Although much has been learned in the past decade about infant pain, this was the first study to explore the relationship between caregivers' beliefs about both infant pain and pain management. The study had somewhat surprising results.

"We found that the caregivers believe more effective pain management should be provided. Obstacles to offering better pain relief now must be addressed," said Porter.

"Infants May Not Receive Adequate Pain Relief, Caregivers Believe," by Diane Duke, Washington University, School of Medicine in St. Louis, October 1997. © 1997 Washingon University School of Medicine; reprinted with permission.

Rating the Pain

The researchers distributed surveys to 467 physicians and nurses in 15 hospital nurseries in St. Louis. Most of the babies they care for are premature or acutely ill. The researchers received 374 completed surveys. The caregivers were asked to rate the painfulness of 12 bedside nursery procedures and how often pharmacological and comfort measures are currently used and should be used for those procedures. The therapeutic and diagnostic procedures included chest tube insertions, heel sticks, circumcisions, IV placements and catheter insertions among others. The respondents also were asked to compare the intensity of infant and adult pain.

Almost 59 percent of the physicians and 64 percent of the nurses believed that infants feel the same amount of pain as adults, and about 27 percent believed infants feel more pain. Only 10 percent believed infants feel less pain than adults.

The caregivers rated nine of the 12 procedures as being at least moderately painful, believing that some procedures were more painful than others. Circumcision and insertion of a chest tube were rated as more painful, whereas airway suctioning and insertion of a feeding tube were rated as less painful.

Analgesics and anesthesia are rarely used, the nurses and physicians reported, even for the most painful procedures. But both physicians and nurses believed that pharmacological agents should be used more often than they currently are, with the highest preference for circumcisions and insertion of chest tubes.

Both nurses and physicians also believe that comfort measures are seldom used. Nurses tended to rate their use of comfort measures, such as swaddling, holding and rocking, slightly higher than physicians did. The caregivers believe that comfort measures should be used more often.

More Comfort Measures Needed

The caregivers also were asked questions about their current position, training, years of experience, gender, parental status and whether they had undergone surgery or had experienced significant pain.

Physicians who said they had experienced significant pain during their lives rated the painfulness of the infants as higher. They also said more drugs are currently given and that more comfort measures should be used.

Similar relationships between personal pain and pain management beliefs were not found among the nurses.

Porter said there are numerous possibilities why caregivers do not use more pain-relieving drugs and comfort measures. Appropriate approved drugs for some of these procedures in infants may not be available. And pain management may not be a priority in job descriptions and is not a priority in medical training. Comfort measures are safe and inexpensive to administer, but the nursing environment may not encourage their use.

"This study confirms that attitudes about infant pain have changed dramatically in the past 20 years, which is very important and positive," Porter said. "At the same time, caregivers believe many of the procedures they perform are painful for the babies and for most procedures, pain relief is inferior. This must place many caregivers in uncomfortable situations," said Porter. "We need to identify the barriers to more effective pain relief for these small patients."

Note: For more information, refer to: Porter FL, Wolf CM, Gold J, Lotsoff D, Miller JP, "Pain and Pain Management in Newborn Infants: A Survey of Physicians and Nurses," *Pediatrics* 100, 626-632, 1997.

— by Diane Duke

Chapter 7

Children with Pain

Getting a shot in the doctor's office. Skinning a knee. Suffering from a headache. In these and other encounters with pain, girls and boys may differ in how they behave, express their pain, and perhaps even how they perceive pain, according to Patricia McGrath, Ph.D., professor of pediatrics and director, Paediatric Pain Program, Child Health Research Institute, University of Western Ontario, London, Ontario.

A child's age, past experience with pain, and family and cultural styles, McGrath said, influences his or her response to new, painful situations. Parents serve as models. Young children often fall down, she observed, and then look at a parent for cues on how to react. In general, the younger the child, the greater his or her overt distress, and the more the child has to be physically restrained, she said, the more painful the experience will be.

Sex differences in pain responses may be apparent but are not always explainable. Boys rate having braces tightened as more severe than do girls, for example, while girls rate having a broken arm as more painful than do boys. Even so, girls, in general, grade many procedures as more painful than boys do. In comparable situations,

This chapter includes text from "Children and Pain," National Institutes of Health, Gender and Pain Conference, April 1998 (available online at http://www1.od.nih.gov/painresearch/genderandpain.children.htm); and "Procedure Pain," an undated fact sheet available online at http://www.nursing.uiowa.edu/sites/PedsPain/Procedure/ProcOver.htm, © University of Iowa College of Nursing, reprinted with permission.

she said, girls are more likely to be fearful and anxious, and boys to be angry.

It sometimes is hard for health professionals, and even parents, to avoid causing children pain when attending to their health. But some strategies, she said, can lessen pain. These include giving children as much control as possible over what is being done to their bodies. A child who needs to provide a blood sample, for example, can chose the finger, and perhaps even stick it, and smear the blood on a slide without help. At home, a child could wash his or her own cuts with soap and water, and put on a bandage.

With age, children inevitably encounter a variety of pains that differ in quality and intensity. Their perspective on pain changes, and they generally become more adept at dealing with pain.

Those who think of childhood as largely a care-free time, however, may be dismayed to learn that in a typical month, a normal, otherwise-healthy child averages about four acute pains related to injuries and diseases—falls, sore throats, sprains—plus one achy pain, such as a headache or stomachache. Pain diaries kept by children show a diverse list of pain-causing experiences: being hit on the head with a golf club, stung by a bee, bitten by a dog, stepping on broken glass.

Many otherwise healthy and pain-free children, more often girls than boys, McGrath said, experience recurrent pain syndromes. These consist of episodes of headaches, abdominal pains, and limb pains as often as three or four times a week. In such instances, the pain usually does not reflect an underlying disease needing medical treatment, she said. The pain by itself is the problem.

Persistent pain problems in childhood may be predisposing factors for more debilitating pain in adulthood. "If we were able to better recognize and manage children's pain problems," McGrath said, "we might be able to prevent some disability in adults."

"In our clinic," she said, "we teach children that what they know, do, and feel, can influence their perception of pain." She and her colleagues try to improve children's understanding and control by giving them age-appropriate information, telling them, for example, that an injection will sting. They explain the rationale for what is happening, and they teach children simple pain-reducing coping strategies, such as active distraction.

Procedure Pain

Holding still: Often when doctors and nurses are trying to find out what is wrong with a boy or girl they have to go through some tests (procedures) to see exactly what is going on. Some procedures (x-rays and scans) aren't painful but require that you hold still, which is hard for young children. Kids may be scared during these procedures. It is perfectly all right to ask for some medicine to help a child be less afraid. Children are often given a medicine named chloral hydrate; it's orange and doesn't taste the best, but works.

Painful Procedures

Some procedures require that the person hold still and are also painful. Two of these are bone marrow aspiration and lumbar puncture. Even though these tests can be painful, doctors and nurses have some ways to numb the area being tested so it won't hurt so much.

Numbing medicines: In the past the only "numbing" medicine that was available was novocaine, the same medicine that the dentists use for dental work. Dentists have an advantage because when they inject into the lining of the mouth they can rub the area before injecting and the needle is not felt. Unfortunately, the same thing does not happen when you inject into skin. When you inject a "caine" (medicines with names that end in "-caine") into skin that isn't broken (intact) it can sting. Either novocaine or Xylocaine can be combined with baking soda (we call it sodium bicarbonate) in a ratio of nine or ten parts to one and the stinging will not occur but the medicine will work.

EMLA: EMLA (eutectic mixture of local anesthetic) is a white cream that comes in a tube that looks like a toothpaste tube. The white EMLA cream is put on the skin one hour before the procedure and covered with a dressing. After one hour the skin will be numb. This has really helped in pediatrics particularly for bone marrow aspirations, lumbar punctures, accessing ports, and starting IVs. It is approved for use when the skin is intact. It is important to remember that you will still be able to feel pressure as the test is being done but you should not feel pain if EMLA cream us used. Because EMLA cream only numbs the skin, sometimes both the cream and novocaine are used if the testing requires going deep into the bone.

General anesthetics: In some settings, children are taken to a room just outside of the operating room and put to sleep for their bone marrow aspirations and lumbar punctures. Several hospitals are using an anesthetic agent called "Propofol-Diprivan" which is a short acting general anesthetic. Children who have had lumbar punctures or bone marrow aspirations performed with this agent usually have no memory of the procedures and generally are not fearful of them. The problems, of course, are getting insurance companies to pay for them and there is risk whenever you put someone to sleep with a general anesthetic.

Sedatives, analgesics, and conscious sedation: A number of other medicines can be used to assist children through procedures. Some medicines help people relax, such as midazolam (Versed), and others, such as fentanyl or morphine, help with the pain. As with any medication, these must be given carefully in doses specific for the person and they must be given under close supervision.

Chapter 8

Pain in the Elderly

Pain and the Elderly

Chronic unrelieved pain is the cause of untold suffering for millions of people worldwide. It has been estimated that approximately 30% of the general population of the U.S. suffers from some form of chronic pain.[1] In a recent study of the general population of the state of Michigan, The Michigan Pain Study, it was found that one in five adults, or about 1.2 million people in Michigan suffer from some form of chronic, ongoing or recurring pain.[2] The elderly, especially those over 80 years of age, are the fastest growing population in the USA,[3] and the elderly report more pain than younger persons. Approximately 2–27% of the elderly report some form of headache,[4] 14–49% report low back pain and 24–71% report some form of joint pain.[5,6] The elderly in extended care facilities report a higher prevalence of pain than the elderly living at home. 71–83% of the elderly in nursing homes report some form of pain, joint pain, back pain, and muscle aches being the most reported pains.[7] Other pain problems that are most prevalent in this population include vertebrogenic pain syndrome from osteoporosis, rheumatoid arthritic pains, post herpetic neuralgia, post thalamic pain syndrome, etc.

This chapter includes text from "Pain and the Elderly" by Elliot Krames, MD. Reprinted with permission from *San Francisco Medicine*, the official publication of the San Francisco Medical Society. And, "Elderly with Dementia Have Trouble Reporting Pain, According to Study" by Diane Duke, Washington University, School of Medicine in St. Louis, February 1997. © 1997 Washingon University School of Medicine; reprinted with permission.

The Evaluation of Pain

The treatment of pain associated with both cancer and non-cancer requires that the pain practitioner first understand and evaluate the nature of the patient's pain, the possible psychological and behavior factors that may influence chronic pain, and the possible treatment modalities that are appropriate for the patient's specific pain syndrome. Chronic pain is highly complex, and because of cognitive issues and changing metabolic issues it may be even more so in the elderly population. Chronic pain is never unidimensional, solely biological or solely psychological; it is almost always multidimensional, involving not only neurophysiological systems, but emotional and behavioral systems as well. Pain should be well assessed and continuously reassessed with treatment.

The Treatment of Pain

The practitioner caring for the elderly person with pain should have familiarity with possible therapies for the treatment of chronic pain in the elderly and should be willing, when necessary, to send these patients to experts in pain medicine for consultation. The tools of the pain practitioner include all of the modalities and therapies, either conservative or invasive, that are used for treating chronic pain syndromes. These tools can be broadly organized as non-invasive and invasive therapies. Non-invasive therapies include cognitive and behavioral therapies, rehabilitational pain medicine, and complimentary pain relieving therapies such acupuncture, acupressure, meditation/relaxation, nutrition, and Qui-gong, etc. The purpose of cognitive-behavioral therapy is to improve self locus of control, to increase awareness and understanding of the painful experience, to promote activity that is not harmful or activating of the painful experience, to increase relaxation time and adopt behavioral patterns that promote healing and reduce repetitive behaviors that perpetuate the chronic painful experience. Interventional pain management includes pharmacologic therapy such as non-opioid analgesics, opioid analgesics, and adjuvant medication, nerve blocking techniques, neuromodulatory or surgical interventions, and neurodestructive interventions.

Cancer Pain Management

In the early 1970s, because of the growing awareness of lay people and healthcare givers alike that it was not acceptable for terminally ill patients to die in extreme pain and suffering, the World Health Organization (WHO), provided guidelines for managing the pain of dying patients. These guidelines were an attempt to obey a recognized medical management principle, the KISS principle ("keep it sweet and simple"), simplifying pain management for cancer patients so that it could be used by technologically advanced as well as technologically deprived societies. Approximately 80–90 percent of patients dying of cancer should have their pain well controlled using these guidelines. Because this approach provides adequate pain management in only 80–90 percent of patients suffering from pain of terminal illness, and because interventional approaches do work, many have proposed the addition of interventional strategies to the WHO guidelines as a "fourth rung" of this ladder. Interventional strategies, as last resort interventions include peripheral and central nerve blocks, sympathetic nerve blocks, epidural steroid injections, continuous epidural, plexus, and spinal analgesia techniques, intrapleural analgesia and neurolytic chemical, thermal and surgical techniques.

The Treatment of Chronic, Non-Malignant Pain

Because there are also multiple noninvasive and invasive modality choices for the treatment of chronic nonmalignant pain, it is suggested that these patients be treated using the treatment continuum suggested by the WHO for cancer patients. Obeying a time honored medical principle of utilizing simple, least invasive, and least costly interventions before using more invasive, highly technological, and more costly interventions, it is suggested that an algorithm of treatment, a pain treatment continuum, that lists available pain therapies by increasing order of both invasiveness and cost, be used for the treatment of chronic pain patients. According to this suggested pain treatment continuum, least invasive and least costly therapies, either in series (utilizing one therapy at a time, abandoning those that do not work, and advancing to more invasive therapies as in climbing a ladder) or in parallel (utilize more than one therapy simultaneously and advancing to more costly and invasive therapies) should be used before more invasive or more costly therapies. When more conservative interventions for the relief of intractable pain fail to provide adequate analgesia, it is important that the practitioner not abandon the patient. Interventional techniques such as nerve blocking, spinal cord stimulation and intraspinal, implantable drug delivery can and do provide analgesia when more conservative therapies have failed.

The Elderly, a Special Case

As a population of pain patients, the elderly are more undertreated than any other group of patients besides infants. Approximately 47–80% of these patients living at home and not institutionalized do not receive any pain care.[8] 16–27% of patients within nursing homes or extended care facilities do not receive any care for their pain complaints.[9]

The reasons for this undertreatment is poorly understood, but clearly physicians and caregivers often find it hard to assess the elderly patient's complaints. Pain, as a subjective complaint, as stated above, is a complex phenomenon. Because of cognitive changes that occur with aging, sometimes, it may be difficult to assess the quality and intensity of pain in this group. The elderly have multiple medical problems and multiple complaints making adequate assessments of pain difficult and confusing for the practitioner. Even with appropriate assessment, this group of patients may, because of memory problems or confusion, present with special treatment issues. They might not understand directions for taking medications, might forget these directions, or just forget to take their medications altogether.

Confounding the cognitive issues in the elderly is the difficulty in assessing the differences between pain and dementia. Pain complaints, in fact, may be the first signs of dementia in the elderly.[10] As this dementia progresses it becomes increasingly important to rely on the assessment of the patient's pain from the caregivers, and not the patient, and oftentimes, caregivers do not believe that the patient is in pain. Just because these patients might not be able to adequately communicate their complaints of pain, the practitioner should never abandon the patient. The patient still hurts and needs redress of his or her suffering.

There are certain pharmacodynamic and kinetic principles that must be remembered when treating the elderly with analgesic medications. There are age-associated changes in the metabolism and clearance rates of agents that are usually used for the treatment of pain. As a group these patients are subject to overdosing of their medications because of a lack of knowledge of these age related changes by physicians who treat them. Special problems with medications that may present because of metabolic and kinetic changes in aging populations include:

- Increased risk of stomach irritation, water retention, hypertension, headache, and kidney disorder with the taking of NSAIDs.

- Quicker onset of action and prolonged time of action of opioids.

- Mental changes and confusion with opioids and local anesthetics.

- Urinary retention, severe constipation and even obstipation
with opioids or antidepressants.

- Severe dizziness, increased risk of falling with antidepressants,
opioids, and anticonvulsants.

In summary, it should be stressed that the elderly, as a group, have
more complaints of pain than younger patients and that there are
special concerns regarding appropriate treatment. Metabolic and
pharmacokinetic changes that come with age make these patients
more vulnerable to overdosing of analgesic agents. The inability to
adequately assess pain in this group, coupled with caregiver's fear of
overdosing them, has often led to the undertreatment of their pain.

1. Bonica JJ. *Chronic non-cancer pain*, In Anderson S, Bond M,
   Mehta M, et al (eds) Lancaster UK, MTP Press, 1987.

2. The Michigan Pain Study: EPIC/MRA 4710 W. Saginaw Hwy.
   Lansing Michigan 48917-2601, 1997.

3. US Department of Commerce Global aging: comparative indicators and future trends. US Department of Commerce, Economics and Statistics Administration, Bureau of the Census,
   Washington, DC. 1991.

4. Lipton RB, Pfeffer D, Newman LC, Solomon S: Headaches in
   the elderly. *J Pain and Symptom Management* 1993 8:87-97.

5. Sternbach RA: Survey of pain in the United States: the
   Nuprin pain report. *Clinical J of pain* 1986 2:49-53.

6. Valkenburg HA: Epidemiological considerations of the geriatric population. *Gerontology* 1988 34(suppl 1):2-10.

7. Ferrel BA, Ferrell BR: Pain in the nursing home. *J of the
   Amer Geriatrics Soc.* 1990 38:409-414.

8. Woo J, Ho SC, Lau J, Leung PC: Musculoskeletal complaints
   and associated consequences in elderly Chinese aged 70 and
   over. *J of Rheum* 1994 21:1927-1931.

9. Roy R and Thomas M: A survey of chronic pain in an elderly population. *Canadian Family Physician* 1986 32:513-516.

10. Kisely S, Tweddle D, Pugh EW: Dementia presenting with sore eyes. *British Journal of Psychiatry* 1992 161:120-121.

—Section by Elliot Krames, MD

Dr. Elliot Krames is Medical Director of Pacific Pain Treatment Centers with offices in San Francisco and Concord. Pacific Pain Treatment Centers provides interdisciplinary care for patients suffering with chronic pain. Pacific Pain Treatment Centers utilizes the expertise of a team of nurses, chronic pain oriented psychologists, physical therapists and occupational therapists. Dr. Krames is a national and internationally known expert in pain medicine and implantable technologies. He is Editor-in-Chief of *NEUROMODULATION*, the official journal of the International Neuromodulation Society and the International Functional Electrical Stimulation Society. He serves on the Boards of the American Academy of Pain Medicine, the International and American Neuromodulation Societies, and the World Institute of Pain. Dr. Krames is chairman of the fellowship committee of the American Board of Pain Medicine.

Elderly with Dementia Have Trouble Reporting Pain, According to Study

According to survey data, most nursing-home patients have problems with pain, one-third are in constant pain and more than half suffer severe pain. A study by School of Medicine at Washington University Medical Center researchers has found that elderly people with dementia are less likely to report pain than other elderly patients.

"This study told us that in the more demented population, people really cannot answer very simple questions about pain. This has never really been documented before," said Fran L. Porter, Ph.D., assistant professor of pediatrics and principal investigator of the study, which was published in the December 1996 issue of the journal *Pain*.

These findings are important because they could impact the effectiveness of pain-management efforts. The medical system relies heavily on verbal reporting to isolate and treat pain problems. Also, Porter said, failure to report pain can delay medical attention and lead to problematic behavior in the elderly.

Porter, who is an infant-pain researcher, said she decided to study pain in the elderly because pain management is difficult in this population, too. She wanted to measure the effects of dementia on the ability to report pain.

"As you get older, there is an increase in illness, and you're more likely to experience pain," she said. "It's a population that may have trouble communicating about pain, especially when you add in dementia."

A pilot-project grant from Washington University's Alzheimer's Disease Research Center (ADRC) supported the research.

Porter and her colleagues studied two groups of people 65 or older—51 cognitively intact people and 44 individuals with varying degrees of dementia. All were participants in a long-term ADRC project that compares aging in normal persons and in persons with dementia.

The researchers measured each participant's physiologic responses—such as heart rate—before, during and after a venipuncture, which draws a vial of blood for testing. For the first phase, each participant sat quietly in a chair for 10 minutes (baseline). Then, a nurse came into the room, cleansed the venipuncture site on the arm, applied a tourniquet and showed the patient the syringe and needle (preparation). The nurse then drew blood. Physiologic responses also were measured for about 10 minutes after the venipuncture. Additionally, participants were asked a series of questions about their anticipated and actual anxiety levels during the procedure.

Porter expected the volunteers' verbal reports to correlate with the physiologic measurements. In the cognitively normal group, heart rate increased greatly during the preparation phase but fell during the actual needle stick.

"So, for them, the disturbing part was the anticipation," Porter said. "But when the needle stick came, they weren't surprised at all and calmed down because they knew what was happening. Their heart rates went back down."

The participants with dementia had a different reaction. They did not use the preparation time to psychologically brace themselves for the needle stick.

"In fact, they may not have even realized there was an impending event," Porter said. "So they were caught off-guard by the painful event and showed an increase in heart rate that stayed high in response to the needle stick."

Using questionnaires, the cognitively normal people rated their fear and anxiety as relatively low. The demented group also reported relatively low anxiety and pain. However, of the patients with moderate dementia, only 40 percent were able to answer the questions. Of the patients with severe dementia, zero percent to 20 percent were able to answer queries about their anxiety and pain.

"If you translate this to a doctor's office, the only tool the doctor has is to ask them questions. The likelihood of them reporting pain is even lower than we thought it was," Porter said.

Toward the end of the study, the researchers also began videotaping the facial expressions of participants during the procedure. The individuals with dementia used twice as many facial actions during the preparation period than the cognitively normal patients. They also were five times more expressive during the venipuncture.

"Our study concluded that even though individuals with dementia did not show the same response as individuals who were cognitively intact, both their behavioral and physiologic responses indicate they were feeling pain," Porter said.

In nursing homes, where many patients are irritable and sometimes show inappropriate emotional reactions, this behavior might signal underlying pain that is not being treated appropriately, Porter said.

"This study is a first attempt to look at whether demented people can tell their caregivers and physicians if they're in pain and to what extent they respond to pain," she said. "Learning more about pain in this population could help with education and awareness in caring for the elderly."

—Section by Diane Duke

Chapter 9

Roadblocks to Pain Relief

Survey of People with Chronic Pain

More than four out of every 10 people with moderate to severe chronic pain have yet to find adequate relief, saying their pain is out of control, according to a survey released by the American Pain Society, the American Academy of Pain Medicine, and Janssen Pharmaceutica. The survey of 805 individuals also revealed a population of sufferers who often don't receive the type of care experts consider necessary—despite the fact that nearly half have switched physicians at least once and more than 50 percent have been in pain for more than five years.

"Many Americans with chronic pain are suffering too much for too long and need more aggressive treatment," says Russell Portenoy, MD, president of the American Pain Society and chairman of the Department of Pain Medicine and Palliative Care at the Beth Israel Medical Center in New York City. "This survey suggests that there are millions of people living with severe uncontrolled pain.

This chapter includes text from "New Survey of People with Chronic Pain Reveals Out-of-Control Symptoms, Impaired Daily Lives," © 1999 American Pain Society. Reprinted with permission of the American Pain Society, American Academy of Pain Management, and Janssen Pharmaceutica. This chapter also includes text from "Chronic Pain in America: Roadblocks to Relief," a study conducted by Roper Starch Worldwide for American Academy of Pain Medicine, American Pain Society, and Janssen Pharmaceutica. © 1999. Reprinted with permission of the American Academy of Pain Medicine, the American Pain Society, and Janssen Pharmaceutica.

This is a great tragedy. Although not everyone can be helped, it is very likely that most of these patients could benefit if provided with state-of-the-art therapies and improved access to pain specialists when needed."

The survey was conducted by Roper Starch Worldwide and sponsored by Janssen Pharmaceutica, a developer of pain treatments, the American Pain Society, and the American Academy of Pain Medicine. All individuals surveyed had experienced pain for at least six months, and described their pain as being a 5 or higher on a scale of 1-10, with 10 being "the worst pain imaginable." The source of their pain was fairly evenly split between arthritis, back disorders, and other causes. (Individuals with cancer were specifically excluded from the survey.)

A majority of all survey respondents reported some difficulty doing such basic activities as sleeping, doing chores at home, and walking. These problems are accentuated among those whose pain is very severe (8, 9, or 10 on the pain scale)—of whom nearly one in five had been forced to visit an emergency room at least once in the past year due to their pain.

Search for a Physician Who Will Help

More than half (56%) of respondents reported suffering from pain for more than five years. Yet only 22% had been referred to a specialized pain treatment program or clinic, which offers a comprehensive, multidisciplinary approach to care. In fact, 49% of those currently being treated for very severe pain were still being seen by a family doctor or internist.

"Pain that persists and impairs a person's ability to be productive and enjoy life often requires evaluation and treatment by a team of health-care professionals who specialize in pain," says Dr. Portenoy. "But too often, patients don't seek out this option because they're not aware of it, and physicians don't refer them."

In their quest for pain relief, almost half (47 percent) of all chronic-pain sufferers surveyed had changed doctors at least once. Among those with very severe pain, almost a third (29 percent) had switched physicians three or more times. The most common reasons for the decision to search for a new doctor were "too much pain" (42%), the perception that their last physician did not know a lot about pain treatment (31%), the belief that their doctor didn't take their pain seriously enough (29%), and the physician's unwillingness to treat their pain aggressively (27%).

Pain Treatments: Too Little Too Late

Despite the fact that "opioid" drugs, such as morphine and the fentanyl skin patch, were rated the most effective treatments by those respondents who had used them, these medications were seldom used.

Only about a quarter (26 percent) of respondents with very severe pain reported taking opioid medications at the time of the survey. Instead, many said they were using less-potent medications such as non-prescription pain relievers. While opioid drugs are not suitable for all patients with moderate to severe pain, experts agree that some patients benefit greatly and that both the public and professionals need more education about their use.

"This survey shows the stigma associated with opioid drugs. Although these drugs can clearly benefit some patients with chronic pain, patients, caregivers, and physicians overestimate the risks and fail to use them appropriately," observes Dr. Portenoy. "Many patients suffer needlessly because of an inappropriate level of concern about long-term reliance on medication in general, and about addiction caused by strong pain medications such as opioids specifically. The input of pain specialists may be helpful when deciding on the best drug therapy for patients with severe chronic pain." Dr. Portenoy also emphasized that medication is only one of many strategies that can be used to treat pain and the disability that may accompany it. Both drug therapy and non-drug approaches may be needed concurrently.

Chronic Pain in America: Roadblocks To Relief

Background: The overall purpose of this study was to identify the barriers or problems individuals face in their efforts to achieve relief from moderate to severe chronic pain. The information will be used to heighten the awareness and understanding of consumers and the medical community on the issue of chronic pain and the need to treat it aggressively.

The study covers how chronic pain impacts quality of life, whether chronic pain sufferers have their pain under control or not, how they are able to get to a control status, whether or not the treatment used goes far enough and what barriers or stigmas are related to pain treatment in general and to the medicine being taken for pain.

Treating Chronic Pain

It is estimated that 9% of the U.S. adult population are suffer from moderate to severe non-cancer related chronic pain.

How effective is the medical profession in meeting the need for pain relief?

Almost all chronic pain sufferers have gone to a doctor for relief of their pain at one time or another. Almost 4 of every 10 are not currently doing so, since they think either there is nothing more a doctor can do, or in one way or another their pain is under control, or they can deal with it themselves.

This is not the case with those having very severe pain; over 7 of every 10 are currently going to a doctor for pain relief. In addition, those with very severe pain are more likely to require emergency room visits, hospitalization, and even psychological counseling or therapy to treat their pain.

Doctors are not a major barrier when a patient asks for a medicine they saw or heard about; in the majority of instances the doctor prescribes it. Similarly, in the majority of instances when a sufferer has been referred to a program or clinic for relief, in the great majority of referrals, their managed care or workman's comp program permitted access.

What medicines do they perceive to be effective in providing relief and what are they taking for their pain?

The majority of chronic pain sufferers believe that over-the-counter medicines (OTCs), narcotic pain relievers, and prescription NSAIDs can be effective in relieving moderate to severe pain. Those with moderate pain are the most likely to say this about OTCs, while those with very severe pain are most likely to say this about narcotic pain relievers.

The more common medicines used for chronic pain are OTCs and prescription NSAIDs regardless of pain severity. However, among those with very severe pain the current use of narcotic pain relievers almost equals that of prescription NSAIDs.

Among those ever using them, narcotic pain relievers are rated significantly higher in providing pain relief than other medicine types among their respective users. Concerns about addiction and side effects, not stigma, are barriers to wider usage.

What role do non-medicinal therapies play?

Medical therapies are not providing sufficient relief, since the majority of chronic pain sufferers, especially those with severe pain, have also turned to non-medicinal therapies. The primary one is a hot/

cold pack. Surprisingly, almost all of the major non-medicinal therapies currently used are perceived as providing more relief by their
users than OTCs, the most widely used medicines; the one exception
are herbs/dietary supplements/vitamins which are perceived as offering the least amount of relief than any medicines or other major non-
medicinal therapies.

The overall favorable perceptions of non-medicinal therapies are
driven by those with moderate pain. Although those with very severe
pain are more likely to use them, they have a significantly lower opinion of their efficacy versus medicinal therapies.

Are chronic pain sufferers receiving universal support?

Chronic pain sufferers report that their closest family members and
friends provide very strong positive support. Doctors are perceived
as being equally supportive taking into account their different relationship with patients; however, among those employed, there is the
perception that their employers are significantly less supportive.

Parameters of Moderate to Severe Chronic Pain

- Chronic pain sufferers have a serious health problem. The majority have pain that is more likely to be severe or very severe
  rather than moderate and is the type that flares up frequently;
  they have had their pain for many years and feel their pain on
  an average 6 out of 7 days a week.

- The more severe their pain, the more likely it is to be constant
  rather than flaring up frequently, to be a long time problem,
  and less likely to be caused by arthritis.

- 55% of chronic pain sufferers say they have their pain under
  control; but, having pain under control varies inversely with the
  severity of the pain. Only 39% of those with very severe pain
  say they have it under control versus 70% of those with moderate pain. It is important to note that control does not vary significantly by age or sex of the sufferer.

- It takes time to get chronic pain under control. Among those
  having their pain under control, it took the majority at least six
  months to reach that point. However, the more severe the pain
  the longer it takes to get it under control; it took at least six
  months for almost 70% of those with very severe pain to reach
  that point versus just over half of those with moderate pain.

- When pain is under control, there is a significant positive improvement in a chronic pain sufferer's emotional well-being.

- Whether or not pain is under control, very severe pain still has a major negative impact on quality of life.

- Whether or not pain is under control, very severe pain still has a major negative impact on a chronic pain sufferer's emotional well-being.

- Chronic pain sufferers perceive positive and helpful support from the people most important to them; however, employers are not as supportive as close family and friends or doctors.

Role of the Medical Profession

- Almost 40% of chronic pain sufferers are not currently going to a doctor for relief of their pain; however, the more severe their pain, the more likely it is being treated by a doctor.

- Chronic pain sufferers, especially those with severe pain, have had a significant number of past year occurrences that required emergency room visits, hospitalization, or counseling for relief of their pain.

- 40% of chronic pain sufferers who ever went to a doctor did so within one month after their pain began; still, at least one fourth wait at least six months after their pain begins before going to a doctor.

- Chronic pain sufferers delay going to a doctor for relief primarily because they under-estimate the problem and think they can see it through.

- Almost one half of all chronic pain sufferers who have ever gone to a doctor for relief of their pain, have found it necessary to change doctors in their search for relief; almost one fourth have changed doctors at least three times for this purpose. The more severe their pain, the more likely they have changed doctors and to have done so more often.

- The primary reasons for changing doctors relate for the most part to how chronic pain sufferers perceive the doctor's attitude toward their pain and the doctor's knowledge about pain and the ability to treat pain.

- Chronic pain sufferers who have never gone to a doctor for pain relief or are not currently going to one believe either there is nothing doctors can do to help, the pain is under control, or that they themselves can either treat it or just live with it. Cost is a significant barrier among those with severe or very severe pain.

- 22% of chronic pain sufferers have asked their doctor for a medicine they saw or heard about to relieve their pain and in the majority of instances doctors prescribe the medicine; only 5% of all sufferers have asked for such a medicine and their doctor refused to prescribe it.

- 22% of chronic pain sufferers have been referred to a specialized treatment program for their pain; only 3% of all chronic pain sufferers were denied access by a managed care gatekeeper or workman's comp program after such a referral.

Perceptions and Use of Medicine Types

- Almost 75% of chronic pain sufferers perceive over-the-counter medicines (OTCs) as being effective in relieving moderate to severe pain; a majority also believe narcotic pain relievers and prescription nonsteroidal anti-inflammatory drugs (NSAIDs) would provide effective relief. The overall favorable perception of OTC efficacy is driven by sufferers having moderate pain.

- Almost all chronic pain sufferers have used OTCs to relieve their pain and over one half have used prescription NSAIDs. Narcotic pain relievers have been tried by just over four of every ten sufferers. Their use, along with prescription NSAIDs, anti-depressants, and anti-seizure drugs, varies directly with the severity of the pain.

- Regardless of pain severity, the most common medicines currently being used are OTCs. Among those with very severe pain, narcotic pain relievers are almost as widely used as prescription NSAIDs. In addition, those with very severe pain are also more likely to use anti-depressants and anti-seizure drugs than those with moderate pain.

- Medicines are being taken at least two times a day; the more severe the pain, the more frequently medicine is being taken.

- Regardless of pain severity, OTCs have been taken almost twice as long for pain relief than any other medicine types. Prescription NSAIDs and narcotic pain relievers have been taken for about the same length of time.

- Narcotic pain relievers are rated significantly higher by their users providing pain relief than is the case with other medicines among their users; OTCs, the more widely used medications for pain relief, receive relatively low ratings on effectiveness among their users compared to narcotic pain relievers and prescription NSAIDs.

- A small, but significant number of chronic pain sufferers have at one time or another turned to alcohol for relief; this occurs more often among middle aged adults and men.

Attitudes toward Narcotic Pain Relievers

- Chronic pain sufferers currently taking narcotic pain relievers differ from other chronic pain sufferers as to the severity of their pain, being less likely to have it under control, changing doctors more often, requiring more intensive treatment at hospitals, taking more pills per day, more likely following their doctor-prescribed regimen and lastly, to being referred to a specialized program/clinic for their pain.

- Although the great majority of chronic pain sufferers react positively when first prescribed a narcotic pain reliever, there are concerns relating to side effects and becoming habit forming; however, there is relatively little concern about what other people think about their use.

- The more common side effects attributed to narcotic pain relievers are drowsiness and dry mouth along with a range of stomach related problems; the most bothersome ones are the ones that occur less frequently such as vomiting, urinary problems, and confusion.

- The majority of chronic pain sufferers ever using narcotic pain relievers never had anyone express a concern about it; among those who hear concerns from others it is likely to be a family member or their doctor. The concerns expressed relate to addiction and, especially among family members, side effects.

- Few chronic pain sufferers believe doctors have ever refused to prescribe a narcotic pain reliever to them for fear of being personally criticized by others.

- The quality of life has improved significantly among those who have their pain under control.

Part Two

Types of Pain and Disorders Characterized by Pain

Chapter 10

Appendicitis

Appendicitis is inflammation of the appendix, a small portion of the large intestine that hangs down from the lower right side. Although the appendix does not seem to serve any purpose, it can still become diseased. If untreated, an inflamed appendix can burst, causing infection and even death. About 1 in 500 people has appendicitis each year.

Appendicitis may occur after a viral infection in the digestive tract or when the tube connecting the large intestine and appendix is blocked by trapped stool. The inflammation can cause infection, a blood clot, or rupture of the appendix. Because of the risk of rupture, appendicitis is considered an emergency. Anyone with symptoms needs to see a doctor immediately. Symptoms include:

- Pain in the right side of the abdomen. The pain usually begins near the navel and moves down and to the right. The pain becomes worse when moving, taking deep breaths, coughing, sneezing, and being touched in the area.

- Nausea.

- Vomiting.

- Constipation.

- Diarrhea.

National Institute of Diabetes and Digestive and Kidney Diseases (NIDDK), NIH Pub. No. 99-4547, November 1999.

- Inability to pass gas.

- Low fever that begins after other symptoms.

- Abdominal swelling.

Not everyone has all symptoms. It is important that people with symptoms of appendicitis not take laxatives or enemas to relieve constipation because these medicines could cause the appendix to burst. People also should not take pain medicine because it can mask symptoms that the doctor needs to know about.

The doctor bases an appendicitis diagnosis on symptoms, a physical exam, blood tests to check for signs of infection such as a high white blood cell count, and urine tests to rule out a urinary tract infection. Some doctors use ultrasound to see whether the appendix looks inflamed. Treatment is surgery to remove the appendix, called appendectomy. Doctors are beginning to use laparoscopic surgery for appendectomy. This technique involves making several tiny cuts in the abdomen and inserting a miniature camera and surgical instruments. The surgeon then removes the appendix with the instruments, so there is no need to make a large incision in the abdomen. People can live a normal life without their appendix—no changes in diet, exercise, or other lifestyle factors are necessary.

Additional Information on Appendicitis

The National Digestive Diseases Information Clearinghouse (NIDDC) collects resource information on digestive diseases for the Combined Health Information Database (CHID) which is produced by health-related agencies of the Federal Government. This database (which is on the internet at http://chid.nih.gov) provides titles, abstracts, and availability information for health information and health education resources.

To provide you with the most up-to-date resources, information specialists at the clearinghouse created an automatic search of CHID. To obtain this information, you may view the results of the automatic search on Appendicitis.

If you wish to perform your own search of the database, you may access the CHID Online web site and search CHID yourself.

Chapter 11

Arthritis

What Is Arthritis?

The word arthritis literally means joint inflammation, but is often used to refer to a group of more than 100 rheumatic diseases that can cause pain, stiffness, and swelling in the joints. These diseases may affect not only the joints but also other parts of the body, including important supporting structures such as muscles, bones, tendons, and ligaments, as well as some internal organs. This chapter focuses on pain caused by two of the most common forms of arthritis—osteoarthritis and rheumatoid arthritis.

What Is Pain?

Pain is the body's warning system, alerting you that something is wrong. The International Association for the Study of Pain defines it as an unpleasant experience associated with actual or potential tissue damage to a person's body. Specialized nervous system cells (neurons) that transmit pain signals are found throughout the skin and other body tissues. These cells respond to things such as injury or tissue damage. For example, when a harmful agent such as a sharp knife comes in contact with your skin, chemical signals travel from neurons in the skin through nerves in the spinal cord to your brain, where they are interpreted as pain.

"Questions and Answers about Arthritis Pain," National Institute of Arthritis and Musculoskeletal and Skin Diseases (NIAMS), January 1998.

Most forms of arthritis are associated with pain that can be divided into two general categories: acute and chronic. Acute pain is temporary. It can last a few seconds or longer but wanes as healing occurs. Some examples of things that cause acute pain include burns, cuts, and fractures. Chronic pain, such as that seen in people with osteoarthritis and rheumatoid arthritis, ranges from mild to severe and can last a lifetime.

How Many Americans Suffer from Arthritis Pain?

Chronic pain is a major health problem in the United States and is one of the most weakening effects of arthritis. More than 40 million Americans suffer from some form of arthritis, and many have chronic pain that limits daily activity. Osteoarthritis is by far the most common form of arthritis, affecting about 16 million Americans, while rheumatoid arthritis, which affects about 2.1 million Americans, is the most crippling form of the disease.

What Causes Arthritis Pain? Why Is It So Variable?

The pain of arthritis may come from different sources. These may include inflammation of the synovial membrane (tissue that lines the joints), the tendons, or the ligaments; muscle strain; and fatigue. A combination of these factors contributes to the intensity of the pain.

The pain of arthritis varies greatly from person to person, for reasons that doctors do not yet understand completely. Factors that contribute to the pain include swelling within the joint, the amount of heat or redness present, or damage that has occurred within the joint. In addition, activities affect pain differently so that some patients note pain in their joints after first getting out of bed in the morning whereas others develop pain after prolonged use of the joint. Each individual has a different threshold and tolerance for pain, often affected by both physical and emotional factors. These can include depression, anxiety, and even hypersensitivity at the affected sites due to inflammation and tissue injury. This increased sensitivity appears to affect the amount of pain perceived by the individual.

How Do Doctors Measure Arthritis Pain?

Pain is a private, unique experience that cannot be seen. The most common way to measure pain is for the doctor to ask you, the patient, about your problems. For example, the doctor may ask you to describe the level of pain you feel on a scale of 1 to 10. You may use words like aching, burning, stinging, or throbbing. These words will give the doctor a clearer picture of the pain you are experiencing.

Since doctors rely on your description of pain to help guide treatment, you may want to keep a pain diary to record your pain sensations. On a daily basis, you can describe the situations that cause or alter the intensity of your pain, the sensations and severity of your pain, and your reactions to the pain. For example: "On Monday night, sharp pains in my knees produced by housework interfered with my sleep; on Tuesday morning, because of the pain, I had a hard time getting out bed. However, I coped with the pain by taking my medication and applying ice to my knees." The diary will give the doctor some insight into your pain and may play a critical role in the management of your disease.

What Will Happen When You First Visit a Doctor for Your Arthritis Pain?

The doctor will usually do the following:

- Take your medical history and ask questions such as: How long have you had this problem? How intense is the pain? How often does it occur? What causes it to get worse? What causes it to get better?

- Review the medications you are using

- Conduct a physical examination

- Take blood and/or urine samples and request necessary laboratory work

- Ask you to get x rays taken or undergo other imaging procedures such as a CAT scan (computerized axial tomography) or MRI (magnetic resonance imaging).

Once the doctor has done these things and reviewed the results of any tests or procedures, he or she will discuss the findings with you and design a comprehensive management approach for the pain caused by your osteoarthritis or rheumatoid arthritis.

Who Can Treat Arthritis Pain?

A number of different specialists may be involved in the care of an arthritis patient—often a team approach is used. The team may include doctors who treat people with arthritis (rheumatologists), surgeons (orthopaedists), and physical and occupational therapists. Their goal is to treat all aspects of arthritis pain and help you learn to manage your pain. The physician, other health care professionals, and you, the patient, all play an active role in the management of arthritis pain.

How Is Arthritis Pain Treated?

Short-Term Relief

There is no single treatment that applies to all people with arthritis, but rather the doctor will develop a management plan designed to minimize your specific pain and improve the function of your joints. A number of treatments can provide short-term pain relief.

- **Medications.** Because people with osteoarthritis have very little inflammation, pain relievers such as acetaminophen (Tylenol*) may be effective. Patients with rheumatoid arthritis generally have pain caused by inflammation and often benefit from aspirin or other nonsteroidal anti-inflammatory drugs (NSAIDs) such as ibuprofen (Motrin or Advil).

- **Heat and cold.** The decision to use either heat or cold for arthritis pain depends on the type of arthritis and should be discussed with your doctor or physical therapist. Moist heat, such as a warm bath or shower, or dry heat, such as a heating pad, placed on the painful area of the joint for about 15 minutes may relieve the pain. An ice pack (or a bag of frozen vegetables) wrapped in a towel and placed on the sore area for about 15 minutes may help to reduce swelling and stop the pain. If you have poor circulation, do not use cold packs.

- **Joint protection.** Using a splint or a brace to allow joints to rest and protect them from injury can be helpful. Your physician or physical therapist can make recommendations.

- **Transcutaneous electrical nerve stimulation (TENS).** A small TENS device that directs mild electric pulses to nerve endings that lie beneath the skin in the painful area may relieve some arthritis pain. TENS seems to work by blocking pain messages to the brain and by modifying pain perception.

- **Massage.** In this pain-relief approach, a massage therapist will lightly stroke and/or knead the painful muscle. This may increase blood flow and bring warmth to a stressed area. However, arthritis-stressed joints are very sensitive so the therapist must be very familiar with the problems of the disease.

- **Acupuncture.** This procedure should only be done by a licensed acupuncture therapist. In acupuncture, thin needles are inserted at specific points in the body. Scientists think that this stimulates the release of natural, pain-relieving chemicals produced by the brain or the nervous system.

Long-Term Relief

Osteoarthritis and rheumatoid arthritis are chronic diseases that may last a lifetime. Learning how to manage your pain over the long term is an important factor in controlling the disease and maintaining a good quality of life. Following are some sources of long-term pain relief.

- **Medications**

    Nonsteroidal anti-inflammatory drugs (NSAIDs). These are a class of drugs including aspirin and ibuprofen that are used to reduce pain and inflammation and may be used for both short-term and long-term relief in people with osteoarthritis and rheumatoid arthritis.

    Disease-modifying anti-rheumatic drugs (DMARDS). These are drugs used to treat people with rheumatoid arthritis who have not responded to NSAIDs. Some of these include methotrexate, hydroxychloroquine, penicillamine, and gold injections. These drugs are thought to influence and correct abnormalities of the immune system responsible for a disease like rheumatoid arthritis. Treatment with these medications requires careful monitoring by the physician to avoid side effects.

    Corticosteroids. These are hormones that are very effective in treating arthritis. Corticosteroids can be taken by mouth or given by injection. Prednisone is the corticosteroid most often given by mouth to reduce the inflammation of rheumatoid arthritis. In both rheumatoid arthritis and osteoarthritis, the doctor also may inject a corticosteroid into the affected joint to stop pain. Because frequent injections may cause damage to the cartilage, they should only be done once or twice a year.

- **Weight reduction.** Excess pounds put extra stress on weight-bearing joints such as the knees or hips. Studies have shown that overweight women who lost an average of 11 pounds substantially reduced the development of osteoarthritis in their knees. In addition, if osteoarthritis has already affected one knee, weight reduction will reduce the chance of it occurring in the other knee.

- **Exercise.** Swimming, walking, low-impact aerobic exercise, and range-of-motion exercises may reduce joint pain and stiffness. In addition, stretching exercises are helpful. A physical therapist can help plan an exercise program that will give you the most benefit. (The National Arthritis and Musculoskeletal and Skin Diseases Information Clearinghouse has a fact sheet on arthritis and exercise. See the end of this chapter for contact information.)

- **Surgery.** In select patients with arthritis, surgery may be necessary. The surgeon may perform an operation to remove the synovium (synovectomy), realign the joint (osteotomy), or in advanced cases replace the damaged joint with an artificial one. Total joint replacement has provided not only dramatic relief from pain but also improvement in motion for many people with arthritis.

What Alternative Therapies May Relieve Arthritis Pain?

Many people seek other ways of treating their disease, such as special diets or supplements. Although these methods may not be harmful in and of themselves, no research to date shows that they help. Nonetheless, some alternative or complementary approaches may help you to cope or reduce some of the stress of living with a chronic illness. If the doctor feels the approach has value and will not harm you, it can be incorporated into your treatment plan. However, it is important not to neglect your regular health care or treatment of serious symptoms.

How Can You Cope with Arthritis Pain?

The long-term goal of pain management is to help you cope with a chronic, often disabling disease. You may be caught in a cycle of pain, depression, and stress. To break out of this cycle, you need to be an active participant with the doctor and other health care professionals in managing your pain. This may include physical therapy, cognitive-behavioral therapy, occupational therapy, biofeedback, relaxation techniques (for example, deep breathing and meditation), and family counseling therapy.

Another technique is to substitute distraction for pain. Focus your attention on things that you enjoy. Imagine a peaceful setting and wonderful physical sensations. Thinking about something that is enjoyable can help you relax and become less stressed. Find something that will make you laugh—a cartoon, a funny movie, or even a new joke. Try to put some joy back into your life. Even a small change in your mental image may break the pain cycle and provide relief.

The Multipurpose Arthritis and Musculoskeletal Diseases Center at Stanford University, supported by the National Institute of Arthritis and Musculoskeletal and Skin Diseases (NIAMS), has developed an Arthritis Self-Help Course that teaches people with arthritis how to take a more active part in their arthritis care. The Arthritis Self-Help Course is taught by the Arthritis Foundation and consists of a 12- to 15-hour program that includes lectures on osteoarthritis and rheumatoid arthritis, exercise, pain management, nutrition, medication, doctor-patient relationships, and nontraditional treatment.

You may want to contact some of the organizations listed at the end of this chapter for additional information on the Arthritis Self-Help Course and on coping with pain, as well as for information on support groups in your area.

Things You Can Do to Manage Arthritis Pain

- Eat a healthy diet
- Get 8 to 10 hours of sleep at night
- Keep a daily diary of pain and mood changes to share with your physician
- Choose a caring physician
- Join a support group
- Stay informed about new research on managing arthritis pain

What Research Is Being Conducted on Arthritis Pain?

NIAMS, part of the National Institutes of Health, is sponsoring research that will increase understanding of the specific ways to diagnose, treat, and possibly prevent arthritis pain.

Recent NIAMS studies show that levels of several neuropeptides (compounds produced by cells of the nervous system), such as substance P, are increased in arthritic joints. Substance P is involved in the transmission of pain signals via the nervous system. At the University of Missouri-Kansas City, researchers are studying effects of substance P in the spines of animals with chronic arthritis. Findings from this study may be used to develop specific drugs for chronic pain such as that associated with arthritis.

NIAMS studies are also looking at other aspects of pain. At the Specialized Center of Research in Osteoarthritis at Rush-Presbyterian-St Luke's Medical Center in Chicago, Illinois, researchers are studying the human knee and analyzing how injury in one joint may affect other joints. In addition, they are analyzing the effect of pain and analgesics on gait (walking) and comparing pain and gait before and after surgical treatment of knee osteoarthritis.

At the University of Maryland Pain Center in Baltimore, NIAMS researchers are evaluating the use of acupuncture on patients with osteoarthritis of the knee. Preliminary findings suggest that traditional Chinese acupuncture is both safe and effective as an additional therapy for osteoarthritis, and it significantly reduces pain and improves physical function.

At Duke University in Durham, North Carolina, NIAMS researchers have developed cognitive-behavioral therapy (CBT) involving both patients and their spouses. The goal of CBT for arthritis pain is to help patients cope more effectively with the long-term demands of a chronic and potentially disabling disease. Researchers are studying whether aerobic fitness, coping abilities, and spousal responses to pain behaviors diminish the patient's pain and disability.

NIAMS-supported research on arthritis pain also includes projects in the Institute's Multipurpose Arthritis and Musculoskeletal Diseases Centers. At the University of California in San Francisco, researchers are studying stress factors, including pain, that are associated with rheumatoid arthritis. Findings from this study will be used to develop patient education programs that will improve a person's ability to deal with rheumatoid arthritis and enhance their quality of life. At the Indiana University School of Medicine in Indianapolis, health care professionals are monitoring joint pain in patients with osteoarthritis and documenting this information. The goal of the project is to improve doctor-patient communication about pain management and increase patient satisfaction.

Where Can You Find More Information on Arthritis Pain?

Arthritis Foundation
1330 West Peachtree Street
Atlanta, GA 30309
Phone: (800) 283-7800 or (404) 965-7537 or call your local chapter, (listed in the telephone directory)
Website: www.arthritis.org

This is the major voluntary organization devoted to arthritis. The Foundation publishes a free brochure, "Coping With Pain," and a monthly magazine for members that provides up-to-date information on all forms of arthritis. The Foundation also can provide addresses and phone numbers for their local chapters and physician and clinic referrals.

Additional resources on pain are included in Chapter 91 near the end of this book.

Note

Brand names included in this text are provided as examples only and their inclusion does not mean that these products are endorsed by the National Institutes of Health or any other Government agency. Also, if a particular brand name is not mentioned, this does not mean or imply that the product is unsatisfactory.

Acknowledgments

The NIAMS gratefully acknowledges the assistance of John H. Klippel, M.D., Clinical Director, National Institute of Arthritis and Musculoskeletal and Skin Diseases; Brian M. Berman, M.D., Director of the Complementary Medicine Program, University of Maryland, School of Medicine; and Laurence A. Bradley, Ph.D., Professor of Medicine/Rheumatology, University of Alabama at Birmingham.

The National Arthritis and Musculoskeletal and Skin Diseases Information Clearinghouse (NAMSIC) is a public service sponsored by the NIAMS that provides health information and information sources, including additional information on arthritis. The NIAMS, a part of the National Institutes of Health (NIH), leads the Federal medical research effort in arthritis and musculoskeletal and skin diseases. The

NIAMS sponsors research and research training throughout the United States as well as on the NIH campus in Bethesda, Maryland, and disseminates health and research information.

Chapter 12

Back Pain

During his 27 years as a hospital corpsman, Richard Mettetal lifted injured people and remained suspended by harness from helicopters for long periods. For the 54-year-old Thurmont, Maryland, resident, the legacy of those years of public service is chronic back pain that has plagued him since 1984.

"It's been so long now, I can't remember when I didn't feel the pain," Mettetal says. "And I'm so angry that I can't do all that I want because of it."

Work-related back pain is among the most common occupational disorders in the United States, according to the National Institute for Occupational Safety and Health in Cincinnati, Ohio. Delay in return to work remains an expensive component in the overall cost of back pain for workers' compensation claims, as well, the institute notes. And back pain is responsible for more loss of work time and increased medical expenses related to treatment than any other ailment, says Robert Shields, M.D., an osteopathic physician practicing general medicine in Plano, Texas.

"This is one of the most common problems I see in my medical practice," he says. "Low back pain strikes 8 out of 10 adults at some point in their lives."

"What to Do When Your Back Is in Pain," by Carol Lewis, *FDA Consumer*, U.S. Food and Drug Administration (FDA), March-April 1998.

Understanding Back Pain

Back pain comes in two forms, acute and chronic, and is most often felt in the lower back. Acute pain comes on suddenly and intensely, usually from doing something you shouldn't be doing or from doing it in the wrong way. The pain usually lasts a short while. Chronic pain is recurring; any little movement can set it in motion and, for whatever reason, it lingers on and on for what can seem like an eternity.

Although back pain is usually preventable, experts claim that 4 out of 5 Americans will experience it at some time in their lives, given that the lower back supports most of the body's weight. The stability of the lower back depends on the integrity of the vertebral bodies and the intervertebral disks.

To understand the many ways you can do injury to your back, consider that each of us has between 24 and 25 bones in and around our backs, including the neck and chest areas, which are held together by ligaments and muscles. Throw in some major nerves, a few disks (which act as shock absorbers), and joints that guide the direction of movement of the spine, and stack them all up, explains Shields. "Expect to twist and bend them in a multitude of directions, and try to imagine what might go wrong."

Shields says you can sprain the ligaments, strain the muscles, rupture the disks, and irritate the joints. While logic would point to injuries from sports or traumatic accidents as the cause of the pain, sometimes the simplest of movements will have painful results. In addition, arthritis, congenital disorders, poor posture, obesity, and psychological problems due to stress can be the source of back pain. Complicating the issue further is the fact that back pain can also directly result from internal problems such as kidney stones, kidney infections, blood clots, or bone loss.

Even with modern technology, however, the exact reason or cause of back pain can be found in very few people, according to the *Clinical Practice Guideline for Understanding Acute Low Back Problems*, published in 1994 by the Department of Health and Human Services' Agency for Health Care Policy and Research. X-ray examinations explain only a small proportion of the nonspecific complaints doctors receive.

Pain Management Options

Mettetal's troubles began 14 years ago when he nearly collapsed from excruciating pain searing down his leg. His initial diagnosis was a ruptured disk. Since then, even with four major surgeries to repair the problems, his pain has only worsened. Out of desperation, he has tried medications, physical therapies, and pain clinics—all in an attempt to restore some semblance of a functional life.

The *Journal of the American Medical Association* concluded in a 1996 surgical back pain study that more than $50 billion is spent on the diagnosis and treatment of back pain in the United States. Since the causes are so varied, what works for one person might fail with another.

For most people, drugs work well to control pain and discomfort. But any medication can have side effects. Back pain experts say that over-the-counter, nonsteroidal anti-inflammatory drugs (NSAIDs)—including acetaminophen (Tylenol), naproxen (Aleve), and ibuprofen (Nuprin, Motrin IB and Advil)—can be of value in reducing the pain. More severe pain may require prescription medications such as oxycodone-release (Oxycontin), acetaminophen with codeine (Tylenol with Codeine), and meperidine (Demerol).

Peter Rheinstein, M.D., director of the medicine staff in FDA's Office of Health Affairs, says the many effective NSAIDs available on the market today means there is less need for narcotics. However, he cautions that all NSAIDs cause gastrointestinal bleeding, and advises that patients suffering from other medical conditions need to consult with their doctors about other treatment options for managing their back pain.

"If you have an ulcer, for example, or are taking a blood thinner," Rheinstein says, "you are at an increased risk for gastrointestinal bleeding and should have your doctor prescribe medication that won't aggravate the ulcer or cause any kind of drug interaction."

Exercise and Physical Therapy

Bed rest was once thought to be an effective treatment for back pain, but recently its therapeutic benefit has been questioned. In a study published in the 1996 issue of *Spine*, Finnish researchers experimented to find out whether exercises to mobilize the back worked better than bed rest. Subjects in the mobility test, who were encouraged to continue normal activities and have no daytime rest, appeared to have better back flexibility by the seventh day than their immobile counterparts, who remained in bed for the duration of the experiment.

"Most people think that a week of bed rest will take away the pain," says David Lehrman, M.D., chief of orthopedic surgery at St. Francis

Hospital and founder of the Lehrman Back Center in Miami. "But that's not so. For every week of bed rest, it takes two weeks to rehabilitate."

Vert Mooney, M.D., professor of orthopedic surgery at the University of California, San Diego School of Medicine, says that bed rest for low back pain should be limited to one day and exercise should begin immediately. He explains that exercises which increase flexibility and tone and strengthen muscles can get back pain sufferers up and around by hydrating disks that become painful from loss of fluid. "Exercise can actually pump fluid back into the disk," Mooney says, "and it is important to keep the patient moving so that the disk remains fully hydrated."

However, FDA's Rheinstein says, "For some people, bed rest is just the most comfortable position for the first couple of days."

Spinal manipulation, or osteopathic manipulative therapy and chiropractic, are therapies commonly practiced for correcting abnormalities that are thought to eventually cause disease and inhibit recovery. Shields uses this type of manual manipulation technique on the majority of his patients. Occasionally, however, the spasm is too great or the muscles are too traumatized—for example, following an automobile accident or a fall—and the pain or swelling must be "calmed down" using a muscle relaxer for a day or two before manipulation.

Surgical Procedures

Doctors recommend back surgery much less often now than in the past, and only for certain conditions that do not improve after other treatments have been tried. FDA has approved or cleared medical devices such as the Intervertebral Body Fusion device, Anterior Spinal Implant, and Posterior Spinal Implant to treat degenerative disk disease and stabilize and fuse the spine.

Implantable spinal cord stimulation devices are another aid in the management of chronic pain of the trunk and limbs. These devices electrically stimulate the spinal cord by discharging a one-time or continuous stream of electrical pulses. The implanted portion of the device consists of a pulse generator (which contains an internal power source similar to that used in a cardiac pacemaker) and lead extensions that are connected to electrodes placed in the spinal canal. The nonimplanted components of the system include the programming device and screening pulse generator, which are controlled by the physician or patient.

Acupuncture

Acupuncture is a centuries-old Chinese healing technique that employs needles placed at specified points on the body. FDA classified acupuncture needles in 1996 as medical devices for "general use" by trained professionals.

The needles are required to have proper labeling, and good manufacturing practices must be followed. Manufacturers must include on the label the statement "for single use only" and provide information about device material sterility and compatibility with the body. The needles must also bear a prescription label restricting use to qualified practitioners as determined by individual states.

Harold Pellerite, assistant to the director of compliance in FDA's Center for Devices and Radiological Health says, "I think today's society is more receptive to alternative medicine. This just points to the need for our agency to be able to have some degree of control over what the American public is exposed to."

Complicating the evaluation of effectiveness of treatment is the fact that most back problems clear spontaneously. How can you tell if the problem was relieved by a particular treatment or if it would have gone away in the same period without treatment? "You really can't," says Shields.

Out of all these options, only two things have given Mettetal any measure of relief—the Spinal Cord Stimulation System and acupuncture. But, as Shields points out, "One of the most important things to keep in mind is that pain is caused by a variety of underlying problems, and it is naive to think that one modality will help improve all back pain."

—by Carol Lewis

Carol Lewis is a writer in FDA's Office of Consumer Affairs.

Chapter 13

Cancer Pain

Understanding the Problem

When many people think of cancer, they think of pain. Today, however, most cancer pain can be controlled or even eliminated. For example, even with advanced cancer, pain can be controlled in 90% to 99% of cases. In nine out of ten cases, physicians can control pain by using pills alone; they do not have to use injections, operations, or other methods. In those few situations in which pain from cancer cannot be eliminated completely, it can be reduced so that the person with advanced cancer can live with it day to day and still accomplish activities that are important to him or her.

People with advanced cancer and their home caregivers must tell the doctors and nurses how pain gets in the way of their everyday activities, such as moving around or dressing. This information is useful to the doctors in evaluating the pain and developing an effective treatment.

It also is important that everyone be open and supportive. Family and friends should make clear that they believe the patient. *Those with pain are the only ones who really know how much pain they are feeling.* If people in pain feel that others do not believe them, they become upset and may even stop reporting their pain accurately, which only makes controlling the pain more difficult.

Because the level of pain medicines takes time to build in the bloodstream, it also usually takes time to get the pain under control. The doctor may need to try different medicines or amounts to see which ones work best. The things you can do on your own to control pain take time to learn as well, but do not give up just because complete control does not happen immediately. Remember, most cancer pain can be controlled.

When the people with pain feel something new, many think it is a sign that the cancer is growing. The pain might not be from the cancer at all, however. For example, treatments can change tissues, either shrinking and swelling them, and this can cause pain. Weight loss or gain also changes tissues and muscles, which again can cause pain. Many things in addition to growth of the cancer itself can produce these new aches and discomforts.

How Doctors Control Cancer Pain

Physicians who treat cancer pain use the Three-Step Analgesic Ladder for Cancer Pain Management, which was developed by the World Health Organization. Doctors usually begin treatment as low as possible on the ladder, working their way up gradually until control of the pain has been achieved.

Step 1 for Mild Pain: Non-narcotic pain medicines

These drugs also are called:

1. Analgesics: Examples are acetaminophen or Tylenol.

2. Nonsteroidal anti-inflammatory drugs: Examples are aspirin and ibuprofen (Motrin or Advil).

3. Adjuvants: These medicines treat specific pain and ease other types of symptoms. Examples are antidepressants such as Elavil, anticonvulsants such as Tegretol or Dilantin, antinausea medicines, and antianxiety medicines such as Xanax, Valium, Ativan, and Atarax or Vistaril.

Step 2 for Moderate Pain: Weak narcotics with other pain medicines

If Step 1 drugs do not work or the pain is rated as moderate, the next rung is used. Weak narcotics are stronger pain relievers and often are prescribed with other medicines such as those listed in Step 1. Examples of weak narcotics are Codeine, Darvon or Darvocet, Empracet, and Wygesic. Darvon, Darvocet, and Wygesic can cause side effects after long use, however, so these generally are not used for long periods. Stronger medicines in this category include Tylox, Percocet, and Percodan.

Step 3 for Severe Pain: Strong narcotics with other pain medicines

The last rung on the ladder describes what category of medicines should be used to control severe pain. A strong narcotic can be either short-acting or long-acting. Morphine, Dilaudid, and Numorphan are examples of strong narcotics that carry an effect lasting from 3 to 4 hours. Methadone also is a strong narcotic, giving 4 to 6 hours of relief. These medicines are available in 12-hour time-release pills as well.

When to Get Professional Help

Emergency Symptoms

Call the doctor or nurse if any of the following conditions exist:

Actions to relieve "breakthrough pain" are not working, and pain continues to be a problem between doses of long-acting medicines (6 to 12 hours of relief expected).

Breakthrough pain is pain that "breaks through" the relief achieved by regularly scheduled, around-the-clock medicines. This type of pain occurs in between the scheduled times for medicine to be taken.

Inability to get up or walk because of pain.

A tumor can press on a nerve and cause severe pain, especially when the person moves. Swelling or inflammation around a tumor also can push on tender tissues and nerves. In these cases, people with cancer will feel severe pain, usually complain, and be unable to get up when lying down or to walk without help.

Inability to sleep because of pain.

Not sleeping well because of discomfort, aches, and pains is a sure sign that something should be done to increase the patient's comfort.

Crying and getting upset about feeling pain.

Look for physical responses to pain: tears, closed eyes, knitted eyebrows, wrinkled forehead, grimaced face, clenched fists, or a stiffened trunk (chest and back) that is held rigidly and moved slowly. When these occur or the patient complains of severe pain, call the doctor or nurse for help immediately.

Unwillingness to move, or muscles that are very tense when moving.

Even if the patient does not complain and tries to act as if nothing is wrong, watch how easily he or she moves. People in pain move with great difficulty, try not to move, and do not do normal, everyday things like getting dressed or out of bed.

A bone sticks out in an unusual way.

Bones can break or fracture more easily as a person ages, and bone cancer also increases the risk of a fracture. If a bone sticks out in a new way, report this even if pain does not immediately follow the event.

Have the answers to the following questions ready when you call the doctor or nurse:

1. How long has the pain been a problem?

2. Where is the pain located? Is it in more than one area?

3. How severe is the pain? Ask the patient to use a number from 0 to 10 to describe or rate the pain, where 0 = none, 5 = moderate, and 10 = worst ever.

4. Is the pain sharp and stabbing or dull and aching?

5. Does the pain burn or feel like an electric shock?

6. Is there any numbness or tingling?

7. How much has the pain interfered with normal activities?

8. Describe any current prescriptions for pain, including:
   Name of medicine(s)
   How much time should go by between doses
   How many pills can be taken at one time

How many doses were taken in the last 2 days

How long does the medicine take to work

How much relief is achieved

How long does the relief last

Is the patient still able to swallow pills

9. What other medicines have been taken, or what else has been done to relieve the pain? What were the results?

When to Get Immediate Professional Help for the Side Effects of Pain Medicine

A drug reaction or narcotic overdose is a different type of emergency related to pain control. If the person with advanced cancer is allergic to a pain medicines or that medicine is too strong, professional help is needed.

Most of the symptoms on the following "call now" list indicate that a drug reaction is causing a problem with the central nervous system, gastrointestinal tract, urinary tract, or skin, and that the body's normal functioning is being severely impaired. The medicine is too strong, or there is an uncommon allergic reaction.

Side effects like those on this list demand immediate action. When you call and report these symptoms, the doctor or nurse most likely will want to see the patient right away, or they will send help to you. After evaluating what is happening, they can give additional medicines to clear any drugs from the body. They also can prescribe other ways to calm the central nervous system and reverse an allergic reaction.

Problems with drug reactions are not very common. When they do happen, however, it is important to get help right away. *Call the doctor or nurse immediately if any of the following symptoms occur*:

- Disturbing hallucinations (hearing or seeing things that are not there).

- Ringing or buzzing in the ears.

- Sudden confusion or being "out of it."

- Severe trembling, uncontrolled muscle movements, or convulsions (seizures).

- Numbness or tingling in the feet or lower legs.

- Unable to hold in urine or stool when this was not a problem in the past.
- Unable to urinate despite feeling the need.
- Unable to have a bowel movement for 2 or 3 days.
- Nausea or vomiting with no relief.
- Hives, itching, skin rash, or swelling of the face.

Have the answers to the following questions ready when you call the doctor or nurse:

1. What pain medicine was taken over the last few days?
2. How much of the medicine was taken?
3. How often was this medicine taken?

Symptoms that Should Be Reported but Do Not Indicate an Emergency

Call the doctor or nurse if any of the following conditions exist:

- No relief after taking pain medicine three times as prescribed.
- Some pain relief is achieved, but significant pain remains 1 or 2 days after starting the medicine or changing either the way it is taken or the amount.
- A new type of pain, pain in new locations, or new pain when moving or sitting.
- Numbness, tingling, or burning sensations that are new.
- Medicines for breakthrough pain are used more than three times a day in addition to the regular pain medicines.
- Tremors or involuntary jerking motions while awake or asleep.
- More pain occurs with movement, such as being lifted or turned in bed.

What You Can Do to Help

Make the best use of pain medicine.

If the pain is not an emergency but the patient needs medicine on a regular basis, be sure you are using the medicine correctly and preventing pain before it becomes severe.

Give the pain medicine at regular times, as prescribed by the doctor.

When pain occurs regularly and not just once or twice a day, give the pain medicine on a consistent schedule. This will keep enough medicine in the bloodstream to control the pain.

Also, encourage the patient not to wait too long to taking the medicine. For example, suppose the pain medicine is prescribed "every 4 to 6 hours as needed." You can give pain medicine anytime after 4 hours. Do not wait longer than 6, however, because the pain then may become so bad that the prescribed amount will not give full relief.

Give the medicine before pain becomes severe.

When pain occurs regularly and not just once or twice a day, control is more difficult. It also takes longer to achieve if pain is allowed to build to a severe level. People need to take pain medicine to avoid a "pain crisis" just like diabetics need to take insulin to avoid a "sugar crisis."

Taking the medicine with the same amount of hours between doses prevents peaks and valleys and keeps a steady supply of medicine in the body. You may even find that you can decrease the amount of medicine given, because the person with pain is more confident that the pain can be controlled.

Continue to give pain medicine during the night.

Try not to go longer than 4 hours without giving medicine during the night, unless the person is taking a medicine like MS Contin (a time-release capsule), which is prescribed to be given every 12 hours, or a drug like Duragesic or Fentanyl, which lasts up to 72 hours. Too much time between shorter-acting pills means that the amount of medicine in the body keeps dropping and the level of pain keeps increasing. In this event, the patient will need more of the medicine to return to the right amount of pain control because he or she waited too long before taking the next dose.

Giving a pill on a regular schedule, even in the middle of the night, will help to prevent breakthrough pain. By adhering strictly to the medication schedule, you are not waiting too long for the next recommended dose.

Sometimes, a "night dose" method is ordered. This means that a larger dose of medicine is given at bedtime to help the patient sleep, but you will still have to give regular doses throughout the night.

Do not suddenly stop the pain medicine if it has been taken for a number of weeks.

If pain medicine is stopped suddenly, the body almost always experiences a "shock." It expects a steadier flow of these medicines into the bloodstream, and withdrawal symptoms can occur in the same way as if one suddenly stopped smoking cigarettes or drinking coffee. Increasing the length of time between doses and taking lower doses allow the body to be weaned off the medicines in a gentle manner. The discomfort of withdrawal, such as shakiness or headache, is less likely to occur or be a problem if the medicine is stopped slowly, over several days, and under the direction of a physician.

Expect that giving pain medicine correctly also will help to relieve other problems that can increase pain, such as muscle tension, lack of sleep, and emotional distress.

Because the patient no longer is battling pain, use of pain medicine restores comfort, helps the patient to rest, and reduces some anxieties. It also helps to relieve other problems that can increase pain, such as muscle tension, lack of sleep, and emotional distress.

Ask the doctor or nurse what to do in the following situations:

1. If the medicine wears off and pain returns (or if pain does not diminish even when the medicine is taken as prescribed) but it is too early for the next does to be taken.

2. If pain causes the patient to wake up at night.

3. If a dose of medicine is accidentally skipped.

Find out whether the prescribed medicine can be crushed by a pharmacist or mixed in a liquid to make it easier for the patient to swallow.

Some medicine, such as MS Contin, should not be crushed, because then all of the medicine will be absorbed at one time. This could be dangerous when the medicine is to be delivered in a time-release fashion. If the patient is having trouble swallowing, the hospice staff will show you other ways to give it.

Understand the Medication Plan

Understanding how and when the doctor and nurse want you to give pain medicine is the key to successful control and prevention.

There are three basic plans that can be followed, and you should ask which the person you are caring for is on:

Plan 1: Take medicine as needed

Know when to give a medicine that is prescribed as "give as needed" (or "give prn"). Pain medicines can be ordered "as needed." For example, the bottle may be labeled "take every 3 to 4 hours as needed" or "take every 6 hours as needed." This means that people with advanced cancer can decide when to take the medicine, but that they should not take it more frequently than the lowest number of hours listed on the instructions. If they need the medicine before this shortest time, discuss the problem with the doctor or nurse. Maybe the dose is not high enough, or maybe the medicine needs to be combined with another, such as Tylenol or aspirin, to prevent the pain.

For example, if the prescription is "take every 3 to 4 hours as needed," people with pain can take the medicine every 3 hours and do so consistently, especially if the pain starts to come back 3 hours after the last dose. Writing down the times at which the person takes the pain medicine helps the doctor or nurse to understand what is happening. They can then see that the medicine is being taken every 3 hours—morning, afternoon, evening, and night—and that the patient is not waiting 4 hours for the next dose. This information is important.

Taking medicine "as needed" also means that the person can take a dose and then wait for the next until the first inkling of pain begins again or they begin an activity that stimulates pain. For example, some people learn exactly what brings on their pain, such as bending or turning for a bath. Taking pain medicine before these activities and 3 hours afterward prevents the pain that could follow these activities.

If pain begins to return after 3, 4, 5, or 6 hours and the medicine is ordered "take as needed," the patient should try taking it with the same number of hours between pills for at least a 2-day period. For example, if the pain returns in 4 hours, he or she should take the pills every 4 hours and not "tough it out" by waiting until 6 or 8 hours have passed.

Plan 2: Take medicine with an equal number of hours between doses

Know when to give a medicine ordered for a certain number of times per day. If medicine is ordered for a certain number of times per day (and not for a certain number of hours), start with the time that the patient wakes up and divide the 24-hour day into equal spaces. For example, if medicine is ordered as "take twice a day" and the person usually wakes at 9:00 a.m., give a dose at 9:00 a.m. and again at 9:00 p.m. The times do not need to be exactly right, but you should try to divide the day into even sections.

If the dose is ordered as "take 4 times a day" and the person wakes at 9:00 a.m., then make sure that a dose is taken at 9:00 a.m., 3:00 p.m., 9:00 p.m., and 3:00 a.m. (or sometime in the middle of the night).

If the dose is ordered as "take 6 times a day" and the person wakes at 9:00 a.m., then make sure that a dose is taken at 9:00 a.m., 1:00 p.m., 5:00 p.m., 9:00 p.m., and during the night at about 1:00 a.m. and 5:00 a.m.

Plan 3: Take extra medicine when pain breaks through before the next dose is due

Treat breakthrough pain to prevent its return. Usually, there is a prescription for just when this happens, or the doctor may advise the patient to take an analgesic medicine if pain returns before it is time to take the strongest pain medicine.

If breakthrough pain is occurring for the first time, make sure that the person is taking the pain medicine as frequently as ordered. Sometimes, taking the medicine more consistently (the same number of hours between doses) and more frequently (for example, if ordered every 4 to 6 hours, then take every 4 hours) will prevent breakthrough pain.

Treat incident pain to help with moving or treatments that cause pain. Medicine for incident pain can be prescribed and taken only as needed between the normally scheduled doses. This dose usually is very small. For example, 2 mg of morphine sulfate can be offered every 2 hours while a patient goes back and forth between home and clinic appointments.

Ask about Changing Prescriptions, Times, and Doses

If the patient is taking the medicine as prescribed but still feels significant pain or is bothered by side effects from the current medication, ask the doctor about other medicines or ways of taking them that might be more helpful.

- Ask about increasing the amount of medicine.

- Ask about shortening the time between doses.

- Ask about taking short-acting or immediate-release narcotics in between long-acting (time-release) narcotic orders (such as taking immediate-release morphine for breakthrough pain).

- Ask about giving the same medicine in a different way
  - Liquid pain medicine.
  - Skin patches.
  - Single injections into muscles.
  - Subcutaneous needles attached under the skin for 3 days.
  - Nasal sprays.
  - Intravenous (IV) lines into large veins.
  - Epidural catheters near the spine.
  - Implanted ports under the skin.
  - IV infusing pumps attached to implanted ports.

- Ask about adding other medicines

- Ask about changing pain medicine.

- Ask about use of radiation therapy for pain.

- Ask about referral to a pain clinic or specialists in pain management.

- Use the hospice staff for help with pain control.

Manage the More Common Side Effects of Pain Medicine

Not all people react the same way to medicine; however, certain side effects are very common. Watch for these, and deal with them early.

- Prevent constipation with stool softeners and laxatives.

- Relieve a dry mouth with crushed ice, hard candy, and frequent rinses with water or products that do not contain alcohol.

- Relieve painful, dry nasal passages by humidifying the air or breathing in moisture from a sink full of warm water.

- Avoid an upset stomach by taking medicine with food or antacids unless instructed otherwise.

- Expect drowsiness.

Managing Pain Medicine

- Set an alarm as a reminder to take the medicine.

- Use a tray with slots for the time of day to hold the medicine.

- Telephone the pharmacy before going to fill the prescription. Some pharmacies do not carry all pain medicines. They may have to "special order" it or send you to another store. Telephone at least 2 days ahead of time.

- Always use the same pharmacy if possible.

- Keep at least a 3-day supply of pain medicine.

- Write the time and dose of pain medicine on a special form or tablet.

Prevent and Control Pain through Methods Other than Medication

- Use warm showers, baths, hot-water bottles, or warm washcloths.

- Use cool washcloths or ice.

- Use physical methods.
    - Position the person carefully with pillows and soft seat cushions.
    - Massage sore spots.
    - Avoid lifting or straining.

- Encourage use of deep breathing exercises.

- Distract the patient with pleasant, involving activities.

- Remind the person to use pleasant and relaxing imagery, daydreams, or pictures in the mind to relax muscles.

- Ask about using biofeedback for muscle relaxation.

- Offer special foot rubs ("reflexology").

- Ask for help with tasks.

- Do activities when the patient feels most comfortable.

- Keep a diary, rate the pain, and note what makes it worse or better.

- Avoid stressful events when possible.

Consider going to a family-caregiver support group or educational session.

To find out where and when local support groups meet, look in the telephone book, which usually has a large section called "Guide to Human Services." Cancer support groups are listed under "Cancer," and groups for family and friends who help anyone with a chronic illness are listed under "Caregivers."

You also can ask medical staff about local support groups. Your local office of the American Cancer Society most likely has a list of support groups; their number is in the white pages of the phone book. In addition, you can ask the hospice staff. If you are not successful in finding a caregivers group, call the Cancer Information Hotline at the National Cancer Institute (1-800-4-CANCER).

Possible Obstacles

"I'm afraid of addiction."

People who take narcotics for pain rarely become addicted. In fact, if their pain is treated effectively, it decreases the risk of addiction.

People who are "addicts" take drugs for a "high," or an altered state of mind. People who take narcotics for cancer pain take them to get relief from physical pain. People who are not addicts before they take narcotics for cancer pain do not become addicts later. Remember, the medicine is being used for controlling pain, not for a psychologic "high," and pain medicines can be stopped in such a way that the person does not experience the effects of withdrawal.

Even if you understand that the person you are caring for is not addicted, others may not. Do not spend a lot of energy trying to change their minds, however. Just tell them that this medicine is part of the medical treatment and is absolutely crucial to the patient's quality of life and ability to do what is most important to him or her.

"I want to 'save' the medicine until the pain is severe."

Taking pain medicine for mild discomfort now does not affect how well it will work in the future, or when the pain gets worse. Do not hold back the pain medicine you should take today simply to "save up" if more is needed later. In fact, it takes more medicine to treat pain that is uncontrolled than it does to prevent the pain from building up in the first place.

People sometimes need to increase their doses, but this does not mean they are becoming "immune" to the medicine or need more and more to control the same level of pain. These people need more because the pain itself has changed. There is no real limit to the dose a person can take for most of these drugs, but if the patient ever does reach such a limit, the doctor can change to a different medicine.

If pain is controlled now, both you and the patient should be less worried about controlling it later, because you know that the medicine works. Also, taking enough medicine now helps the person with pain to relax and preserve his or her strength.

"No one wants to hear about my pain."

The person with pain should understand that family and friends may seem uninterested because they feel helpless. Doctors and nurses who specialize in pain, such as those in a pain clinic or hospice, understand. Talk to them if you are feel alone with these problems.

"Only people who are dying take morphine."

Morphine is not reserved for those who are dying. It is an effective medicine for many types of cancer pain, and taking it does not mean that a person is near death. Morphine is used to control chronic pain during all phases of the disease. Some people go back to work and do their regular daily activities precisely because the morphine is so effective and lets them return to pain-free lives.

"If I give him his medicine and he dies, would it be the drug that killed him?"

Pain medicine leads to comfort. When death comes, it is because of the disease, not the medicine. If a person gets "too much," he or she usually will just sleep very deeply. Physicians also can order a drug that will cancel the narcotic in the blood and help to wake the person. Giving or not giving the pain medicine only changes the level of comfort, not the effects of the disease.

Carrying Out and Adjusting Your Plan

Carrying out Your Plan

Relieving pain and making the person you are helping comfortable is a challenge. If you follow the suggestions in this plan and work closely with hospice and home health staff, then you will be doing everything you can. Persist, and set the goal as being "pain free."

Checking on Results

Keep track of the level of pain. You can do this by asking the patient how severe the pain is, but use the same terms each time you do this. That way, you will be able to compare one time with another, and this will help you to evaluate how effective your pain control program is as well as to notice any changes. For example, you might want to use "worst ever," "severe," "bad," "moderate," "mild," and "none at all," and the patient can choose which fits best or even say that it is "between" (for example, "It is between 'severe' and 'bad'"). Another way is to think of a 10-inch ruler, where 10 is the worst pain ever, 5 is moderate pain, and 0 is no pain; then, the person can give you a number to fit the pain.

If these ratings are to be meaningful, the patient must understand that you fully accept his or her ratings. Pain can be judged only by the person who has it. The person with advanced cancer has to feel that you trust and accept what he or she says about the pain—or the patient either will not cooperate or will give incorrect information.

If Your Plan Does Not Work

If the pain is growing worse even after you have followed the strategies in this plan, speak with the doctor or nurse. Say what you have done to deal with the problem, and ask for guidance. Continue watching for symptoms that indicate immediate professional help is needed. Do not give up! Most cancer pain can be relieved, and the person you are caring for deserves to be comfortable.

If you feel the medical staff is not listening to your concerns or is unable to provide adequate pain control, ask for a referral to a cancer pain specialist. These are physicians who specialize in such pain and usually can be found at cancer centers, or they may be local physicians involved with hospice care.

Chapter 14

Carpal Tunnel Syndrome

In recent years, reports of repetitive motion injuries have risen dramatically in workplaces across the country. These problems, frequently termed "Cumulative Trauma Disorders" are being reported at alarming rates in all types of workplaces—from meatpacking plants to newspaper pressrooms. According to the Bureau of Labor Statistics, "disorders associated with repeated trauma" account for about 60% of all occupational illnesses. Of all these disorders, carpal tunnel syndrome is the condition most frequently reported.

What Is Carpal Tunnel Syndrome (CTS)?

The carpal tunnel receives its name from the eight bones in the wrist, called carpals, that form a tunnellike structure. The tunnel is filled with flexor tendons which control finger movement. It also provides a pathway for the median nerve to reach sensory cells in the hand. Repetitive flexing and extension of the wrist may cause a thickening of the protective sheaths which surround each of the tendons. The swollen tendon sheaths, or tenosynovitis, apply increased pressure on the median nerve and produce Carpal Tunnel Syndrome (CTS).

National Institute for Occupational Safety and Health (NIOSH), Document #705001, June 1997.

What Are the Symptoms of CTS?

The symptoms of CTS often first appear as painful tingling in one or both hands during the night, frequently painful enough to disturb sleep. Accompanying this is a feeling of uselessness in the fingers, which are sometimes described as feeling swollen, even though little or no swelling is apparent. As symptoms increase, tingling may develop during the day, commonly in the thumb, index, and ring fingers. A decreased ability and power to squeeze things may follow. In advanced cases, the thenar muscle at the base of the thumb atrophies, and strength is lost.

Many patients with CTS are unable to differentiate hot from cold by touch, and experience an apparent loss of strength in their fingers. They appear clumsy in that they have trouble performing simple tasks such as tying their shoes or picking up small objects.

What Causes CTS?

As stated earlier, swelling of the tendons that line the carpal tunnel causes CTS. Although there are many reasons for developing this swelling of the tendon, it can result from repetitive and forceful movements of the wrist during work and leisure activities. Research conducted by the National Institute for Occupational Safety and Health (NIOSH) indicates that job tasks involving highly repetitive manual acts, or necessitating wrist bending or other stressful wrist postures, are connected with incidents of CTS or related problems. The use of vibrating tools also may contribute to CTS. Moreover, it is apparent that this hazard is not confined to a single industry or job but occurs in many occupations—especially those in the manufacturing sector. Indeed, jobs involving cutting, small parts assembly, finishing, sewing, and cleaning seem predominantly associated with the syndrome. The factor common in these jobs is the repetitive use of small hand tools.

How Large a Problem Is CTS?

In the past ten years, more and more cases of workers afflicted with CTS have been reported in medical literature. One reason for this increase may be that automation and job specialization have fragmented workers' tasks to the point where a given job may involve only a few manipulations performed thousands of times per workday. Increased awareness of work-related risk factors in the onset of CTS is reflected in the growing number of requests for health hazard evaluations (HHEs) received by NIOSH to investigate such suspected problems. NIOSH received about three times as many HHE requests related to hand and wrist pain in 1992 as compared to 1982.

Prevention

NIOSH recommendations for controlling carpal tunnel syndrome have focused on ways to relieve awkward wrist positions and repetitive hand movements, and to reduce vibration from hand tools. NIOSH recommends redesigning tools or tool handles to enable the user's wrist to maintain a more natural position during work. Other recommendations have involved modified layouts of work stations. Still other approaches include altering the existing method for performing the job task, providing more frequent rest breaks, and rotating workers across jobs. As a means of prevention, tool and process redesign are preferable to administrative means such as job rotation.

The frequency and severity of CTS can be minimized through training programs that increase worker awareness of symptoms and prevention methods, and through proper medical management of injured workers.

Treatment

Treatment of CTS may involve surgery to release the compression on the median nerve and/or use of anti-inflammatory drugs and hand splinting to reduce tendon swelling in the carpal tunnel. Such medical interventions have met with mixed success, especially when an affected person must return to the same working conditions.

Current NIOSH Research

NIOSH continues to investigate musculoskeletal disorders, including cumulative trauma disorders (CTDs) such as CTS, in many work environments and will make its research information available as investigations are finalized.

Additional Information

Additional NIOSH information about musculoskeletal disorders is available from the toll-free CDC Fax Information Service (1-888-232-3299); request fax document # 705005. NIOSH has also developed several publications that provide a description of NIOSH research on CTDs, including carpal tunnel syndrome, and practical ways to identify and evaluate musculoskeletal disorders. Copies of these publications, *Cumulative Trauma Disorders in the Workplace Bibliography* and *Elements of Ergonomics Programs*, are available free-of-charge from the NIOSH Publications Office while supplies last.

National Institute for Occupational Safety and Health (NIOSH)
Phone: 1-800-35-NIOSH (1-800-356-4674)
Fax: (513) 533-8573
E-mail: pubstaft@cdc.gov

Chapter 15

Central Pain Syndrome

Introduction to Central Pain

Central Pain is the name for a pain syndrome which occurs when injury to the central nervous system is insufficient to cause numbness but sufficient to cause central sensitization of the pain system.

An injured motor nerve simply carries less current. Injured pain nerves, paradoxically, do exactly the opposite: they increase their signal. It is not a simple increase, however. They eventually gain the power to influence uninjured neighbor neurons, which begin autonomous firing.

The process can become so violent that the thalamus, the brain pain center, records "bursts" of impulses from these injured nerves. After sufficient bombardment threatens neuron death in the thalamus, it "shuts down." Central Pain apparently occurs at this point. It is as if the entire pain system is acting like a nerve ending. Ungated pain signals thus reach the cortex (part of the brain), causing unbearable suffering.

This chapter includes text excerpted from two documents written by David Berg with medical advice and consultation from Kenneth McHenry, MD, "Introduction to Central Pain: The Pain Beyond Pain," © 2001 David Berg, reprinted with permission; and, "Guessing at the Cause of Central Pain: A Primer on What We Think We Know," © 2002 David Berg, reprinted with permission. The full text of both documents, which includes descriptions of ongoing research and a more complete discussion of biochemical processes, is available online at http://www.painonline.org.

Pain nerves were designed to do their best work in the face of injury. This differs from motor nerves, which put the body to rest with injury by decreasing their function. It is difficult to get some clinicians, born and bred on "motor think" to adjust to "pain think." There are features of Central Pain which may seem unexpected.

Among these unexpected features are the following:

- The stimulus which usually causes the most unbearable aspects of Central Pain is the evoked pain of light touch, especially light touch which is persistent and occlusive. Such patients may wear abbreviated clothing to avoid textures rubbing on the skin.

- The burning pain, which light touch evokes, does not occur when the stimulus is first applied, but after time, (similar to the way the pain of sunburn occurs well after the UV injury). This is called slow summation and is a temporal (time-limited) phenomenon. In other words, spontaneous burning is not always capable of being evoked. Very limited data suggest that dysesthesia (burning pain) also displays spatial summation, which means as larger areas are covered with touch, the magnitude of burning becomes greater. The dysesthesia is of a greater magnitude where touch sensation is poorest.

- Central Pain also displays a hyperpathia (an amplified response to pain that continues after the thing that prompted the pain is removed). Sharp hyperpathia tends to occur most where sensation is most retained.

Because these patients have decreased touch sensation, including decreased sense to very light painful stimulus, Central Pain hyperpathia has been termed to have a "delay." This is an unfortunate term since it has nothing to do with time. It appears to have been adopted because hyperpathia is often coexistent with dysesthesia, which has a true temporal delay. With hyperpathia, there is a level of noxious stimulus which is not perceived. This is actually a heightened threshold to pain, not a temporal delay. The heightened threshold is very difficult to test for because it is so easily exceeded. Once the threshold has been exceeded, or when pain is first perceived, the pain response overshoots and responds violently. This is called delay with overshoot. The stimulus may be sharpness, heat, or cold. It is more common for heat to stimulate hyperpathic response in those with profound motor loss (plegics), while it is more common for cold or sharpness to generate hyperpathia in those who retain some motor function (paretics).

114

"Delay with overshoot" is generally considered a synonym of hyperpathia, but it is not really the same since hypersensitivity to pain can occur in those with normal nervous systems (such as sunburn). Only those with nerve injury can perceive hyperpathia long-term. The testing has not been done to determine how neuropathic hyperpathia (injured nervous system) is similar to or different from nociceptive hyperpathia (normal nervous system). Hyperpathia also occurs in the viscera (gut), but is displayed there as a feeling of overfulness, almost to exploding, like very severe distention with flatus. Similarly, a full bladder can be unbearable. The "fullness" is evoked in an inconsistent pattern by dietary intake. Patients often can affect its course by choice and timing of food/water intake or elimination.

- Light touch which is perceived in Central Pain has a "tingly" quality to it. This may be thought of as similar to the "tingle" of a lip touched while it is returning from dental anesthesia, or like the tingle of limbs falling "asleep." It is however, quite painful, "like needles." It is the most intense of the central pains but does not cause the most suffering. This tingle can be pronounced, compelling the attention of the patient, or it can exist in a minor form. Patients nearly always compare it to a limb which has fallen asleep and is regaining feeling. It has been called "circulatory pain."

  A Central Pain patient who is paying very close attention may be able to respond fairly well to light touch, creating a false impression for the hasty examiner that the patient does not have diminished touch sensation.

- Clinicians are often impressed at what good historians normal patients can be regarding pain, but the opposite can be expected pertaining to pain which the patient knows is not normal pain, yet is severe. Central Pain, in its fully developed form, is persistent torture. Humans chronically tortured often become alienated and withdrawn. It is so severe that, lacking a vocabulary, they may be very poor historians and may be reluctant to reveal the inroads the pain has made into their humanity. Poor verbal skills may also be impacted by the thalamic shutdown in this disease, making it difficult to prioritize and stick to the appropriate comments, with the appropriate emphasis, in the flow of conversation. The vagueness and strangeness of the symptoms are also factors in poor descriptive performance.

The Lowest Common Denominator of Central Pain

Because the disease has so many aspects, we are indebted to Dr. David Bowsher for finding the lowest common denominator. Of all the symptoms, he has identified the three which allow for simple diagnosis:

- Burning pain, often with a paradoxical component of cold, made worse by light touch or the rubbing of clothing.

Central Pain has definite thermal aspects. This is usually a narrow window of relative comfort in ambient temperatures and onset of burning with temperature change, either hot or cold. Alternatively, thermal aspects may manifest as an unusual sensitivity to heat, generally at the distal parts of a limb. Thermal aspects are omitted from these criteria because they are also seen in ciguatera poisoning (from a particular kind of fish).

In general, it appears that the more sensation retained, the broader display of Central Pain symptoms. Those with a greater retention of neural function (for example, quadriparetics) seem more likely to display a greater range of symptoms and also seem to have more problems enduring the pain. Notwithstanding this, very severe pain may be found in quadriplegics, although it tends to have fewer dimensions.

Guessing at the Cause of Central Pain

No one comprehends Central Pain well enough to fit all the pieces together, not to mention the fact that many pieces are missing and that scientists don't always agree about the meaning of the pieces we do have. This section attempts to summarize much of what is currently known about central pain and the research that shows promise. Since the experts do not agree, we have chosen in some parts to follow our interpretation of the general scheme of things as described by Tony Yaksh, a pharmacologist and researcher at the University of California, San Diego who has done much important work toward discovering the processes behind Central Pain, and in mentoring other researchers.

Difficulties in Diagnosing and Treating Central Pain

Many pain clinics find it hard to admit that there is currently no satisfactory treatment for Central Pain. It is worth pointing out that it is almost certainly not possible to tell which type of pain is present by using electrical test devices (which supposedly reach different nerve types with different wave patterns) or by procaine infusions (which supposedly block different nerve types at given concentrations), regardless of how impressive these tests may appear.

Since administration of the "caines" (for example, procaine and lidocaine) for prolonged times carries high risk of stopping the heart and since the levels of these drugs necessary to block brain sodium channels is probably well above toxic levels in most Central Pain patients, the attempts to determine Central Pain with these drugs is scientifically unsound. We are also concerned that this may represent an opportunistic chance for clinics to sell services to third-party payers, such as insurance companies, who seek a way to claim that the patient is well, in spite of their very serious condition. If so, this would be wrong indeed and the courts should reject any claim of evaluation based on lidocaine infusion. Many central pain patients receive no benefit from lidocaine or any other drug.

As Dejerine and Roussy stated nearly 100 years ago, traditional pain relievers are of no benefit in Central Pain. Also, the symptoms are so complex that a hysteric could never imagine them. For example, hysterics nearly always claim complete numbness in an affected area, while Dejerine and Roussy found that Central Pain patients report only a partial loss of sensation, along with the burning pain. Furthermore, Central Pain patients have some form of injury to the central nervous system, which causes them distress in addition to their Central Pain. Even quadriplegics who are affected by Central Pain often state that their pain is much more disabling than the paralysis.

Neuroanatomy

In the brain the gray matter is on the outside. This is the cortex and is supposedly where we do our conscious thinking. The inner brain has insulation on its nerve fibers, which causes it to be more whitish in color; hence, the term white matter.

In the cord the gray matter is mostly in the center of the cord, with insulated fibers of white matter tending to occupy the outer part of the cord. Medulla means "middle" in Latin. The spinal medulla is the spinal cord, which sits in the middle of the spinal canal, which is made of bone. Several layers surround the cord. These layers, going in order from inside out are the pia, the arachnoid (where spinal fluid is), and the dura, which is the outermost enclosing layer of the cord. The epidural space is outside the dura.

Pain nerves are a subset of sensory nerves. Pain nerves are named according to their diameter and whether or not they have insulation.

117

A-beta nerves are fatter and insulated. They can respond to lighter stimulus as well as heavy stimulus and are associated with wide dynamic range neurons (WDR neurons), which are nerve cells that can respond to weak or strong stimulus.

Nerve scientists like to divide pain neurons into separate categories. These categories are mechanoreceptors (pressure), thermoreceptors (temperature), and chemoreceptors (chemical). The thinnest nerve cells are C-fibers and have no insulation. They are very slow and require lots of stimulation to fire. A-delta fibers are slightly larger and have some insulation. C-fibers are present in all areas except the dentin of the teeth and are capable of feeling pain that is not particularly well localized, although they can sensitize the A-beta fibers, which are precise in locating the origin of the pain. This phenomenon may explain the 20 – 30 second delay in evocation of touch pain in central pain patients; time for C-fibers to sensitize surrounding nerve fibers.

A cross section of the spinal cord looks like a more or less oval structure. Now imagine an "X" painted across the oval. The arms of the "X" that point toward the back are the sensory nerves entering on either side from the dorsal root ganglion just outside the spine, which is a swollen sort of gathering place for the different types of nerves to join before coming into the cord. The arms of the "X" that point toward the front are motor and other nerves going out to the body. Signals coming in are called "afferent." Signals going out from the cord to the body are called "efferent."

On either side at the back of the cord is an entry point where the nerves of the body go into the cord at each spinal level, from the cervical area (neck) down to the lower levels, including the lumbar nerves. The cord ends at the lumbar levels and the nerves below that, like the sacral, sort of dangle like the tail of a horse (called the "cauda equina"). Each spinal level is numbered, for example, C-1 or L-4 tells you which spinal level is receiving or sending information in that nerve.

Pain scientists are very interested in the organization of afferent nerves entering the cord. The big, fast A-beta fibers go deep into the cord. The layers (or lamina) are numbered beginning at the outside. Their predominance deep in the cord is why A-betas are sometimes called Lamina V cells for quick identification, although they do things in other lamina as well. The thin, slow C-fibers terminate at one of the outermost areas, called the gelatinosa, or Lamina II. In normal people the C-fibers and A-beta fibers don't talk to each other much, but in nerve injury pain they do little else, probably because the interneurons have been altered in the course of Central Pain to allow it. Scientists aren't sure about the intermediate sized A-deltas but they think they possess some of the characteristics of both the thick A-betas and the thin C-fibers.

Pain is considered a crossed pathway, because fibers entering the cord on one side form connections, called synapses, with cells on the other side of the cord before ascending to the lower brain and then the thalamus, where the brain identifies where the sensation came from on the body. Once fibers are inside the cord they have many connections with interneurons, which modify the signal going to the nerve cell as the signal travels up the cord to the brain. The big center in the brain that receives pain input is the thalamus. The thalamus processes pain signals before sending them on to the cortex, or gray matter, which forms the outer portion of the brain.

Pain goes to at least two primary areas of the brain. The main one runs like a stripe across the top of the brain along the ridge (post central gyrus or somatosensory cortex I) and right behind a trough (the central sulcus) that also runs crosswise of the brain about at the top of your head. The main motor cortex also runs along the front of that fold, but sinks deep into the fold.

The Emotional Component of Pain

Pain also has an emotional component. The experts don't agree on whether or not the emotional component can really be considered separate from the pain component. Some view and study them separately, and others feel that they are inexorably connected.

Although much of this anatomy is now being challenged and updated as scientists advance their knowledge, it has been fashionable until recently to say that the fibers we have been discussing tell the brain about the presence and quality of pain, but that the emotional aspects of pain travel up a different path to the brain, along the course of marginal cells. The marginal cells are second order neurons to the C-fibers. Second order means they are the second nerve cell (neuron) to carry the pain signal, after they receive the signal from the nerves that send messages to the spinal cord.

The marginal cells don't seem to care where the pain is coming from, just that it is present and they tell the emotional centers in the brain that they better decide what to do about the pain. Marginal cells are few in number and carry little discriminative information. These cells seem to connect to the anterior cingulum, a part of the brain toward the front. In the days of prefrontal lobotomies, pain patients still

119

had pain after lobotomy but they had less emotion about it. Some think this is because the lobotomy also removed the cingulum.

Chemistry

Now we get to the really complex stuff, the chemistry of pain. Proteins are composed of amino acids. Peptides are a type of protein that is made of little short chains of amino acids. Peptides are fine tuners, or modifiers, of the pain message.

Chemicals that affect nerve transmission are called neurotransmitters. Where one nerve joins another at the synapse, little packets of chemical form and there are receptor sites or neuron channels where these neurotransmitters bind to cause an effect on the other side of the gap. Released neurotransmitters enter the gap between the nerves and then find receptor sites specific to them on the other side of the gap, in the closest end of the next higher order nerve cell.

Genes in the nerve cell chromosomes produce neurotransmitter proteins. With chronic pain, the expression (protein production) of your genes changes and chemicals are made in the wrong proportions. This causes too much excitation of pain nerves. These excitatory chemicals act on ion channels or receptors in the cell membranes or travel up the neuron and excite the connections (synapses) up the line toward the brain, and also travel down the nerve to excite the nerve endings out on the body surface. Strangely, if the nerve is injured too badly to do this, it can become a "pain cell martyr" as it were, and the neighboring uninjured nerve cells may begin to make these chemicals in sympathy and distribute them up or down the pain pathway. Marshall Devor calls this "crossed afterdischarge."

Another class of chemicals affecting pain are catecholamines. You probably know one of them already, adrenalin (also called norepinephrine), and you should know it makes the heart beat faster and causes things to get worked up. The sympathetic nervous system is part of the autonomic or unconscious nerves, which supply things like internal organs and blood vessels. The sympathetic catecholamines are divided into Alpha 1 and Alpha 2. Chemicals that stimulate Alpha 2 receptors are said to quiet the sympathetic nervous system when it is part of the pain state. Not all scientists agree on this point.

Aspartate is an amino acid. When we find it in receptor sites on the receiving end of a synapse it has been modified and deposited as N-methyl-D-aspartate (NMDA). NMDA is very quiet unless the pain signal is massive. It then becomes activated and makes matters much, much worse. Glutamate and glycine are excitatory amino acids.

Gamma amino butyric acid (GABA) is an inhibitory neurotransmitter substance. GABA inhibits pain signals. Glutamate and glycine excite pain signals. There is not enough GABA present when nerve injury pain is occurring, and at the same time there is too much glutamate.

The Body's All-Purpose Battery

A battery stores energy chemically. The energy comes from the voltage difference at the positive and negative ends of the battery. If something connects the two ends, the current flow will try to equalize the voltage and that flowing current supplies electrical energy. Once the energy is released, the battery has to be replaced.

The body uses high-energy phosphate bonds for energy storage. In the body's "all purpose" battery arrangement, phosphates attach to adenosine. The bonds can be removed and the energy passed to another chemical by attaching a phosphate to (phosphorylating) the new substance, which is done by kinase enzymes. For example, if substance "X" has a phosphate attached, it is called phospho "X" or "p-X," meaning it is phosphorylated and ready to rumble. To the energy supplier adenosine are attached, one, two, or even three high-energy phosphate batteries. This means there can be adenosine monophosphate, diphosphate or triphosphate (the three compounds are abbreviated AMP, ADP, and ATP).

Many chemical reactions can happen only if phosphate bonds supply energy. The result is that wherever phosphorylation is taking place in the body, more energy is going to be available to make chemical reactions happen. Remember that word, "phosphorylation," but you can just think "battery power" if you want to. If you were fighting central pain you would not want phosphorylation to occur, because it would be excitatory and you want to quiet things in the pain system, so excess phosphorylation in pathways that excite pain nerves is *bad*. You'll remember that glutamate excites pain signals and GABA inhibits or quiets pain signals. Many chemicals in nerve cells are inert and do not function unless a phosphate attaches to them. For example, glucose (sugar) is relatively inert, but if something attaches a phosphate bond to it, it becomes glucose 6 phosphate, which is very reactive.

The substances that attach phosphate energy packets to cells are enzymes called kinases. Currently, pain researchers believe that mitogen-activated protein kinase (MAPK) is at the center of the cascade of events causing nerve injury pain. MAPK is bad if you have

121

central pain because it really cranks out excitatory chemicals. Medicines controlling MAPK could be a whole new class of pain drug.

Types of Pain

If you touch something hot and drop it quickly enough, you stop hurting. If you contact it long enough, you get a burn. Once you have a burn, if you touch the area, even with something that isn't hot, the skin will feel a burn. This is called primary hyperalgesia, which means heightened pain. It is referred to as primary because it is in the area of original injury.

Any pain caused by a normally nonpainful stimulus is called allodynia. If skin is hyperalgesic, you may get allodynia. Hyperalgesia refers to pain in a normal nerve. If the nerve is injured then this is called *hyperpathia* and it acts in a particular way. Heightened sensation *outside* the area of injury is called secondary hyperalgesia. Any pain from a normally nonpainful stimulus is allodynia. Pain in an area other than the area touched is called allachesthesia. Hyperpathia, allodynia, and dysesthesia are all part of the pain abnormalities experienced in Central Pain.

If you isolate a C-fiber nerve and pinch it, you cause a firing that is received by the spinal cord neurons. If you pinch it hard enough, the firing continues for 30 minutes or more. At first, it was thought that this was because the C-fiber had been injured and this was responsible for the continued firing. The pH of the area around the injury drops to the acid range and may go as low as 6 or even 5 in some circumstances (7.4 is normal). These chemicals together have a synergistic effect on firing of the C-fibers. Together they are more potent than any single one alone. What is very interesting is that a C-fiber has specific receptors to bind these chemicals. For example, the prostanoids (of which the prostaglandins are best known) have specific receptors called EP and IP receptors. The injury pattern and chain of receptors devoted to the exciter chemicals is organized and is often very specific.

These same compounds normally have *no* effect on the big A-beta fibers. The smaller A-deltas may respond if they are of the type called "chemically sensitive," but we think the A-betas are indifferent to chemically induced pain. Strong pain means pain where the pain fibers fire at high frequency. What if you graph the firing intensity (frequency of firing) of C-fibers in relation to the intensity of an applied stimulus (how hard you are pinching)? If tissue injury chemicals are present, not only can they cause spontaneous firing, they also increase the slope of pain response so that each increment in stimulus causes an even greater increment in the frequency at which the C-fibers fire. This means the pain ramps up quickly on an ever-steeper curve. *Intensity of pain is ultimately defined by the frequency at which the nerves fire, not the strength with which they fire.*

Now let's return to the WDR neuron. This is the second order neuron in the cord that connects with both low threshold fibers and high threshold fibers. If we stimulate every second or two, we get a certain firing rate in the WDR neuron. If we continue the stimulation long enough and then shut it off, the WDR neuron will still continue to fire because of the sensitization of C-fibers by tissue injury chemicals described above. The repetitive firing by WDR neurons due to C-fibers sensitization is called *windup*. Overstimulation of A-betas alone does *not* give windup. Windup is very important. Try to remember it.

Now these A-betas that connect to WDR neurons are usually very precise about informing the brain about exactly where the painful stimulus was applied, but they have connections, or collateral synapses, with other A-betas connected to WDR neurons. Normally, stimulation in a small area of skin only reaches the one WDR neuron that supplies it. However, if A-beta cross-talk occurs, the patient will feel pain in a wide area because the high frequency firing sends out signals to other A-betas, which would normally not fire. The ability to localize pain decreases but the intensity and durability of the pain signal increases.

At this point, even a modest stimulation in the area of skin supplied by these neighboring neurons will give a strong pain response. Note that this supersensitization in WDR neurons, which results in allodynia is now being driven by A-betas, the big boys who are bad news to the brain when it comes to pain. Some A-delta, smaller slow conducting fibers, may be able to drive windup if the stimulus is of the type the fiber was specifically designed for, such as thermoreceptors, but this has not been proven. For now we will say windup comes from A-betas that have been sensitized by C-fibers.

The Significance of Delay

People with peripheral pain display the evoked or augmented pain from touch *immediately*, while those with central pain have a *delay*, usually a matter of 20 – 30 seconds before the pain evokes above its spontaneous, normal, level. This is an important diagnostic distinction that allows clinical differentiation between peripheral and central nerve injury pain. S. Weir Mitchell used the same test to differentiate the site of injury in nerve pain as early as 1872.

123

We have called this delay in evocation *temporal summation* or *slow summation*, a kind of central version of peripheral windup. Doctors who are not experienced with Central Pain may think the delay means the patient is faking, since they are used to seeing the immediate pain in peripheral neuropathy. Actually, the delay for evocation is proof that the patient has Central Pain.

Quick vs. Long-lasting Pain

When Substance P (an excitatory peptide) is released into the gap between neuron endings it acts on the other side of the gap, on the next higher order of neuron, at what are called non-NMDA receptors. The glutamate causes a *quick* firing by acting on AMPA and kainate receptors (AMPA/kainite receptors in the second order neuron). Substance P is able to cause a much *longer lasting* firing by acting on neurokinin (NK1) receptors. So, glutamate = quick pain and Substance P = long lasting pain.

Intense Pain

NMDA is also buried in the nerve cell on the other side of the gap, but normally it is unable to fire. It remains quiet. Some researchers believe this arrest is caused by magnesium in the receptor. Newer research by Woolf and others suggests a different mechanism, but the effect is the same. When sufficient sensitization has taken place from release of excitatory chemicals, the magnesium is supposedly washed out and then the NMDA, which is capable of truly large pain signals, can be acted on by glutamate. Note that considerable sensitization must have occurred to kick the NMDA receptors into action, but they can really get the job done when stirred from their deep sleep by Substance P, together with the actions of glutamate. NMDA is not your friend if you have Central Pain.

GABA

Most of the work of the brain and central nervous system is to inhibit, whether from pain or anything else. It has been demonstrated in animal models that simple loss of interneurons that respond to the inhibitory chemicals GABA or glycine (called GABAergic and glycinergic neurons) is sufficient to generate a constant severe pain state, through loss of inhibition. *Some researchers feel that loss of GABA through nerve injury is a major cause of central pain.*

Chapter 16

Chest Pain

Facts about Angina

What is angina?

Angina pectoris ("angina") is a recurring pain or discomfort in the chest that happens when some part of the heart does not receive enough blood. It is a common symptom of coronary heart disease (CHD), which occurs when vessels that carry blood to the heart become narrowed and blocked due to atherosclerosis.

Angina feels like a pressing or squeezing pain, usually in the chest under the breast bone, but sometimes in the shoulders, arms, neck, jaws, or back. Angina is usually precipitated by exertion. It is usually relieved within a few minutes by resting or by taking prescribed angina medicine.

What brings on angina?

Episodes of angina occur when the heart's need for oxygen increases beyond the oxygen available from the blood nourishing the heart. Physical exertion is the most common trigger for angina. Other

This chapter includes text from "Facts about Angina," National Heart, Lung, and Blood Institute (NHLBI), NIH Pub. No. 95-2890, September 1995; "Frequently Asked Questions about Heart Attack," an undated NHLBI fact sheet available at www.nhlbi.nih.gov/actintime/faq/faq.htm (accesssed October 2001); and "Women and Heart Attack, an undated NHLBI fact sheet available at www.nhlbi.nih.gov/actintime/haws/women.htm (accessed October 2001).

triggers can be emotional stress, extreme cold or heat, heavy meals, alcohol, and cigarette smoking.

Does angina mean a heart attack is about to happen?

An episode of angina is not a heart attack. Angina pain means that some of the heart muscle in not getting enough blood temporarily—for example, during exercise, when the heart has to work harder. The pain does *not* mean that the heart muscle is suffering irreversible, permanent damage. Episodes of angina seldom cause permanent damage to heart muscle.

In contrast, a heart attack occurs when the blood flow to a part of the heart is suddenly and permanently cut off. This causes permanent damage to the heart muscle. Typically, the chest pain is more severe, lasts longer, and does not go away with rest or with medicine that was previously effective. It may be accompanied by indigestion, nausea, weakness, and sweating. However, the symptoms of a heart attack are varied and may be considerably milder.

When someone has a repeating but stable pattern of angina, an episode of angina does not mean that a heart attack is about to happen. Angina means that there is underlying coronary heart disease. Patients with angina are at an increased risk of heart attack compared with those who have no symptoms of cardiovascular disease, but the episode of angina is not a signal that a heart attack is about to happen. In contrast, when the pattern of angina changes—if episodes become more frequent, last longer, or occur without exercise—the risk of heart attack in subsequent days or weeks is much higher.

A person who has angina should learn the pattern of his or her angina—what causes an angina attack, what it feels like, how long episodes usually last, and whether medication relieves the attack. If the pattern changes sharply or if the symptoms are those of a heart attack, one should get medical help immediately, perhaps best done by seeking an evaluation at a nearby hospital emergency room.

Is all chest pain "angina?"

No, not at all. Not all chest pain is from the heart, and not all pain from the heart is angina. For example, if the pain lasts for less than 30 seconds or if it goes away during a deep breath, after drinking a glass of water, or by changing position, it almost certainly is *not* angina and should not cause concern. But prolonged pain, unrelieved by rest and accompanied by other symptoms may signal a heart attack.

How is angina diagnosed?

Usually the doctor can diagnose angina by noting the symptoms and how they arise. However one or more diagnostic tests may be needed to exclude angina or to establish the severity of the underlying coronary disease. These include the electrocardiogram (ECG) at rest, the stress test, and x- rays of the coronary arteries (coronary "arteriogram" or "angiogram").

The ECG records electrical impulses of the heart. These may indicate that the heart muscle is not getting as much oxygen as it needs ("ischemia"); they may also indicate abnormalities in heart rhythm or some of the other possible abnormal features of the heart. To record the ECG, a technician positions a number of small contacts on the patient's arms, legs, and across the chest to connect them to an ECG machine.

For many patients with angina, the ECG at rest is normal. This is not surprising because the symptoms of angina occur during stress. Therefore, the functioning of the heart may be tested under stress, typically exercise. In the simplest stress test, the ECG is taken before, during, and after exercise to look for stress related abnormalities. Blood pressure is also measured during the stress test and symptoms are noted.

A more complex stress test involves picturing the blood flow pattern in the heart muscle during peak exercise and after rest. A tiny amount of a radioisotope, usually thallium, is injected into a vein at peak exercise and is taken up by normal heart muscle. A radioactivity detector and computer record the pattern of radioactivity distribution to various parts of the heart muscle. Regional differences in radioisotope concentration and in the rates at which the radioisotopes disappear are measures of unequal blood flow due to coronary artery narrowing, or due to failure of uptake in scarred heart muscle.

The most accurate way to assess the presence and severity of coronary disease is a coronary angiogram, an x-ray of the coronary artery. A long thin flexible tube (a "catheter") is threaded into an artery in the groin or forearm and advanced through the arterial system into one of the two major coronary arteries. A fluid that blocks x-rays (a "contrast medium" or "dye") is injected. X-rays of its distribution show the coronary arteries and their narrowing.

How is angina treated?

The underlying coronary artery disease that causes angina should be attacked by controlling existing "risk factors." These include high blood pressure, cigarette smoking, high blood cholesterol levels, and excess weight. If the doctor has prescribed a drug to lower blood pressure, it should be taken as directed. Advice is available on how to eat to control weight, blood cholesterol levels, and blood pressure. A physician can also help patients to stop smoking. Taking these steps reduces the likelihood that coronary artery disease will lead to a heart attack.

Most people with angina learn to adjust their lives to minimize episodes of angina, by taking sensible precautions and using medications if necessary.

Usually the first line of defense involves changing one's living habits to avoid bringing on attacks of angina. Controlling physical activity, adopting good eating habits, moderating alcohol consumption, and not smoking are some of the precautions that can help patients live more comfortably and with less angina. For example, if angina comes on with strenuous exercise, exercise a little less strenuously, but do exercise. If angina occurs after heavy meals, avoid large meals and rich foods that leave one feeling stuffed. Controlling weight, reducing the amount of fat in the diet, and avoiding emotional upsets may also help.

Angina is often controlled by drugs. The most commonly prescribed drug for angina is nitroglycerin, which relieves pain by widening blood vessels. This allows more blood to flow to the heart muscle and also decreases the work load of the heart. Nitroglycerin is taken when discomfort occurs or is expected. Doctors frequently prescribe other drugs, to be taken regularly, that reduce the heart's workload. Beta blockers slow the heart rate and lessen the force of the heart muscle contraction. Calcium channel blockers are also effective in reducing the frequency and severity of angina attacks.

What if medication fails to control angina?

Doctors may recommend surgery or angioplasty if drugs fail to ease angina or if the risk of heart attack is high. Coronary artery bypass surgery is an operation in which a blood vessel is grafted onto the blocked artery to bypass the blocked or diseased section so that blood can get to the heart muscle. An artery from inside the chest (an "internal mammary" graft) or long vein from the leg (a "saphenous vein" graft) may be used.

Balloon angioplasty involves inserting a catheter with a tiny balloon at the end into a forearm or groin artery. The balloon is inflated briefly to open the vessel in places where the artery is narrowed. Other catheter techniques are also being developed for opening narrowed coronary arteries, including laser and mechanical devices applied by means of catheters.

Can a person with angina exercise?

Yes. It is important to work with the doctor to develop an exercise plan. Exercise may increase the level of pain-free activity, relieve stress, improve the heart's blood supply, and help control weight. A person with angina should start an exercise program only with the doctor's advice. Many doctors tell angina patients to gradually build up their fitness level—for example, start with a 5-minute walk and increase over weeks or months to 30 minutes or 1 hour. The idea is to gradually increase stamina by working at a steady pace, but avoiding sudden bursts of effort.

What is the difference between "stable" and "unstable" angina?

It is important to distinguish between the typical stable pattern of angina and "unstable" angina.

Angina pectoris often recurs in a regular or characteristic pattern. Commonly a person recognizes that he or she is having angina only after several episodes have occurred, and a pattern has evolved. The level of activity or stress that provokes the angina is somewhat predictable, and the pattern changes only slowly. This is "stable" angina, the most common variety.

Instead of appearing gradually, angina may first appear as a very severe episode or as frequently recurring bouts of angina. Or, an established stable pattern of angina may change sharply; it may by provoked by far less exercise than in the past, or it may appear at rest. Angina in these forms is referred to as "unstable angina" and needs prompt medical attention.

The term "unstable angina" is also used when symptoms suggest a heart attack but hospital tests do not support that diagnosis. For example, a patient may have typical but prolonged chest pain and poor response to rest and medication, but there is no evidence of heart muscle damage either on the electrocardiogram or in blood enzyme tests.

Are there other types of angina?

There are two other forms of angina pectoris. One, long recognized but quite rare, is called Prinzmetal's or variant angina. This type is caused by vasospasm, a spasm that narrows the coronary artery and lessens the flow of blood to the heart. The other is a recently discovered type of angina called microvascular angina. Patients with this condition experience chest pain but have no apparent coronary artery blockages. Doctors have found that the pain results from poor function of tiny blood vessels nourishing the heart as well as the arms and legs. Microvascular angina can be treated with some of the same medications used for angina pectoris.

Frequently Asked Questions about Heart Attack

How would I know if I were having a heart attack?

Often, it is not easy to tell. But there are symptoms people may have. These are: an uncomfortable pressure, squeezing, fullness, or pain in the center of the chest that lasts more than a few minutes, or goes away and comes back; discomfort in other areas of the upper body, which may be felt in one or both arms, the back, neck, jaw, or stomach; shortness of breath, which often occurs with or before chest discomfort; and other symptoms such as breaking out in a cold sweat, nausea, or light-headedness. When in doubt, check it out! Call 9-1-1. Don't wait more than a few minutes—5 at most. Call right away.

What is angina and how is it different from a heart attack?

An episode of angina is *not* a heart attack. However, people with angina report having a hard time telling the difference between angina symptoms and heart attack symptoms. Angina is a recurring pain or discomfort in the chest that happens when some part of the heart does not receive enough blood temporarily. A person may notice it during exertion (such as in climbing stairs). It is usually relieved within a few minutes by resting or by taking prescribed angina medicine. People who have been diagnosed with angina have a greater risk of a heart attack than do other people.

I'd rather wait until I'm sure something's really wrong. What's the rush anyway?

Clot-busting drugs and other artery-opening treatments work best when given within the first hour after a heart attack starts. The first hour also is the most risky time during a heart attack—it's when your heart might stop suddenly. Responding fast to your symptoms really increases your chance of surviving.

So how quickly should I act?

If you have any heart attack symptoms, call 9-1-1 immediately. Don't wait for more than a few minutes—5 at most—to call 9-1-1.

Why should I bother? If I'm going to die, there's not much I can do about it anyway, is there?

That's not true. There is something that can be done about a heart attack. Doctors have clot-busting drugs and other artery-opening procedures that can stop or reverse a heart attack, if given quickly. These drugs can limit the damage to the heart muscle by removing the blockage and restoring blood flow. Less heart damage means a better quality of life after a heart attack.

Given that these new therapies are available, it's very sad to know that so many people cannot receive these treatments because they delay too long before seeking care. The greatest benefits of these therapies are gained when patients come in early (preferably within the first hour of the start of their symptoms).

Emergency medical personnel cause such a commotion. Can't I just have my wife/husband/friend/coworker take me to the hospital?

Emergency medical personnel—also called EMS, for emergency medical services—bring medical care to you. For example, they bring oxygen and medications. And they can actually restart someone's heart if it stops after they arrive. Your wife/husband/friend/coworker can't do that, or help you at all if they are driving. In the ambulance, there are enough people to give you the help you need and get you to the hospital right away.

I'm not sure I can remember all this. What can I do to make it easier for me?

You can make a plan and discuss it in advance with your family, your friends, your coworkers and, of course, your doctor. Then you can rehearse this plan, just like a fire drill. Keep it simple. Know the warning signs. Keep information—such as what medications you're taking—in one place. If you have any symptoms of a heart attack for a few minutes (no more than 5), call the EMS by dialing 9-1-1 right away.

I carry nitroglycerin pills all the time for my heart condition. If I have heart attack symptoms, shouldn't I try them first?

Yes, if your doctor has prescribed nitroglycerin pills, you should follow your doctor's orders. If you are not sure about how to take your nitroglycerin when you get chest pain, check with your doctor.

What about taking an aspirin like we see on television?

You should not delay calling 9-1-1 to take an aspirin. Studies have shown that people sometimes delay seeking help if they take an aspirin (or other medicine). Emergency department personnel will give people experiencing a heart attack an aspirin as soon as they arrive. So, the best thing to do is to call 9-1-1 immediately and let the professionals give the aspirin.

Women and Heart Attack

If you're a woman, you may not believe you are as vulnerable to a heart attack as men—but you are. Women account for nearly half of all heart attack deaths. Heart disease is the number one killer of both women and men.

There are differences in how women and men respond to a heart attack. Women are less likely than men to believe they're having a heart attack and more likely to delay in seeking emergency treatment.

Further, women tend to be about 10 years older than men when they have a heart attack. They are more likely to have other conditions, such as diabetes, high blood pressure, and congestive heart failure—making it all the more vital that they get proper treatment fast.

Women should learn the heart attack warning signs. These are:

- Pain or discomfort in the center of the chest.

- Pain or discomfort in other areas of the upper body, including the arms, back, neck, jaw, or stomach.

- Other symptoms, such as a shortness of breath, breaking out in a cold sweat, nausea, or light-headedness.

As with men, women's most common heart attack symptom is chest pain or discomfort. But women are somewhat more likely than men to experience some of the other common symptoms, particularly shortness of breath, nausea/vomiting, and back or jaw pain.

If you feel heart attack symptoms, do not delay. Remember, minutes matter! Do not wait for more than a few minutes—5 minutes at most—to call 9-1-1. Your family will benefit most if you seek fast treatment.

Additional Resources

"Facts about Blood Cholesterol" (revised 1994), NIH Publication No. 94-2696

"Facts about Coronary Heart Disease" (reprinted 1993), NIH Publication No. 93-2265

"Facts about Heart Failure" (reprinted 1995), NIH Publication No. 95-923

"Facts about Heart Disease and Women: So You Have Heart Disease," NIH Publication No. 95-2645

"High Blood Pressure and What You Can Do about It," No. 55-222A

"So You Have High Blood Cholesterol" (revised 1993), NIH Publication No. 93-2922

"Step by Step: Eating to Lower Your High Blood Cholesterol" (revised 1994), NIH Publication No. 94-2920

For Further Information

National Heart, Lung, and Blood Institute
Information Office
P.O. Box 30105
Bethesda, MD 20892-0105
Phone: (301) 592-8573

Chapter 17

Complex Regional Pain Syndrome

What Is Complex Regional Pain Syndrome (CRPS)?

Complex Regional Pain Syndrome (CRPS) is a chronic pain condition. A patient with CRPS has pain as well as changes in blood flow, sweating, and swelling in the painful area. Sometimes the condition leads to changes in the skin, bones, and other tissues. It may also become hard for a patient with CRPS to move the painful body part.

The patient's arms or legs are usually involved, but CRPS may affect any part of the body, such as the face or trunk. In some patients, many different areas of the body are affected. CRPS can be progressive (meaning that it gets worse at one site or spreads to other sites), or it can stay the same for a long time or even improve on its own.

CRPS usually develops after an injury. The injury may be to the skin, bone, joints, or tissue. This type of CRPS has been called reflex sympathetic dystrophy. CRPS can also develop after any type of injury to major nerves. This type has been called causalgia. The injury that leads to CRPS may be only minor, and sometimes a patient cannot remember any injury or event that caused CRPS to start.

Who Gets CRPS?

Like all human beings, patients who develop CRPS have had many other injuries that did not become CRPS. Patients want to know: "Why

"Complex Regional Pain Syndrome," Department of Pain Medicine and Palliative Care at Beth Israel Medical Center, online at www.stoppain.org. © 2000 Continuum Health Partners, Inc.; reprinted with permission.

did this injury result in my getting CRPS?" Unfortunately, no one knows the answer to this question. Experts say that it might happen because:

- The chance of getting it might run in the family

- There is some type of stress in the person's life at the time of injury

- The injured body part is not being used for a long time (either because it is in a cast or sling, or because the person is protecting it and not moving it normally)

What Is Happening in the Body to Cause CRPS?

Until recently, doctors thought that CRPS always involved a problem in the sympathetic nervous system (a set of nerves that control the size of blood vessels, sweating, and many other bodily functions).

They now think that only some patients with CRPS have these sympathetic nervous system problems. Pain that comes from problems in the sympathetic nerves is called "sympathetically-maintained pain," or SMP. The only way a doctor can find out if a patient has SMP is to do a sympathetic nerve block. (Sympathetic nerve blocks are injections of a numbing drug, called a local anesthetic, into different sites in the body). A person suffering from CRPS can be said to have SMP only if he or she has good pain relief from a sympathetic block.

If SMP does not explain the pain in most patients with CRPS, what is the cause of the pain? Experts agree that there are problems in the peripheral nervous system (the nerves in the body) and the central nervous system (the brain and spinal cord) of patients with CRPS, but the details are not known. There are other factors that could be involved in the development of CRPS because they directly affect the activity of the nervous system, muscles and bones. Examples of these factors are emotional issues or stress and not using a painful body part.

Diagnosing and Treating CRPS

A doctor makes the diagnosis of CRPS based on how a patient describes his or her symptoms and from what the doctor finds when he gives the patient a physical exam. The patient does not have to have a nerve block to get a diagnosis of CRPS. Laboratory tests or tests such as X-rays or bone scans are usually not needed to make the diagnosis, either.

Symptoms Needed to Make the Diagnosis of CRPS

These are the symptoms that doctors use to decide whether or not a patient has CRPS:

Pain that is constant or almost constant, with:

- pain caused by things that do not usually cause pain, such as clothing, wind, cold or a light touch to the skin (called "allodynia"), and/or

- severe pain when only a slight pain would be expected, such as when a doctor lightly pricks the skin with a pin (called "hyper-algesia")

Having some of the following in the painful area:

- swelling

- changes in skin color (mottled, purple-bluish, red)

- skin temperature that is not normal (either hotter or colder than other areas)

- either more or less sweating in the area

Other Symptoms

The following symptoms are also commonly experienced by CRPS patients:

- Problems moving the painful body part

- Tremors ("shakes")

- Depression or anxiety (common to all chronic pain disorders)

- Sleep problems (common to all chronic pain disorders)

Trophic Changes

Some patients with CRPS have changes in the area of the pain that are known as "trophic changes." These include:

- Wasting away of the skin, tissues, or muscle

- Thinning of the bones

- Changes in how the hair or nails grow, including thickening or thinning of hair or brittle nails

It is important to know that every patient with CRPS has different signs and symptoms. Also, a patient's symptoms and signs can change from minute-to-minute or hour-to-hour.

Treatments

No single treatment, such as a pill or nerve block, can cure CRPS, but many CRPS patients do find that their pain and other symptoms get much better with the right therapies. CRPS can improve when patients:

- get treatments that lessen the pain (such as nerve blocks, medicines, and other treatments),
- take part in a physical therapy program, and
- get helpful psychological treatments (such as stress management skills).

Every patient with CRPS responds differently to each therapy—what works well for one patient may not work at all for another. Because of this, doctors may need to try many different medical therapies in different combinations. It is often best for patients with CRPS to see pain specialists, who are experienced in taking care of patients with difficult pain problems.

Drugs

Doctors might prescribe drugs like anti-inflammatory drugs, corticosteroids, antidepressants, anticonvulsants, calcitonin,or opioids for patients with CRPS. Patients may have to take several different drugs together to get the best pain relief.

Sympathetic Block

Sympathetic nerve blocks include stellate ganglion nerve blocks, lumbar sympathetic nerve blocks and Bier blocks. For all of these blocks, doctors inject numbing drugs (called "local anesthetics") in different nerves. For the Beir block, a drug is injected into a vein after a cuff is inflated. The cuff keeps the drug in the painful area, so the drug only affects the tissues in that area. Doctors may also use a phentolamine infusion, in which a drug is given intravenously (through an IV). Phentolamine infusions are thought to have a similar effect as a sympathetic nerve block.

Most patients with CRPS should receive at least one sympathetic block because some patients will have dramatic pain relief. If a sympathetic block does not provide good pain relief, the patient should probably stop getting them.

Sympathectomy

Some patients with CRPS have good pain relief from sympathetic nerve blocks, but the pain relief does not last long. For these patients, doctors might suggest a sympathectomy (killing the sympathetic nerves leading to the painful body part, either by using surgery or chemicals). Some patients get longer pain relief after the sympathectomy, but others do not. Also, there is the slight chance that patients who get a sympathectomy for CRPS of the leg might develop a new pain syndrome, called post-sympathectomy syndrome.

Other Treatments

Some patients get pain relief from acupuncture and transcutaneous electrical nerve stimulation (TENS). With acupuncture, needles are placed in specific areas on the skin to help relieve pain. With TENS, patients carry a small, box-shaped device that sends electrical impulses into the body through electrodes. These electrical impulses interfere with pain signals.

Sometimes, pain specialists recommend that a patient try a treatment called spinal cord stimulation, or dorsal column stimulation. This treatment provides low-voltage electrical stimulation by placing an electrode inside the spine. Pain specialists also sometimes recommend that a patient try intraspinal infusion. Intraspinal infusion means that medications are given through a catheter going directly into the spine. Drugs that prevent or treat pain (called "analgesic medications"), such as morphine, can be given in low doses through the catheter.

Physical/Occupational Therapy

Physical and occupational therapists can help patients with CRPS begin a program of stretching, strengthening, and aerobic conditioning. The goal of this program is to help the patient get back range of motion, strength and motor control. Physical and occupational therapists might also try treatments like warm and cold baths, ultrasound, or electric stimulation.

"Desensitization" is another important treatment that can be used to help with allodynia (pain caused by things that do not normally cause pain, such as clothing, wind, cold or a light touch to the skin). The patient's painful skin is rubbed with different materials, starting with soft, light textures and proceeding to rough, irritating surfaces. Gradually, the painful skin gets used to the rough textures, until the patient can easily deal with the touch of clothing, bed sheets, towels, etc.

Chapter 18

Earache (Otitis Media)

What Is Otitis Media?

Otitis media is an infection or inflammation of the middle ear. This inflammation often begins when infections that cause sore throats, colds, or other respiratory or breathing problems spread to the middle ear. These can be viral or bacterial infections. Seventy-five percent of children experience at least one episode of otitis media by their third birthday. Almost half of these children will have three or more ear infections during their first three years. It is estimated that medical costs and lost wages because of otitis media amount to $5 billion (Gates GA, Cost-effectiveness considerations in otitis media treatment, *Otolaryngol Head Neck Surg,* 114 (4), April 1996, 525–530) a year in the United States. Although otitis media is primarily a disease of infants and young children, it can also affect adults.

How Do We Hear?

The ear consists of three major parts: the outer ear, the middle ear, and the inner ear. The outer ear includes the pinna—the visible part of the ear—and the ear canal. The outer ear extends to the tympanic membrane or eardrum, which separates the outer ear from the middle ear. The middle ear is an air-filled space that is located behind the eardrum. The middle ear contains three tiny bones, the malleus, incus,

"Otitis Media," National Institute on Deafness and Other Communication Disorders (NIDCD), NIH Pub. No. 97-4216, updated October 2000.

and stapes, which transmit sound from the eardrum to the inner ear. The inner ear contains the hearing and balance organs. The cochlea contains the hearing organ which converts sound into electrical signals which are associated with the origin of impulses carried by nerves to the brain where their meanings are appreciated.

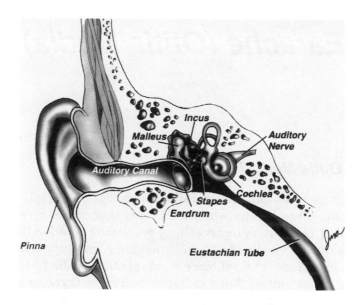

Figure 18.1. *The Ear. (Illustration provided by the National Institute on Deafness and Other Communication Disorders.)*

Why Are More Children Affected by Otitis Media Than Adults?

There are many reasons why children are more likely to suffer from otitis media than adults. First, children have more trouble fighting infections. This is because their immune systems are still developing. Another reason has to do with the child's eustachian tube. The eustachian tube is a small passageway that connects the upper part of the throat to the middle ear. It is shorter and straighter in the child than in the adult. It can contribute to otitis media in several ways.

The eustachian tube is usually closed but opens regularly to ventilate or replenish the air in the middle ear. This tube also equalizes middle ear air pressure in response to air pressure changes in the environment. However, a eustachian tube that is blocked by swelling of its lining or plugged with mucus from a cold or for some other reason cannot open to ventilate the middle ear. The lack of ventilation may allow fluid from the tissue that lines the middle ear to accumulate. If the eustachian tube remains plugged, the fluid cannot drain and begins to collect in the normally air-filled middle ear.

One more factor that makes children more susceptible to otitis media is that adenoids in children are larger than they are in adults. Adenoids are composed largely of cells (lymphocytes) that help fight infections. They are positioned in the back of the upper part of the throat near the eustachian tubes. Enlarged adenoids can, because of their size, interfere with the eustachian tube opening. In addition, adenoids may themselves become infected, and the infection may spread into the eustachian tubes.

Bacteria reach the middle ear through the lining or the passageway of the eustachian tube and can then produce infection, which causes swelling of the lining of the middle ear, blocking of the eustachian tube, and migration of white cells from the bloodstream to help fight the infection. In this process the white cells accumulate, often killing bacteria and dying themselves, leading to the formation of pus, a thick yellowish-white fluid in the middle ear. As the fluid increases, the child may have trouble hearing because the eardrum and middle ear bones are unable to move as freely as they should. As the infection worsens, many children also experience severe ear pain. Too much fluid in the ear can put pressure on the eardrum and eventually tear it.

What Are the Effects of Otitis Media?

Otitis media not only causes severe pain but may result in serious complications if it is not treated. An untreated infection can travel from the middle ear to the nearby parts of the head, including the brain. Although the hearing loss caused by otitis media is usually temporary, untreated otitis media may lead to permanent hearing impairment. Persistent fluid in the middle ear and chronic otitis media can reduce a child's hearing at a time that is critical for speech and language development. Children who have early hearing impairment from frequent ear infections are likely to have speech and language disabilities.

143

How Can Someone Tell if a Child Has Otitis Media?

Otitis media is often difficult to detect because most children affected by this disorder do not yet have sufficient speech and language skills to tell someone what is bothering them. Common signs to look for are:

- unusual irritability
- difficulty sleeping
- tugging or pulling at one or both ears
- fever
- fluid draining from the ear
- loss of balance
- unresponsiveness to quiet sounds or other signs of hearing difficulty such as sitting too close to the television or being inattentive.

Can Anything Be Done to Prevent Otitis Media?

Specific prevention strategies applicable to all infants and children such as immunization against viral respiratory infections or specifically against the bacteria that cause otitis media are not currently available. Nevertheless, it is known that children who are cared for in group settings, as well as children who live with adults who smoke cigarettes, have more ear infections. Therefore, a child who is prone to otitis media should avoid contact with sick playmates and environmental tobacco smoke. Infants who nurse from a bottle while lying down also appear to develop otitis media more frequently. Children who have been breast-fed often have fewer episodes of otitis media. Research has shown that cold and allergy medications such as antihistamines and decongestants are not helpful in preventing ear infections. The best hope for avoiding ear infections is the development of vaccines against the bacteria that most often cause otitis media. Scientists are currently developing vaccines that show promise in preventing otitis media. Additional clinical research must be completed to ensure their effectiveness and safety.

How Does a Child's Physician Diagnose Otitis Media?

The simplest way to detect an active infection in the middle ear is to look in the child's ear with an otoscope, a light instrument that allows the physician to examine the outer ear and the eardrum. Inflammation of the eardrum indicates an infection. There are several ways that a physician checks for middle ear fluid. The use of a special type of otoscope called a pneumatic otoscope allows the physician to blow a puff of air onto the eardrum to test eardrum movement. (An eardrum with fluid behind it does not move as well as an eardrum with air behind it.)

A useful test of middle ear function is called tympanometry. This test requires insertion of a small soft plug into the opening of the child's ear canal. The plug contains a speaker, a microphone, and a device that is able to change the air pressure in the ear canal, allowing for several measures of the middle ear. The child feels air pressure changes in the ear or hears a few brief tones. While this test provides information on the condition of the middle ear, it does not determine how well the child hears. A physician may suggest a hearing test for a child who has frequent ear infections to determine the extent of hearing loss. The hearing test is usually performed by an audiologist, a person who is specially trained to measure hearing.

How Is Otitis Media Treated?

Many physicians recommend the use of an antibiotic (a drug that kills bacteria) when there is an active middle ear infection. If a child is experiencing pain, the physician may also recommend a pain reliever. Following the physician's instructions is very important. Once started, the antibiotic should be taken until it is finished. Most physicians will have the child return for a followup examination to see if the infection has cleared. Unfortunately, there are many bacteria that can cause otitis media, and some have become resistant to some antibiotics. This happens when antibiotics are given for coughs, colds, flu, or viral infections where antibiotic treatment is not useful. When bacteria become resistant to antibiotics, those treatments are then less effective against infections. This means that several different antibiotics may have to be tried before an ear infection clears. Antibiotics may also produce unwanted side effects such as nausea, diarrhea, and rashes. (See Note below.)

Once the infection clears, fluid may remain in the middle ear for several months. Middle ear fluid that is not infected often disappears after 3 to 6 weeks. Neither antihistamines nor decongestants are recommended as helpful in the treatment of otitis media at any stage in the disease process. Sometimes physicians will treat the child with an antibiotic to hasten the elimination of the fluid. If the fluid persists for more than 3 months and is associated with a loss of hearing, many physicians suggest the insertion of "tubes" in the affected ears. This operation, called a myringotomy, can usually be done on an outpatient basis by a surgeon, who is usually an otolaryngologist (a physician who specializes in the ears, nose, and throat). While the child is asleep under general anesthesia, the surgeon makes a small opening in the child's eardrum. A small metal or plastic tube is placed into the opening in the eardrum. The tube ventilates the middle ear and helps keep the air pressure in the middle ear equal to the air pressure in the environment. The tube normally stays in the eardrum for 6 to 12 months, after which time it usually comes out spontaneously. If a child has enlarged or infected adenoids, the surgeon may recommend removal of the adenoids at the same time the ear tubes are inserted. Removal of the adenoids has been shown to reduce episodes of otitis media in some children, but not those who are under 4 years of age. Research, however, has shown that removal of a child's tonsils does not reduce occurrences of otitis media. Tonsillotomy and adenoidectomy may be appropriate for reasons other than middle ear fluid.

Hearing should be fully restored once the fluid is removed. Some children may need to have the operation again if the otitis media returns after the tubes come out. While the tubes are in place, water should be kept out of the ears. Many physicians recommend that a child with tubes wear special ear plugs while swimming or bathing so that water does not enter the middle ear.

What Research Is Being Done on Otitis Media?

Several avenues of research are being explored to further improve the prevention, diagnosis, and treatment of otitis media. For example, research is better defining those children who are at high risk for developing otitis media and conditions that predispose certain individuals to middle ear infections. Emphasis is being placed on discovering the reasons why some children have more ear infections than other children. The effects of otitis media on children's speech and language development are important areas of study, as is research to develop more accurate methods to help physicians detect middle ear infections. How the defense molecules and cells involved with immunity respond to bacteria and viruses that often lead to otitis media is also under investigation. Scientists are evaluating the success of certain drugs currently being used for the treatment of otitis media and are examining new drugs that may be more effective, easier to administer, and better at preventing new infections. Most important, research is leading to the availability of vaccines that will prevent otitis media.

Note

There is ongoing scientific discussion about the use and potential overuse of antibiotic therapy for otitis media. For further information, please note the following publications.

Berman S, Byrns PJ, Bondy J, Smith PJ, Lezotte D. Otitis media-related antibiotic prescribing patterns, outcomes, and expenditures in a pediatric Medicaid population. *Pediatrics*. 4 Oct 1997. 100(4): 585-592.

Culpepper L, Froom J. Routine antimicrobial treatment of acute otitis media: is it necessary? *JAMA*. 26 Nov 1997. 278(20): 1643-1645.

Dagan R, Leibovitz E, Leiberman A, Yagupsky P. Clinical significance of antibiotic resistance in acute otitis media and implication of antibiotic treatment on carriage and spread of resistant organisms. *Pediatr Infect Dis J*. 19 May 2000. 19 (5 Suppl): S57-S65.

Dowell SF, Butler JC, Giebink GS, Jacobs MR, Jernigan D, Musher DM, Rakowsky A, Schwartz B. Acute otitis media: management and surveillance in an era of pneumococcal resistance—a report from the Drug-Resistant Streptococcus pneumoniae Therapeutic Working Group. *Pediatr Infect Dis J*. Jan 1999. 18(1): 1-9.

Glasziou PP, Hayem M, Del Mar CB. Antibiotics for acute otitis media in children. *Cochrane Database Syst Rev*. 2000. 2: CD000219.

Kozyrskyj AL, Hildes-Ripstein GE, Longstaffe SE, Wincott JL, Sitar DS, Klassen TP, Moffatt ME. Treatment of acute otitis media with a shortened course of antibiotics: a meta-analysis. *JAMA*. 3 Jun 1998. 279(21): 1736-1742.

Maw R, Wilks J, Harvey I, Peters TJ, Golding J. Early surgery compared with watchful waiting for glue ear and effect on language development in preschool children: a randomised trial. *Lancet*. 20 Mar 1999. 353 (9157): 960-963.

Otitis Media with Effusion in Young Children, Clinical Practice Guideline No. 12, AHCPR Publication No. 94-0622. Agency for Healthcare Research and Quality, Rockville, MD. July 1994.

Pichichero ME. Acute otitis media: part II. Treatment in an era of increasing antibiotic resistance. *Am Fam Physician*. 15 April 2000. 61(8): 2410-2416.

Rosenfeld RM, Vertrees JE, Carr J, Cipolle RJ, Uden DL, Giebink GS, Canafax DM. Clinical efficacy of antimicrobial drugs for acute otitis media: metaanalysis of 5400 children from thirty-three randomized trials. *J Pediatric*s. Mar 1994. 124(3): 355-367.

Stine AR. Is amoxicillin more effective than placebo in treating acute otitis media in children younger than 2 years? *J Fam Pract*. May 2000. 49(5): 465-6.

Where Can I Get Additional Information?

Agency for Healthcare Research and Quality Publications Clearinghouse
2101 E. Jefferson Street, Suite 501
Rockville, MD 20852
Phone: (800) 358–9295 or (301) 594–1364
Website: www.ahrq.gov

American Academy of Otolaryngology–Head and Neck Surgery
One Prince Street
Alexandria, VA 22314
Phone: (703) 519–1589
TTY: (703) 519–1585
Fax: (703) 299–1125
E-mail: webmaster@entnet.org
Website: www.entnet.org

American Academy of Pediatrics
141 Northwest Point Boulevard
Elk Grove Village, IL 60007–1098
Phone: (847) 434–4000
Fax: (847) 434–8000
Website: www.aap.org

American Speech-Language-Hearing Association
10801 Rockville Pike
Rockville, MD 20852
Phone: (800) 638–8255 or (301) 897–3279
TTY (301) 897–0157
Fax: (301) 897–7355
E-mail: actioncenter@asha.org
Website: www.asha.org

Chapter 19

Fibromyalgia

What Is Fibromyalgia?

Fibromyalgia is a chronic disorder characterized by widespread musculoskeletal pain, fatigue, and multiple tender points. "Tender points" refers to tenderness that occurs in precise, localized areas, particularly in the neck, spine, shoulders, and hips. People with this syndrome may also experience sleep disturbances, morning stiffness, irritable bowel syndrome, anxiety, and other symptoms.

How Many People Have Fibromyalgia?

According to the American College of Rheumatology, fibromyalgia affects 3 to 6 million Americans. It primarily occurs in women of child-bearing age, but children, the elderly, and men can also be affected.

What Causes Fibromyalgia?

Although the cause of fibromyalgia is unknown, researchers have several theories about causes or triggers of the disorder. Some scientists believe that the syndrome may be caused by an injury or trauma. This injury may affect the central nervous system. Fibromyalgia may

This chapter includes text from "Questions and Answers About Fibromyalgia," National Institute of Arthritis and Musculoskeletal and Skin Diseases (NIAMS), December 1999; and "Fibromyalgia Research: Challenges and Opportunities" NIAMS, December 1999.

be associated with changes in muscle metabolism, such as decreased blood flow, causing fatigue and decreased strength. Others believe the syndrome may be triggered by an infectious agent such as a virus in susceptible people, but no such agent has been identified.

How Is Fibromyalgia Diagnosed?

Fibromyalgia is difficult to diagnose because many of the symptoms mimic those of other disorders. The physician reviews the patient's medical history and makes a diagnosis of fibromyalgia based on a history of chronic widespread pain that persists for more than 3 months. The American College of Rheumatology (ACR) has developed criteria for fibromyalgia that physicians can use in diagnosing the disorder. According to ACR criteria, a person is considered to have fibromyalgia if he or she has widespread pain in combination with tenderness in at least 11 of 18 specific tender point sites.

How Is Fibromyalgia Treated?

Treatment of fibromyalgia requires a comprehensive approach. The physician, physical therapist, and patient may all play an active role in the management of fibromyalgia. Studies have shown that aerobic exercise, such as swimming and walking, improves muscle fitness and reduces muscle pain and tenderness. Heat and massage may also give short-term relief. Antidepressant medications may help elevate mood, improve quality of sleep, and relax muscles. Patients with fibromyalgia may benefit from a combination of exercise, medication, physical therapy, and relaxation.

What Research Is Being Conducted on Fibromyalgia?

The National Institute of Arthritis and Musculoskeletal and Skin Diseases (NIAMS) is sponsoring research that will increase understanding of the specific abnormalities that cause and accompany fibromyalgia with the hope of developing better ways to diagnose, treat, and prevent this disorder.

Recent NIAMS studies show that abnormally low levels of the hormone cortisol may be associated with fibromyalgia. At Brigham and Women's Hospital in Boston, Massachusetts, and at the University of Michigan Medical Center in Ann Arbor, researchers are studying regulation of the function of the adrenal gland (which makes cortisol) in fibromyalgia. People whose bodies make inadequate amounts of cortisol experience many of the same symptoms as people with fibromyalgia. It is hoped that these studies will increase understanding about fibromyalgia and may suggest new ways to treat the disorder.

NIAMS research studies are looking at different aspects of the disorder. At the University of Alabama in Birmingham, researchers are concentrating on how specific brain structures are involved in the painful symptoms of fibromyalgia. At George Washington University in Washington, DC, scientists are investigating the causes of a post-Lyme disease syndrome as a model for fibromyalgia. Some patients develop a fibromyalgia-like condition following Lyme disease, an infectious disorder associated with arthritis and other symptoms.

NIAMS-supported research on fibromyalgia also includes several projects at the Institute's Multipurpose Arthritis and Musculoskeletal Diseases Centers. Researchers at these centers are studying individuals who do not seek medical care, but who meet the criteria for fibromyalgia. (Potential subjects are located through advertisements in local newspapers asking for volunteers with widespread pain or aching.) Other studies at the Centers are attempting to uncover better ways to manage the pain associated with the disorder through behavioral interventions such as relaxation training.

In March 1998, NIAMS and several other National Institutes of Health (NIH) institutes and offices issued a Request for Proposals to promote research studies of fibromyalgia. As a result of this request, NIAMS and its partners funded 15 new fibromyalgia projects totaling more than $3.6 million.

Support of fundamental research is extremely important in fibromyalgia as well as in many disorders characterized by pain and sleep abnormalities, and many disciplines of medical research contribute to the knowledge base in understanding these symptoms. Since it is impossible to know with certainty which area will produce the next important discovery, the community of science, of which the National Institute of Arthritis and Musculoskeletal and Skin Diseases (NIAMS) is a part, has to be open to all ideas. Discoveries can come from research funded in a variety of areas. For example, the National Institutes of Health (NIH) supports pain research at different levels—from the gene, molecule, cell, and organ to the human organism itself. NIH spends more than $75 million on pain research, which is conducted and supported by 15 institutes, centers, and offices. While this figure would not be reported as funding for fibromyalgia research specifically, certain aspects of pain research are applicable to understanding fibromyalgia.

Examples of NIAMS-supported clinical research in fibromyalgia include comparing pain mechanisms in this disorder and low back pain; determining if aerobic exercise benefits patients with fibromyalgia through the action of the hypothalamus and pituitary and adrenal glands; and studying neuroendocrine changes in fibromyalgia and irritable bowel syndrome. The Institute is also funding a new clinical trial to determine the effectiveness of combining two antidepressants in treating the disorder.

In addition, NIAMS is currently funding research projects related to the role of behavioral factors in fibromyalgia. Investigators are evaluating the effects of two of the most promising nonpharmacologic interventions for fibromyalgia: cognitive behavioral therapy for pain management and physical exercise training. This study is designed to test the hypothesis that combining cognitive behavioral therapy and physical training will be more effective than cognitive behavioral therapy or exercise alone. If the cognitive and exercise interventions have synergistic effects in fibromyalgia patients, future studies could evaluate this combination in patients with other rheumatic diseases, or in those with stroke or burn injuries who are experiencing pain during exercise/rehabilitation regimens.

Providing social support and education about one's disease or disorder has been shown to be an effective means for improving the health care status of individuals with chronic diseases. Studies are currently underway focusing on patients with fibromyalgia to advance understanding of how social support and education interventions may be helpful to these patients as well.

The NIAMS supports and encourages outstanding basic and clinical research that increases the understanding of fibromyalgia. However, much more research needs to be done before fibromyalgia can be successfully treated or prevented.

Why Is Behavioral Research Important to Understanding Fibromyalgia?

Behavioral and social sciences research is an important area of investigation at NIH and cuts across a wide range of research topics. NIAMS has long supported behavioral research related to many rheumatic and musculoskeletal conditions. Behavioral and social factors are significant contributors to health and illness, frequently interact with biological factors to influence health outcomes, and represent critical avenues for treatment and prevention.

Behavioral and social sciences research encompasses a wide array of disciplines. The field employs a variety of methodological approaches including surveys and questionnaires, interviews, randomized clinical trials, direct observation, physiological manipulation and recording, descriptive methods, laboratory and field experiments, standardized tests, economic analyses, statistical modeling, ethnography, and evaluation. In addition, several key crosscutting themes are characteristic of social and behavioral sciences research. These include an emphasis on theory-driven research; the search for general principles of behavioral and social functioning; the importance ascribed to a developmental, life-span perspective; an emphasis on individual variation and variation across sociodemographic categories such as gender, age, and sociocultural status; and a focus on both the social and biological context of behavior.

Behavioral and social sciences research is important to understanding how to better treat some of the clinically challenging symptoms that are experienced by fibromyalgia patients. Research opportunities include behavioral research on all aspects of fibromyalgia, including the relationships among disturbed sleep, inactivity, pain, and depression that are often observed in patients with fibromyalgia, and the development of innovative approaches for treatment.

How Are Fibromyalgia Grants Selected for Funding by NIAMS?

NIAMS currently supports research on fibromyalgia through investigator-initiated research projects, Institute-solicited studies (funded in response to a request for applications [RFA]), and Multipurpose Arthritis and Musculoskeletal Diseases Research Centers. In general, most of the research projects funded by NIH are unsolicited investigator-initiated grants. NIAMS has made awards in the area of fibromyalgia for projects resulting from both solicited and unsolicited applications.

Applications submitted to NIH go through a two-step peer review system. The design of this system is such that applications from researchers are reviewed first by study sections for their scientific merit. Applications for research on fibromyalgia may be reviewed by the Chronic Fatigue Syndrome Special Emphasis Panel or by other relevant panels, depending on the expertise required. The second level of review is each Institute's advisory council, which assesses the relevance and priority of proposed projects, and makes recommendations on funding particular meritorious applications.

Primary consideration for funding is scientific merit. This is determined during the review process and is reflective of the soundness and innovativeness of the approach, the qualifications of the investigators, the potential significance of the work, and the overall research environment. This process is used throughout NIH for applications in all diseases and areas of science. The reviewers are asked to evaluate the significance of the research proposal in terms of improving understanding of an area of research or disease, advancing scientific knowledge, learning about the mechanisms that cause symptoms and signs of disease, or developing new treatments or prevention strategies.

Research Initiatives

New Directions in Pain Research—Program Announcement. In September 1998, NIAMS joined 10 other NIH components in issuing a program announcement (PA) entitled "New Directions in Pain Research." The purpose of the PA is to inform the scientific community of broad, shared interests in pain research across the various components of the NIH, and to stimulate and encourage a wide range of basic, translational, and patient-oriented clinical studies on pain. Applications are encouraged to study pain throughout the life span from the perspectives of molecular genetics; transcriptional controls; signal transduction, including cellular/molecular mechanisms; innovative imaging technologies; plasticity; and hormonal or gender influences. The goal of the PA is to advance the development of novel pain interventions, treatments, and management strategies.

Basic and Clinical Research on Fibromyalgia—Request for Applications. In March 1998, NIAMS issued an RFA to promote research studies and exploratory/developmental projects to advance understanding of fibromyalgia and related disorders and provide critical new knowledge needed for the treatment and prevention of the syndrome. Several NIH institutes and offices joined NIAMS in issuing this RFA. These include the National Institute of Dental and Craniofacial Research (NIDCR), which has an interest in pain and the relationship between temporomandibular disorders and fibromyalgia; the National Institute of Neurological Disorders and Stroke (NINDS), which has an interest in pain research; and three offices within the NIH Office of the Director: the National Center for Complementary and Alternative Medicine, the Office of Research on Women's Health, and the Office of Behavioral and Social Sciences Research.

In addition to the announcement being listed in the usual manner on the world wide web in the *NIH Guide to Grants and Contracts*,

NIAMS distributed over 1,600 copies of the announcement to individual investigators and organizations to stimulate an interest in fibromyalgia research. NIAMS grantees in fibromyalgia, arthritis, and muscle diseases, as well as in the Centers program, received copies, as did grantees NIH-wide in the fields of chronic pain, chronic fatigue syndrome, sleep, neuroendocrinology, and other related fields.

As a result of the RFA, NIAMS and its sister institutes and offices funded 15 new fibromyalgia projects—totaling more than $3.6 million—in 1999.

Acupuncture Clinical Trials—Program Announcement. In February 1998, the NIH Office of Alternative Medicine (now the National Center for Complementary and Alternative Medicine), along with six NIH institutes, including NIAMS and NINDS, and the Agency for Health Care Policy and Research, issued a PA entitled "Acupuncture Clinical Trial Pilot Grants." The objective of the PA is to increase the quality of clinical research evaluating the efficacy of acupuncture for the treatment or prevention of disease and accompanying symptoms. Back pain, cancer, fibromyalgia, temporomandibular disorders, HIV/AIDS, and reflex sympathetic dystrophy are among the diseases and conditions identified in the PA.

NIH Pain Research Consortium—Conferences. The NIH-wide Pain Research Consortium encourages information sharing and collaborative research efforts, provides coordination of pain research across all NIH components, and ensures that results of NIH-sponsored pain research are widely communicated. A major goal of the Consortium is to coordinate efforts across the many NIH components to develop a better understanding of what causes pain, so better treatments are available to people with painful disorders such as fibromyalgia. The Consortium sponsored a symposium entitled "New Directions in Pain Research" on November 20-21, 1997, and a second conference entitled "Gender and Pain" on April 7-8, 1998.

Molecular Biology and Genetics of Sleep and Sleep Disorders—Request for Applications. In fiscal year 1997, NIAMS awarded two grants submitted in response to an RFA issued by the National Heart, Lung, and Blood Institute, NIAMS, and several other NIH institutes. The NIAMS grants are basic research studies and focus on rest and long-term memory consolidation in fruit flies and on the genetics of sleep and rest behavior in mice.

The Neuroscience and Endocrinology of Fibromyalgia: A Scientific Workshop. In July 1996, NIAMS and several other NIH organizations sponsored a scientific workshop that explored advances in the neuroscience and endocrinology of fibromyalgia. The workshop focused on chronic pain, neuroendocrinology, and sleep disorders associated with fibromyalgia. What made this workshop so unusual and effective was its design, which brought together researchers in the basic sciences of chronic pain, neuroendocrinology, circadian rhythms, and sleep disorders—all challenges for patients with fibromyalgia. These experts in basic research were joined by clinicians who treat patients with fibromyalgia and by a significant number of patients themselves. This multidisciplinary workshop helped to identify research needs and opportunities, and the gaps in understanding of this clinically challenging condition.

The summary report of the workshop presentations and discussion was published in *Arthritis and Rheumatism*, Vol. 40, No. 11, November 1997. Publication of the summary of the workshop in this peer-reviewed journal provides for wide distribution of the discussion of research opportunities to the scientific community with interest in this disorder. The workshop also led to the March 1998 RFA described previously.

Fibromyalgia Advocate on Institute Advisory Council. A leading advocate for fibromyalgia, the Advisory Council, which includes both scientific and public members, meets three times a year and provides valuable input to the Institute's priority-setting process.

Where Can People Get More Information about Fibromyalgia?

Arthritis Foundation
1330 West Peachtree Street
Atlanta, GA 30309
Phone: (404) 872-7100
Phone: (800) 283-7800 or call your local chapter (listed in the telephone directory)
Website: http://www.arthritis.org

This is the main voluntary organization devoted to all forms of arthritis. The Foundation publishes a pamphlet on fibrositis. Single copies are free with a self-addressed stamped envelope. The Foundation also can provide physician referrals.

Fibromyalgia Network
P.O. Box 31750
Tucson, AZ 85751-1750
Phone: (800) 853-2929

Fibromyalgia Partnership (formerly Fibromyalgia Association of Greater Washington)
140 Zinn Way
Linden, VA 22642-5609
Phone: (866) 725-4404 (toll free)
Fax: (540) 622-2998
Website: http://www.fmpartnership.org

National Fibromyalgia Awareness Campaign (NFAC)
2415 N. River Trail Road
Suite 200
Orange, CA 92865
Phone: (714) 921-0150
Fax: (714) 921-8139

These are the main organizations devoted to fibromyalgia. They publish newsletters and provide pamphlets on the disease.

Additional resources for people suffering with pain can be found in Chapter 91.

Keywords

Analgesic: A medication or treatment that relieves pain.

Arthritis: Literally means joint inflammation, but is often used to indicate a group of more than 100 rheumatic diseases. These diseases affect not only the joints but also other connective tissues of the body, including important supporting structures such as muscles, tendons, and ligaments, as well as the protective covering of internal organs.

Autoimmune disease: One in which the immune system destroys or attacks the patient's own body tissue.

Cartilage: A tough, resilient tissue that covers and cushions the ends of the bones and absorbs shock.

Chronic disease: An illness that lasts for a long time.

Collagen: The main structural protein of skin, tendon, bone cartilage, and connective tissues.

Connective tissue: The supporting framework of the body and its internal organs.

Fibromyalgia: Sometimes called fibrositis, a chronic disorder that causes pain and stiffness throughout the tissues that support and move the bones and joints. Pain and localized tender points occur in the muscles, particularly those that support the neck, spine, shoulders, and hips. The disorder includes widespread pain, fatigue, and sleep disturbances.

Fibrous capsule: A tough wrapping of tendons and ligaments that surrounds the joint.

Flare: A period in which disease symptoms reappear or become worse.

Genetic marker: A specific tissue type or gene, similar to a blood type, that is passed on from parents to their children. Some genetic markers are linked to certain rheumatic diseases.

Immune response: The reaction of the immune system against foreign substances. When this reaction occurs against substances or tissues within the body, it is called an autoimmune reaction.

Immune system: A complex system that normally protects the body from infections. It combines groups of cells, the chemicals that control them, and the chemicals they release.

Inflammation: A characteristic reaction of tissues to injury or disease. It is marked by four signs: swelling, redness, heat, and pain.

Joint: A junction where two bones meet. Most joints are composed of cartilage, joint space, fibrous capsule, synovium, and ligaments.

Joint space: The volume enclosed within the fibrous capsule and synovium.

Ligaments: Bands of cordlike tissue that connect bone to bone.

Muscle: A structure composed of bundles of specialized cells that, when stimulated by nerve impulses, contract and produce movement.

Myopathies: Inflammatory and noninflammatory diseases of muscle.

Myositis: Inflammation of a muscle.

Nonsteroidal anti-inflammatory drugs (NSAIDs): A group of drugs, such as aspirin and aspirin-like drugs, used to reduce inflammation that causes joint pain, stiffness, and swelling.

Raynaud's phenomenon: A circulatory condition associated with spasms in the blood vessels of the fingers and toes causing them to change color. After exposure to cold, these areas turn white, then blue, and finally red.

Remission: A period during which symptoms of disease are reduced (partial remission) or disappear (complete remission).

Sicca syndrome: A condition manifested by dry eyes and dry mouth.

Sleep disorder: One in which a person has difficulty achieving restful, restorative sleep. In addition to other symptoms, patients with fibromyalgia usually have a sleep disorder.

Synovium: A tissue that surrounds and protects the joints. It produces synovial fluid that nourishes and lubricates the joints.

Tender points: Specific locations on the body that are painful, especially when pressed.

Tendons: Fibrous cords that connect muscle to bone.

Vasculitis: Inflammation in the blood vessels. It may occur throughout the body.

Chapter 20

Gout

Questions and Answers about Gout

This chapter contains general information about gout. It describes what gout is and how it develops. It also explains how gout is diagnosed and treated. At the end is a list of key words to help you understand the terms used in this chapter. If you have further questions after reading this information, you may wish to discuss them with your doctor.

What is gout?

Gout is one of the most painful rheumatic diseases. It results from deposits of needle-like crystals of uric acid in the connective tissue, joint spaces, or both. These deposits lead to inflammatory arthritis, which causes swelling, redness, heat, pain, and stiffness in the joints. Arthritis is a term that is often used to refer to the more than 100 different rheumatic diseases that affect the joints, muscles, and bones, and may also affect other connective tissues. Gout accounts for about 5 percent of all cases of arthritis. Pseudogout, also a crystal-induced arthritis, is a condition with similar symptoms that results from deposits of calcium pyrophosphate dihydrate crystals in the joints. It is sometimes called calcium pyrophosphate deposition disease, crystal deposition disease, or chondrocalcinosis.

"Questions and Answers about Gout," National Institute of Arthritis and Musculoskeletal and Skin Diseases (NIAMS), January 1999.

Uric acid is a substance that results from the breakdown of purines or waste products in the body. Normally, uric acid is dissolved in the blood and passes through the kidneys into the urine, where it is eliminated. If the body increases its production of uric acid or if the kidneys do not eliminate enough uric acid from the body, levels build up (a condition called hyperuricemia). Hyperuricemia may also result when a person eats too many high-purine foods, such as liver, dried beans and peas, anchovies, and gravies. Hyperuricemia is not a disease and by itself is not dangerous. However, if excess uric acid crystals form as a result of hyperuricemia, gout can develop. The excess crystals build up in the joint spaces, causing inflammation. Deposits of uric acid, called tophi, can appear as lumps under the skin around the joints and at the rim of the ear. In addition, uric acid crystals can also collect in the kidneys and cause kidney stones.

For many people, gout initially affects the joints in the big toe, a condition called podagra. Sometime during the course of the disease, gout will affect the big toe in about 75 percent of patients. Gout can also affect the instep, ankles, heels, knees, wrists, fingers, and elbows. The disease can progress through four stages:

- **Asymptomatic (without symptoms) hyperuricemia.** In this stage, a person has elevated levels of uric acid in the blood but no other symptoms. The tendency to develop gout, however, is present. A person in this stage does not usually require treatment.

- **Acute gout, or acute gouty arthritis.** In this stage, hyperuricemia has caused the deposit of uric acid crystals in joint spaces. This leads to a sudden onset of intense pain and swelling in the joints, which may also be warm and very tender. An acute attack commonly occurs at night and can be triggered by stressful events, alcohol or drugs, or another acute illness. Early attacks usually subside within 3 to 10 days, even without treatment, and the next attack may not occur for months or even years. Over time, however, attacks can last longer and occur more frequently.

- **Interval or intercritical gout.** This is the period between acute attacks. In this stage, a person does not have any symptoms and has normal joint function.

- **Chronic tophaceous gout.** This is the most disabling stage of gout and usually develops over a long period, such as 10 years. In this stage, the disease has caused permanent damage to the affected joints and sometimes to the kidneys. With proper treatment, most people with gout do not progress to this advanced stage.

What causes gout?

A number of risk factors are related to the development of hyperuricemia and gout:

- Genetics may play a role in determining a person's risk, since six to 18 percent of people with gout have a family history of the disease.

- Being overweight increases the risk of developing hyperuricemia and gout because excessive food intake increases the body's production of uric acid.

- Excessive use of alcohol can lead to hyperuricemia because it interferes with the removal of uric acid from the body.

- Eating too many foods that are rich in purines can cause or aggravate gout.

- An enzyme defect that interferes with the way the body breaks down purines causes gout in a small number of people.

- Exposure to lead in the environment can cause gout.

Some people are at risk for high levels of uric acid in body fluids because of certain medicines they take or other conditions they may have. For example, the following types of medicines can lead to hyperuricemia because they reduce the body's ability to remove uric acid:

- Diuretics, which decrease the amount of uric acid passed in the urine. Many people take diuretics for hypertension, edema, or cardiovascular disease.

- Salicylates, or medicines made from salicylic acid, such as aspirin.

- The vitamin niacin, also called nicotinic acid.

- Cyclosporine, a medicine used to control the body's rejection of transplanted organs.

- Levodopa, a medicine used to treat Parkinson's disease.

Who is likely to develop gout?

Gout occurs in approximately 275 out of every 100,000 people. Men are more likely to develop gout than women, and men aged 40 to 50 are most commonly affected. Women rarely develop gout before menopause. The disease affects men and women differently: Men tend to develop gout at an earlier age than women, and alcohol is more often associated with the development of the disease in men. Gout is rare in children and young adults.

Signs and Symptoms of Gout

- Hyperuricemia
- Presence of uric acid crystals in joint fluid
- More than one attack of acute arthritis
- Arthritis that develops in one day
- Attack of arthritis in only one joint, usually the toe, ankle, or knee
- A painful joint that is swollen, red, and warm

How is gout diagnosed?

Gout may be difficult for doctors to diagnose because the symptoms may be vague and often mimic other conditions. Although most people with gout have hyperuricemia at some time during the course of their disease, it may not be present during an acute attack. In addition, hyperuricemia alone does not mean that a person has gout. In fact, most people with hyperuricemia do not develop the disease.

To confirm a diagnosis of gout, doctors typically test the fluid in the joint, called synovial fluid, by using a needle to draw a sample of fluid from a person's inflamed joint. The doctor places some of the fluid on a slide and looks for monosodium urate crystals under a microscope. If the person has gout, the doctor will almost always see crystals. Their absence, however, does not completely rule out the diagnosis. Doctors may also find it helpful to examine joint or tophi deposits to diagnose gout. A doctor who suspects a joint infection may check for the presence of bacteria.

How is gout treated?

With proper treatment, most people with gout are able to control their symptoms and live normal lives. Gout can be treated with one or a combination of therapies. Treatment goals are to ease the pain associated with acute attacks, prevent future attacks, and avoid the formation of new tophi and kidney stones.

The most common treatments for an acute attack of gout are high doses of nonsteroidal anti-inflammatory drugs (NSAIDs) and injections of corticosteroid drugs into the affected joint. NSAIDs reduce the inflammation caused by deposits of uric acid crystals. The NSAIDs most commonly prescribed for gout are indomethacin (Indocin) and naproxen (Anaprox, Naprosyn), which are taken by mouth (orally) every day. Patients usually begin to improve within a few hours of treatment, and the attack goes away completely within a few days.

Note: Brand names included in this text are provided as examples only, and their inclusion does not mean that these products are endorsed by the National Institutes of Health or any other Government agency. Also, if a particular brand name is not mentioned, this does not mean that the product is unsatisfactory.

When NSAIDs do not control symptoms, the doctor may consider using colchicine. This drug is most effective when taken within the first 12 hours of an acute attack. Doctors can give colchicine by mouth (usually every hour until symptoms go away), or they can inject it directly into a vein (intravenously). When taken by mouth, colchicine frequently causes diarrhea.

For some people, the doctor may prescribe either NSAIDs or oral colchicine in small daily doses to prevent future attacks. If attacks continue and tophi develop, however, the doctor may prescribe medicine to treat hyperuricemia, most commonly allopurinol (Zyloprim) and probenecid (Benemid).

What can people with gout do to stay healthy?

- To help prevent future attacks, take the medicines your doctor prescribes. Carefully follow instructions about how much medicine to take and when to take it. Acute gout is best treated when symptoms first occur.

- Tell your doctor about all the medicines and vitamins you take. He or she can tell you if any of them increase your risk of hyperuricemia.

- Plan followup visits with your doctor to evaluate your progress.

- Maintain a healthy, balanced diet; avoid foods that are high in purines; and drink plenty of fluids, especially water. Fluids help remove uric acid from the body.

- Exercise regularly and maintain a healthy body weight. Lose weight if you are overweight.

What research is being conducted to help people with gout?

Scientists are studying whether other NSAIDs are effective in treating gout and are analyzing new compounds to develop safe, effective medicines to treat gout and other rheumatic diseases. For example, researchers are testing to determine whether fish oil supplements reduce the risk of gout. They are also studying the structure of the enzymes that break down purines in the body, in hopes of achieving a better understanding of the enzyme defects that can cause gout.

Where can people find more information about gout?

Arthritis Foundation
1330 West Peachtree Street
Atlanta, GA 30309
Phone: (404) 872–7100
Phone: (800) 283–7800, or call your local chapter (listed in the telephone directory)
Website: http://www.arthritis.org/

This is the main voluntary organization devoted to arthritis. The foundation publishes free pamphlets on many types of arthritis and a monthly magazine for members that provides up-to-date information on arthritis. The foundation also provides physician and clinic referrals.

National Arthritis and Musculoskeletal and Skin Diseases Information Clearinghouse (NAMSIC)
National Institutes of Health
1 AMS Circle
Bethesda, MD 20892–3675
Phone: (301) 495–4484
TTY: (301) 565–2966
Fax: (301) 718–6366
Website: http://www.niams.nih.gov/

This clearinghouse, a public service sponsored by the National Institute of Arthritis and Musculoskeletal and Skin Diseases (NIAMS), provides information about various forms of arthritis and rheumatic diseases. The clearinghouse distributes patient and professional education materials and also refers people to other sources of information.

Acknowledgments

The NIAMS gratefully acknowledges the assistance of John H. Klippel, M.D., NIAMS; N. Lawrence Edwards, M.D., of the University of Florida in Gainesville; and Lawrence Ryan, M.D., of the Medical College of Wisconsin, in the preparation and review of this information.

Key Words

Arthritis: Literally means joint inflammation. It is a general term for more than 100 conditions known as rheumatic diseases. These diseases affect not only the joints, but also other parts of the body, including important supporting structures, such as muscles, tendons, and ligaments, as well as some internal organs.

Cartilage: A tough, resilient tissue that covers and cushions the ends of the bones and absorbs shock.

Colchicine: A medicine used to treat gout. It may be given by mouth (orally) or injected directly into a vein (intravenously).

Connective tissue: The supporting framework of the body and its internal organs.

Corticosteroids: Potent anti-inflammatory hormones that are made naturally in the body or synthetically for use as drugs. The most commonly prescribed corticosteroid is prednisone.

Crystal-induced arthritis: An accumulation of crystalline material in various parts of the body, especially the joints. Gout and pseudogout are examples of crystal-induced arthritis.

Gout: A type of arthritis caused by the body's reaction to needle-like crystals that accumulate in joint spaces. This reaction causes inflammation and extreme pain in the affected joint, most commonly the big toe. The crystals are formed from uric acid. Gout is caused by either increased production of uric acid or failure of the body to eliminate uric acid.

Hyperuricemia: Increased amount of uric acid in the blood.

Inflammation: A characteristic reaction of tissues to injury or disease. It is marked by four signs: swelling, redness, heat, and pain.

Joint: A junction where two bones meet. Most joints are composed of cartilage, joint space, fibrous capsule, synovium, and ligaments.

Joint space: The volume enclosed within the fibrous capsule.

Ligaments: Bands of cordlike tissue that connect bone to bone.

Nonsteroidal anti-inflammatory drugs (NSAIDs): A group of drugs, such as aspirin and aspirin-like drugs, used to reduce the inflammation that causes joint pain, stiffness, and swelling.

Pseudogout: Similar to gout; however, the crystals in the synovial fluid are composed of calcium pyrophosphate dihydrate and not uric acid. As in gout, the crystals in the joint space cause an intense inflammatory reaction in the joint.

Purines: Components of all human tissue that break down to form uric acid. Purines are also found in many foods in varying amounts.

Rheumatic diseases: A general term that refers to more than 100 conditions that affect joints, muscles, bones, and other connective tissues.

Synovial fluid: A substance found around the joints that nourishes and lubricates them.

Tendons: Fibrous cords of tissue that connect muscle to bone.

Tophus (plural tophi): A hard deposit of crystalline uric acid that may appear as a lump just under the skin, particularly around the joints and at the rim of the ear.

Uric acid: An organic substance that results from the breakdown of purines or waste products in the body. It is dissolved in the blood and passes through the kidneys into the urine, where it is eliminated. Most patients with gout have high levels of uric acid in their blood. If the concentration of uric acid in the tissues rises above normal levels, crystals can form in the joints and cause inflammation.

Uric acid crystals: Caused by high concentrations of uric acid. When uric acid crystals form in the blood, they can collect in connective tissue, joints, and kidneys. Some kidney stones are made of uric acid.

Chapter 21

Headache

Introduction

An estimated 45 million Americans experience chronic headaches. For at least half of these people, the problem is severe and sometimes disabling. It can also be costly: headache sufferers make over 8 million visits a year to doctor's offices. Migraine victims alone lose over 157 million workdays because of headache pain.

Why Does It Hurt?

What hurts when you have a headache? The bones of the skull and tissues of the brain itself never hurt, because they lack pain-sensitive nerve fibers. Several areas of the head can hurt, including a network of nerves which extends over the scalp and certain nerves in the face, mouth, and throat. Also sensitive to pain, because they contain delicate nerve fibers, are the muscles of the head and blood vessels found along the surface and at the base of the brain.

The ends of these pain-sensitive nerves, called nociceptors, can be stimulated by stress, muscular tension, dilated blood vessels, and other triggers of headache. Once stimulated, a nociceptor sends a message up the length of the nerve fiber to the nerve cells in the brain, signaling that a part of the body hurts. The message is determined

Excerpted from "Headache: Hope Through Research," National Institute of Neurological Disorders and Stroke (NINDS). Originally printed in 1996; updated July 2001. The full text of this document is available online at http://www.ninds.nih.gov/health_and_medical/pubs/headache_htr.htm.

by the location of the nociceptor. A person who suddenly realizes "My toe hurts," is responding to nociceptors in the foot that have been stimulated by the stubbing of a toe.

A number of chemicals help transmit pain-related information to the brain. Some of these chemicals are natural painkilling proteins called endorphins, Greek for "the morphine within." One theory suggests that people who suffer from severe headache and other types of chronic pain have lower levels of endorphins than people who are generally pain free.

When Should You See a Physician?

Not all headaches require medical attention. Some result from missed meals or occasional muscle tension and are easily remedied. But some types of headache are signals of more serious disorders, and call for prompt medical care. These include:

- Sudden, severe headache
- Sudden, severe headache associated with a stiff neck
- Headache associated with fever
- Headache associated with convulsions
- Headache accompanied by confusion or loss of consciousness
- Headache following a blow on the head
- Headache associated with pain in the eye or ear
- Persistent headache in a person who was previously headache free
- Recurring headache in children
- Headache which interferes with normal life

A headache sufferer usually seeks help from a family practitioner. If the problem is not relieved by standard treatments, the patient may then be referred to a specialist—perhaps an internist or neurologist. Additional referrals may be made to psychologists.

What Tests Are Used to Diagnose Headache?

Diagnosing a headache is like playing Twenty Questions. Experts agree that a detailed question-and-answer session with a patient can often produce enough information for a diagnosis. Many types of headaches have clear-cut symptoms which fall into an easily recognizable pattern.

Patients may be asked: How often do you have headaches? Where is the pain? How long do the headaches last? When did you first develop headaches? The patient's sleep habits and family and work situations may also be probed.

Most physicians will also obtain a full medical history from the patient, inquiring about past head trauma or surgery, eye strain, sinus problems, dental problems, difficulties with opening and closing of the jaw, and the use of medications. This may be enough to suggest strongly that the patient has migraine or cluster headaches. A complete and careful physical and neurological examination will exclude many possibilities and the suspicion of aneurysm, meningitis, or certain brain tumors. A blood test may be ordered to screen for thyroid disease, anemia, or infections which might cause a headache.

A test called an electroencephalogram (EEG) may be given to measure brain activity. EEG's can indicate a malfunction in the brain, but they cannot usually pinpoint a problem that might be causing a headache. A physician may suggest that a patient with unusual headaches undergo a computed tomographic (CT) scan and/or a magnetic resonance imaging (MRI) scan. The scans enable the physician to distinguish, for example, between a bleeding blood vessel in the brain and a brain tumor, and are important diagnostic tools in cases of headache associated with brain lesions or other serious disease. CT scans produce X-ray images of the brain that show structures or variations in the density of different types of tissue. MRI scans use magnetic fields and radio waves to produce an image that provides information about the structure and biochemistry of the brain.

If an aneurysm—an abnormal ballooning of a blood vessel—is suspected, a physician may order a CT scan to examine for blood and then an angiogram. In this test, a special fluid which can be seen on an X-ray is injected into the patient and carried in the bloodstream to the brain to reveal any abnormalities in the blood vessels there.

A physician analyzes the results of all these diagnostic tests along with a patient's medical history and examination in order to arrive at a diagnosis.

Headaches are diagnosed as

- Vascular

- Muscle contraction (tension)

- Traction

- Inflammatory

Vascular headaches—a group that includes the well-known migraine—are so named because they are thought to involve abnormal function of the brain's blood vessels or vascular system. Muscle contraction headaches appear to involve the tightening or tensing of facial and neck muscles. Traction and inflammatory headaches are symptoms of other disorders, ranging from stroke to sinus infection. Some people have more than one type of headache.

What Are Migraine Headaches?

The most common type of vascular headache is migraine. Migraine headaches are usually characterized by severe pain on one or both sides of the head, an upset stomach, and at times disturbed vision.

Former basketball star Kareem Abdul-Jabbar remembers experiencing his first migraine at age 14. The pain was unlike the discomfort of his previous mild headaches.

"When I got this one I thought, *'This* is a headache'," he says. "The pain was intense and I felt nausea and a great sensitivity to light. All I could think about was when it would stop. I sat in a dark room for an hour and it passed."

Symptoms of Migraine

Abdul-Jabbar's sensitivity to light is a standard symptom of the two most prevalent types of migraine-caused headache: *classic* and *common.*

The major difference between the two types is the appearance of neurological symptoms 10 to 30 minutes before a classic migraine attack. These symptoms are called an aura. The person may see flashing lights or zigzag lines, or may temporarily lose vision. Other classic symptoms include speech difficulty, weakness of an arm or leg, tingling of the face or hands, and confusion.

The pain of a classic migraine headache may be described as intense, throbbing, or pounding and is felt in the forehead, temple, ear, jaw, or around the eye. Classic migraine starts on one side of the head but may eventually spread to the other side. An attack lasts 1 to 2 pain-wracked days.

Common migraine—a term that reflects the disorder's greater occurrence in the general population—is not preceded by an aura. But some people experience a variety of vague symptoms beforehand, including mental fuzziness, mood changes, fatigue, and unusual retention of fluids. During the headache phase of a common migraine, a person may have diarrhea and increased urination, as well as nausea and vomiting. Common migraine pain can last 3 or 4 days.

Both classic and common migraine can strike as often as several times a week, or as rarely as once every few years. Both types can occur at any time. Some people, however, experience migraines at predictable times—for example, near the days of menstruation or every Saturday morning after a stressful week of work.

The Migraine Process

Research scientists are unclear about the precise cause of migraine headaches. There seems to be general agreement, however, that a key element is blood flow changes in the brain. People who get migraine headaches appear to have blood vessels that overreact to various triggers.

Scientists have devised one theory of migraine which explains these blood flow changes and also certain biochemical changes that may be involved in the headache process. According to this theory, the nervous system responds to a trigger such as stress by causing a spasm of the nerve-rich arteries at the base of the brain. The spasm closes down or constricts several arteries supplying blood to the brain, including the scalp artery and the carotid or neck arteries.

As these arteries constrict, the flow of blood to the brain is reduced. At the same time, blood-clotting particles called platelets clump together—a process which is believed to release a chemical called serotonin. Serotonin acts as a powerful constrictor of arteries, further reducing the blood supply to the brain.

Reduced blood flow decreases the brain's supply of oxygen. Symptoms signaling a headache, such as distorted vision or speech, may then result, similar to symptoms of stroke.

Reacting to the reduced oxygen supply, certain arteries within the brain open wider to meet the brain's energy needs. This widening or dilation spreads, finally affecting the neck and scalp arteries. The dilation of these arteries triggers the release of pain-producing substances called prostaglandins from various tissues and blood cells. Chemicals which cause inflammation and swelling, and substances which increase sensitivity to pain, are also released. The circulation of these chemicals and the dilation of the scalp arteries stimulate the pain-sensitive nociceptors. The result, according to this theory: a throbbing pain in the head.

Women and Migraine

Although both males and females seem to be equally affected by migraine, the condition is more common in adult women. Both sexes may develop migraine in infancy, but most often the disorder begins between the ages of 5 and 35.

The relationship between female hormones and migraine is still unclear. Women may have "menstrual migraine"—headaches around the time of their menstrual period—which may disappear during pregnancy. Other women develop migraine for the first time when they are pregnant. Some are first affected after menopause.

The effect of oral contraceptives on headaches is perplexing. Scientists report that some women with migraine who take birth control pills experience more frequent and severe attacks. However, a small percentage of women have fewer and less severe migraine headaches when they take birth control pills. And normal women who do not suffer from headaches may develop migraines as a side effect when they use oral contraceptives. Investigators around the world are studying hormonal changes in women with migraine in the hope of identifying the specific ways these naturally occurring chemicals cause headaches.

Triggers of Headache

Although many sufferers have a family history of migraine, the exact hereditary nature of this condition is still unknown. People who get migraines are thought to have an inherited abnormality in the regulation of blood vessels.

"It's like a cocked gun with a hair trigger," explains one specialist. "A person is born with a potential for migraine and the headache is triggered by things that are really not so terrible."

These triggers include stress and other normal emotions, as well as biological and environmental conditions. Fatigue, glaring or flickering lights, changes in the weather, and certain foods can set off migraine. It may seem hard to believe that eating such seemingly harmless foods as yogurt, nuts, and lima beans can result in a painful migraine headache. However, some scientists believe that these foods and several others contain chemical substances, such as tyramine, which constrict arteries—the first step of the migraine process. Other scientists believe that foods cause headaches by setting off an allergic reaction in susceptible people.

While a food-triggered migraine usually occurs soon after eating, other triggers may not cause immediate pain. Scientists report that people can develop migraine not only during a period of stress but also afterwards when their vascular systems are still reacting. For example, migraines that wake people up in the middle of the night are believed to result from a delayed reaction to stress.

Other Forms of Migraine

In addition to classic and common, migraine headache can take several other forms.

Patients with *hemiplegic migraine* have temporary paralysis on one side of the body, a condition known as hemiplegia. Some people may experience vision problems and vertigo—a feeling that the world is spinning. These symptoms begin 10 to 90 minutes before the onset of headache pain.

In *ophthalmoplegic migraine*, the pain is around the eye and is associated with a droopy eyelid, double vision, and other problems with vision.

Basilar artery migraine involves a disturbance of a major brain artery at the base of the brain. Preheadache symptoms include vertigo, double vision, and poor muscular coordination. This type of migraine occurs primarily in adolescent and young adult women and is often associated with the menstrual cycle.

Benign exertional headache is brought on by running, lifting, coughing, sneezing, or bending. The headache begins at the onset of activity, and pain rarely lasts more than several minutes.

Status migrainosus is a rare and severe type of migraine that can last 72 hours or longer. The pain and nausea are so intense that people who have this type of headache must be hospitalized. The use of certain drugs can trigger status migrainosus. Neurologists report that many of their status migrainosus patients were depressed and anxious before they experienced headache attacks.

Headache-free migraine is characterized by such migraine symptoms as visual problems, nausea, vomiting, constipation, or diarrhea. Patients, however, do not experience head pain. Headache specialists have suggested that unexplained pain in a particular part of the body, fever, and dizziness could also be possible types of headache-free migraine.

How Is Migraine Headache Treated?

During the Stone Age, pieces of a headache sufferer's skull were cut away with flint instruments to relieve pain. Another unpleasant remedy used in the British Isles around the ninth Century involved drinking "the juice of elderseed, cow's brain, and goat's dung dissolved in vinegar." Fortunately, today's headache patients are spared such drastic measures.

Drug therapy, biofeedback training, stress reduction, and elimination of certain foods from the diet are the most common methods of preventing and controlling migraine and other vascular headaches. Joan, the migraine sufferer, was helped by treatment with a combination of an antimigraine drug and diet control.

Regular exercise, such as swimming or vigorous walking, can also reduce the frequency and severity of migraine headaches. Joan found that whirlpool and yoga baths helped her relax.

During a migraine headache, temporary relief can sometimes be obtained by applying cold packs to the head or by pressing on the bulging artery found in front of the ear on the painful side of the head.

Drug Therapy

There are two ways to approach the treatment of migraine headache with drugs: prevent the attacks, or relieve symptoms after the headache occurs.

For infrequent migraine, drugs can be taken at the first sign of a headache in order to stop it or to at least ease the pain. People who get occasional mild migraine may benefit by taking aspirin or acetaminophen at the start of an attack. Aspirin raises a person's tolerance to pain and also discourages clumping of blood platelets. Small amounts of caffeine may be useful if taken in the early stages of migraine. But for most migraine sufferers who get moderate to severe headaches, and for all cluster headache patients (see section "Besides Migraine, What Are Other Types of Vascular Headaches?"), stronger drugs may be necessary to control the pain.

Several drugs for the prevention of migraine have been developed in recent years, including serotonin agonists which mimic the action of this key brain chemical. One of the most commonly used drugs for the relief of classic and common migraine symptoms is sumatriptan, which binds to serotonin receptors. For optimal benefit, the drug is taken during the early stages of an attack. If a migraine has been in progress for about an hour after the drug is taken, a repeat dose can be given.

Physicians caution that sumatriptan should not be taken by people who have angina pectoris, basilar migraine, severe hypertension, or vascular, or liver disease.

Another migraine drug is ergotamine tartrate, a vasoconstrictor which helps counteract the painful dilation stage of the headache. Other drugs that constrict dilated blood vessels or help reduce blood vessel inflammation also are available.

For headaches that occur three or more times a month, preventive treatment is usually recommended. Drugs used to prevent classic and common migraine include methysergide maleate, which counteracts blood vessel constriction; propranolol hydrochloride, which stops blood vessel dilation; amitriptyline, an antidepressant; valproic acid, an anticonvulsant; and verapamil, a calcium channel blocker.

Antidepressants called MAO inhibitors also prevent migraine. These drugs block an enzyme called monoamine oxidase which normally helps nerve cells absorb the artery-constricting brain chemical, serotonin. MAO inhibitors can have potentially serious side effects—particularly if taken while ingesting foods or beverages that contain tyramine, a substance that constricts arteries.

Many antimigraine drugs can have adverse side effects. But like most medicines they are relatively safe when used carefully and under a physician's supervision. To avoid long-term side effects of preventive medications, headache specialists advise patients to reduce the dosage of these drugs and then stop taking them as soon as possible.

Biofeedback and Relaxation Training

Drug therapy for migraine is often combined with biofeedback and relaxation training. Biofeedback refers to a technique that can give people better control over such body function indicators as blood pressure, heart rate, temperature, muscle tension, and brain waves. *Thermal biofeedback* allows a patient to consciously raise hand temperature. Some patients who are able to increase hand temperature can reduce the number and intensity of migraines. The mechanisms underlying these self-regulation treatments are being studied by research scientists.

"To succeed in biofeedback," says a headache specialist, "you must be able to concentrate and you must be motivated to get well."

A patient learning thermal biofeedback wears a device which transmits the temperature of an index finger or hand to a monitor. While the patient tries to warm his hands, the monitor provides feedback either on a gauge that shows the temperature reading or by emitting a sound or beep that increases in intensity as the temperature increases. The patient is not told how to raise hand temperature, but is given suggestions such as "Imagine your hands feel very warm and heavy."

"I have a good imagination," says one headache sufferer who traded in her medication for thermal biofeedback. The technique decreased the number and severity of headaches she experienced.

In another type of biofeedback called *electromyographic* or *EMG training*, the patient learns to control muscle tension in the face, neck, and shoulders.

Either kind of biofeedback may be combined with relaxation training, during which patients learn to relax the mind and body.

Biofeedback can be practiced at home with a portable monitor. But the ultimate goal of treatment is to wean the patient from the machine. The patient can then use biofeedback anywhere at the first sign of a headache.

The Antimigraine Diet

Scientists estimate that a small percentage of migraine sufferers will benefit from a treatment program focused solely on eliminating headache-provoking foods and beverages.

Other migraine patients may be helped by a diet to prevent low blood sugar. Low blood sugar, or hypoglycemia, can cause headache. This condition can occur after a period without food: overnight, for example, or when a meal is skipped. People who wake up in the morning with a headache may be reacting to the low blood sugar caused by the lack of food overnight.

Treatment for headaches caused by low blood sugar consists of scheduling smaller, more frequent meals for the patient. A special diet designed to stabilize the body's sugar-regulating system is sometimes recommended.

For the same reason, many specialists also recommend that migraine patients avoid oversleeping on weekends. Sleeping late can change the body's normal blood sugar level and lead to a headache.

Besides Migraine, What Are Other Types of Vascular Headaches?

After migraine, the most common type of vascular headache is the toxic headache produced by fever. Pneumonia, measles, mumps, and tonsillitis are among the diseases that can cause severe toxic vascular headaches. Toxic headaches can also result from the presence of foreign chemicals in the body. Other kinds of vascular headaches include "clusters," which cause repeated episodes of intense pain, and headaches resulting from a rise in blood pressure.

Chemical Culprits

Repeated exposure to nitrite compounds can result in a dull, pounding headache that may be accompanied by a flushed face. Nitrite, which dilates blood vessels, is found in such products as heart medicine and dynamite, but is also used as a chemical to preserve meat. Hot dogs and other processed meats containing sodium nitrite can cause headaches.

Eating foods prepared with monosodium glutamate (MSG) can result in headache. Soy sauce, meat tenderizer, and a variety of packaged foods contain this chemical which is touted as a flavor enhancer.

Headache can also result from exposure to poisons, even common household varieties like insecticides, carbon tetrachloride, and lead. Children who ingest flakes of lead paint may develop headaches. So may anyone who has contact with lead batteries or lead-glazed pottery.

Artists and industrial workers may experience headaches after exposure to materials that contain chemical solvents. These solvents, like benzene, are found in turpentine, spray adhesives, rubber cement, and inks.

Drugs such as amphetamines can cause headaches as a side effect. Another type of drug-related headache occurs during withdrawal from long-term therapy with the antimigraine drug ergotamine tartrate.

Jokes are often made about alcohol hangovers but the headache associated with "the morning after" is no laughing matter. Fortunately, there are several suggested treatments for the pain. The hangover headache may also be reduced by taking honey, which speeds alcohol metabolism, or caffeine, a constrictor of dilated arteries. Caffeine, however, can cause headaches as well as cure them. Heavy coffee drinkers often get headaches when they try to break the caffeine habit.

Cluster Headaches

Cluster headaches, named for their repeated occurrence over weeks or months at roughly the same time of day or night in clusters, begin as a minor pain around one eye, eventually spreading to that side of the face. The pain quickly intensifies, compelling the victim to pace the floor or rock in a chair. "You can't lie down, you're fidgety," explains a cluster patient. "The pain is unbearable." Other symptoms include a stuffed and runny nose and a droopy eyelid over a red and tearing eye.

Cluster headaches last between 30 and 45 minutes. But the relief people feel at the end of an attack is usually mixed with dread as they await a recurrence. Clusters may mysteriously disappear for months or years. Many people have cluster bouts during the spring and fall. At their worst, chronic cluster headaches can last continuously for years.

Cluster attacks can strike at any age but usually start between the ages of 20 and 40. Unlike migraine, cluster headaches are more common in men and do not run in families.

Studies of cluster patients show that they are likely to have hazel eyes and that they tend to be heavy smokers and drinkers. Paradoxically, both nicotine, which constricts arteries, and alcohol, which dilates them, trigger cluster headaches. The exact connection between these substances and cluster attacks is not known.

Despite a cluster headache's distinguishing characteristics, its relative infrequency and similarity to such disorders as sinusitis can lead to misdiagnosis. Some cluster patients have had tooth extractions, sinus surgery, or psychiatric treatment in futile efforts to cure their pain.

Research studies have turned up several clues as to the cause of cluster headache, but no answers. One clue is found in the thermograms of untreated cluster patients, which show a "cold spot" of reduced blood flow above the eye.

The sudden start and brief duration of cluster headaches can make them difficult to treat; however, research scientists have identified several effective drugs for these headaches. The antimigraine drug sumatriptan can subdue a cluster, if taken at the first sign of an attack. Injections of dihydroergotamine, a form of ergotamine tartrate, are sometimes used to treat clusters. Corticosteroids also can be used, either orally or by intramuscular injection.

Some cluster patients can prevent attacks by taking propranolol, methysergide, valproic acid, verapamil, or lithium carbonate.

Another option that works for some cluster patients is rapid inhalation of pure oxygen through a mask for 5 to 15 minutes. The oxygen seems to ease the pain of cluster headache by reducing blood flow to the brain.

In chronic cases of cluster headache, certain facial nerves may be surgically cut or destroyed to provide relief. These procedures have had limited success. Some cluster patients have had facial nerves cut only to have them regenerate years later.

Painful Pressure

Chronic high blood pressure can cause headache, as can rapid rises in blood pressure like those experienced during anger, vigorous exercise, or sexual excitement.

The severe "orgasmic headache" occurs right before orgasm and is believed to be a vascular headache. Since sudden rupture of a cerebral blood vessel can occur, this type of headache should be evaluated by a doctor.

What Are Muscle-Contraction Headaches?

It's 5:00 p.m. and your boss has just asked you to prepare a 20-page briefing paper. Due date: tomorrow. You're angry and tired and the more you think about the assignment, the tenser you become. Your teeth clench, your brow wrinkles, and soon you have a splitting *tension headache*.

Tension headache is named not only for the role of stress in triggering the pain, but also for the contraction of neck, face, and scalp muscles brought on by stressful events. Tension headache is a severe but temporary form of muscle-contraction headache. The pain is mild to moderate and feels like pressure is being applied to the head or neck. The headache usually disappears after the period of stress is over. Ninety percent of all headaches are classified as tension/muscle contraction headaches.

By contrast, chronic muscle-contraction headaches can last for weeks, months, and sometimes years. The pain of these headaches is often described as a tight band around the head or a feeling that the head and neck are in a cast. "It feels like somebody is tightening a giant vise around my head," says one patient. The pain is steady, and is usually felt on both sides of the head. Chronic muscle-contraction headaches can cause sore scalps—even combing one's hair can be painful.

In the past, many scientists believed that the primary cause of the pain of muscle-contraction headache was sustained muscle tension. However, a growing number of authorities now believe that a far more complex mechanism is responsible.

Occasionally, muscle-contraction headaches will be accompanied by nausea, vomiting, and blurred vision, but there is no preheadache syndrome as with migraine. Muscle-contraction headaches have not been linked to hormones or foods, as has migraine, nor is there a strong hereditary connection.

Research has shown that for many people, chronic muscle-contraction headaches are caused by depression and anxiety. These people tend to get their headaches in the early morning or evening when conflicts in the office or home are anticipated.

Emotional factors are not the only triggers of muscle-contraction headaches. Certain physical postures that tense head and neck muscles—such as holding one's chin down while reading—can lead to head and neck pain. So can prolonged writing under poor light, or holding a phone between the shoulder and ear, or even gum-chewing.

More serious problems that can cause muscle-contraction headaches include degenerative arthritis of the neck and temporomandibular joint dysfunction, or TMD. TMD is a disorder of the joint between the temporal bone (above the ear) and the mandible or lower jaw bone. The disorder results from poor bite and jaw clenching.

Treatment for muscle-contraction headache varies. The first consideration is to treat any specific disorder or disease that may be causing the headache. For example, arthritis of the neck is treated with anti-inflammatory medication and TMD may be helped by corrective devices for the mouth and jaw.

Acute tension headaches not associated with a disease are treated with analgesics like aspirin and acetaminophen. Stronger analgesics, such as propoxyphene and codeine, are sometimes prescribed. As prolonged use of these drugs can lead to dependence, patients taking them should have periodic medical checkups and follow their physicians' instructions carefully.

Nondrug therapy for chronic muscle-contraction headaches includes biofeedback, relaxation training, and counseling. A technique called cognitive restructuring teaches people to change their attitudes and responses to stress. Patients might be encouraged, for example, to imagine that they are coping successfully with a stressful situation. In progressive relaxation therapy, patients are taught to first tense and then relax individual muscle groups. Finally, the patient tries to relax his or her whole body. Many people imagine a peaceful scene—such as lying on the beach or by a beautiful lake. Passive relaxation does not involve tensing of muscles. Instead, patients are encouraged to focus on different muscles, suggesting that they relax. Some people might think to themselves, *relax* or *my muscles feel warm*.

People with chronic muscle-contraction headaches my also be helped by taking antidepressants or MAO inhibitors. Mixed muscle-contraction and migraine headaches are sometimes treated with barbiturate compounds, which slow down nerve function in the brain and spinal cord.

People who suffer infrequent muscle-contraction headaches may benefit from a hot shower or moist heat applied to the back of the neck. Cervical collars are sometimes recommended as an aid to good posture. Physical therapy, massage, and gentle exercise of the neck may also be helpful.

When is Headache a Warning of a More Serious Condition?

Like other types of pain, headaches can serve as warning signals of more serious disorders. This is particularly true for headaches caused by traction or inflammation.

Traction headaches can occur if the pain-sensitive parts of the head are pulled, stretched, or displaced, as, for example, when eye muscles are tensed to compensate for eyestrain. Headaches caused by inflammation include those related to meningitis as well as those resulting from diseases of the sinuses, spine, neck, ears, and teeth. Ear and tooth infections and glaucoma can cause headaches. In oral and dental disorders, headache is experienced as pain in the entire head, including the face. These headaches are treated by curing the underlying problem. This may involve surgery, antibiotics, or other drugs.

Characteristics of the various types of more serious traction and inflammatory headaches vary by disorder:

- *Brain tumor*. Brain tumors are diagnosed in about 11,000 people every year. As they grow, these tumors sometimes cause headache by pushing on the outer layer of nerve tissue that covers the brain or by pressing against pain-sensitive blood vessel walls. Headache resulting from a brain tumor may be periodic or continuous. Typically, it feels like a strong pressure is being applied to the head. The pain is relieved when the tumor is treated by surgery, radiation, or chemotherapy.

- *Stroke*. Headache may accompany several conditions that can lead to stroke, including hypertension or high blood pressure, arteriosclerosis, and heart disease. Headaches are also associated with completed stroke, when brain cells die from lack of sufficient oxygen.

  Many stroke-related headaches can be prevented by careful management of the patient's condition through diet, exercise, and medication.

  Mild to moderate headaches are associated with transient ischemic attacks (TIAs), sometimes called "mini-strokes," which result from a temporary lack of blood supply to the brain. The head pain occurs near the clot or lesion that blocks blood flow. The similarity between migraine and symptoms of TIA can cause problems in diagnosis. The rare person under age 40 who suffers a TIA may be misdiagnosed as having migraine; similarly, TIA-prone older patients who suffer migraine may be misdiagnosed as having stroke-related headaches.

- *Spinal tap*. About one-fourth of the people who undergo a lumbar puncture or spinal tap develop a headache. Many scientists

183

believe these headaches result from leakage of the cerebrospinal fluid that flows through pain-sensitive membranes around the brain and down to the spinal cord. The fluid, they suggest, drains through the tiny hole created by the spinal tap needle, causing the membranes to rub painfully against the bony skull. Since headache pain occurs only when the patient stands up, the "cure" is to remain lying down until the headache runs its course—anywhere from a few hours to several days.

- *Head trauma.* Headaches may develop after a blow to the head, either immediately or months later. There is little relationship between the severity of the trauma and the intensity of headache pain. In most cases, the cause of the headache is not known. Occasionally the cause is ruptured blood vessels which result in an accumulation of blood called a hematoma. This mass of blood can displace brain tissue and cause headaches as well as weakness, confusion, memory loss, and seizures. Hematomas can be drained to produce rapid relief of symptoms.

- *Temporal arteritis.* Arteritis, an inflammation of certain arteries in the head, primarily affects people over age 50. Symptoms include throbbing headache, fever, and loss of appetite. Some patients experience blurring or loss of vision. Prompt treatment with corticosteroid drugs helps to relieve symptoms.

- *Meningitis and encephalitis.* Meningitis and encphalitis headaches are caused by infections of meninges—the brain's outer covering—and in encephalitis, inflammation of the brain itself.

- *Trigeminal neuralgia.* Trigeminal neuralgia, or tic douloureux, results from a disorder of the trigeminal nerve. This nerve supplies the face, teeth, mouth, and nasal cavity with feeling and also enables the mouth muscles to chew. Symptoms are headache and intense facial pain that comes in short, excruciating jabs set off by the slightest touch to or movement of trigger points in the face or mouth. People with trigeminal neuralgia often fear brushing their teeth or chewing on the side of the mouth that is affected. Many trigeminal neuralgia patients are controlled with drugs, including carbamazepine. Patients who do not respond to drugs may be helped by surgery on the trigeminal nerve.

- *Sinus infection.* In a condition called acute sinusitis, a viral or bacterial infection of the upper respiratory tract spreads to the membrane which lines the sinus cavities. When one or more of these cavities are filled with fluid from the inflammation, they become painful. Treatment of acute sinusitis includes antibiotics, analgesics, and decongestants. Chronic sinusitis may be caused by an allergy to such irritants as dust, ragweed, animal hair, and smoke. Research scientists disagree about whether chronic sinusitis triggers headache.

What Causes Headache in Children?

Like adults, children experience the infections, trauma, and stresses that can lead to headaches. In fact, research shows that as young people enter adolescence and encounter the stresses of puberty and secondary school, the frequency of headache increases.

Migraine headaches often begin in childhood or adolescence. According to recent surveys, as many as half of all schoolchildren experience some type of headache.

Children with migraine often have nausea and excessive vomiting. Some children have periodic vomiting, but no headache—the so-called abdominal migraine. Research scientists have found that these children usually develop headaches when they are older.

Physicians have many drugs to treat migraine in children. Different classes that may be tried include analgesics, antiemetics, anticonvulsants, beta-blockers, and sedatives. A diet may also be prescribed to protect the child from foods that trigger headache. Sometimes psychological counseling or even psychiatric treatment for the child and the parents is recommended.

Childhood headache can be a sign of depression. Parents should alert the family pediatrician if a child develops headaches along with other symptoms such as a change in mood or sleep habits. Antidepressant medication and psychotherapy are effective treatments for childhood depression and related headache.

For More Information

The National Institute of Neurological Disorders and Stroke, a component of the National Institutes of Health, is the leading Federal supporter of research on disorders of the brain and nervous system. The Institute also sponsors an active public information program and can answer questions about diagnosis, treatment, and research related to headache.

For information on neurological disorders or research programs funded by the National Institute of Neurological Disorders and Stroke, contact the Institute's Brain Resources and Information Network (BRAIN) at:

BRAIN
P.O. Box 5801
Bethesda, Maryland 20824
Phone: (301) 496-5751
Phone: (800) 352-9424
Website: http://www.ninds.nih.gov

Private voluntary organizations that offer information and services to those affected by headache include the following:

American Council for Headache Education (ACHE)
19 Mantua Road
Mt. Royal, NJ 08061
Phone: (856) 423-0258
Website: http://www.achenet.org

This organization is a nonprofit patient/health professional partnership dedicated to advancing treatment and management of headache and to raising the public awareness of headache as a valid, biologically based illness. ACHE offers headache brochures, a quarterly newsletter, the book *Migraine: The Complete Guide*, assistance through in-person support groups, and support via the Internet and commercial on-line service providers.

National Headache Foundation
428 W. St. James Place, 2nd Floor
Chicago, IL 60614-2750
Phone: (773) 388-6399
Phone: (888) 643-5552
Website: http://www.headaches.org

The foundation promotes research and public education, publishes a newsletter, and offers many publications including a state-by-state list of physician members, a headache chart, a handbook, brochures, and fact sheets.

Chapter 22

Heartburn

Gastroesophageal reflux disease, or GERD, occurs when the lower esophageal sphincter (LES) does not close properly, and stomach contents splash back, or reflux, into the esophagus. The LES is a ring of muscle at the bottom of the esophagus that acts like a camera shutter between the esophagus and stomach. The esophagus carries food from the mouth to the stomach.

When refluxed stomach acid touches the lining of the esophagus, it causes a burning sensation in the chest or throat called heartburn. The fluid may even be tasted in the back of the mouth, and this is called acid indigestion. Occasional heartburn is common but does not necessarily mean one has GERD. Heartburn that occurs more than twice a week may be considered GERD, which can eventually lead to more serious health problems.

Anyone, including infants, children, and pregnant women, can have GERD.

What Are the Symptoms of GERD?

The main symptoms are persistent heartburn and acid regurgitation. Some people have GERD without heartburn. Instead, they experience pain in the chest, hoarseness in the morning, or trouble

"Heartburn, Hiatal Hernia, and Gastroesophageal Reflux Disease (GERD)," National Institute of Diabetes and Digestive and Kidney Diseases (NIDDK), NIH Pub. No. 02-0882, November 2001.

swallowing. You may feel like you have food stuck in your throat or like you are choking or your throat is tight. GERD can also cause a dry cough and bad breath.

GERD in Children

Recent studies (Nelson SP, Chen EH, Syniar GM, Christoffel KK. Prevalence of symptoms of gastroesophageal reflux during infancy. *Archives of Pediatric and Adolescent Medicine.* 1997;151:569-572.) show that GERD is common and often overlooked in infants and children. It can cause repeated vomiting, coughing, and other respiratory problems. Children's immature digestive systems are usually to blame, and most infants grow out of GERD by the time they are one year old. Still, you should talk to your child's doctor if the problem occurs regularly and causes discomfort. Your doctor may recommend simple strategies for avoiding reflux, like burping the infant several times during feeding or keeping the infant in an upright position for 30 minutes after feeding. If your child is older, the doctor may recommend avoiding:

- sodas that contain caffeine
- chocolate and peppermint
- spicy foods like pizza
- acid foods like oranges or tomatoes
- fried and fatty foods

Avoiding food 2 to 3 hours before bed may also help. The doctor may recommend that the child sleep with head raised. If these changes do not work, the doctor may prescribe medicine for your child. In rare cases, a child may need surgery.

What Causes GERD?

No one knows why people get GERD. A hiatal hernia may contribute. A hiatal hernia occurs when the upper part of the stomach is above the diaphragm, the muscle wall that separates the stomach from the chest. The diaphragm helps the LES keep acid from coming up into the esophagus. When a hiatal hernia is present, it is easier for the acid to come up. In this way, a hiatal hernia can cause reflux. A hiatal hernia can happen in people of any age; many otherwise healthy people over 50 have a small one.

Other factors that may contribute to GERD include:

- alcohol use
- overweight
- pregnancy
- smoking

Also, certain foods can be associated with reflux events, including:

- citrus fruits
- chocolate
- drinks with caffeine
- fatty and fried foods
- garlic and onions
- mint flavorings
- spicy foods
- tomato-based foods, like spaghetti sauce, chili, and pizza

How Is GERD Treated?

If you have had heartburn or any of the other symptoms for a while, you should see your doctor. You may want to visit an internist, a doctor who specializes in internal medicine, or a gastroenterologist, a doctor who treats diseases of the stomach and intestines. Depending on how severe your GERD is, treatment may involve one or more of the following lifestyle changes and medications or surgery.

Lifestyle Changes

- If you smoke, stop.
- Do not drink alcohol.
- Lose weight if needed.
- Eat small meals.
- Wear loose-fitting clothes.
- Avoid lying down for 3 hours after a meal.
- Raise the head of your bed 6 to 8 inches by putting blocks of wood under the bedposts—just using extra pillows will not help.

189

Medications

Your doctor may recommend over-the-counter antacids, which you can buy without a prescription, or medications that stop acid production or help the muscles that empty your stomach.

Antacids: Antacids, such as Alka-Seltzer, Maalox, Mylanta, Pepto-Bismol, Rolaids, and Riopan, are usually the first drugs recommended to relieve heartburn and other mild GERD symptoms. Many brands on the market use different combinations of three basic salts—magnesium, calcium, and aluminum—with hydroxide or bicarbonate ions to neutralize the acid in your stomach. Antacids, however, have side effects. Magnesium salt can lead to diarrhea, and aluminum salts can cause constipation. Aluminum and magnesium salts are often combined in a single product to balance these effects.

Calcium carbonate antacids, such as Tums, Titralac, and Alka-2, can also be a supplemental source of calcium. They can cause constipation as well.

Foaming agents: Foaming agents, such as Gaviscon, work by covering your stomach contents with foam to prevent reflux. These drugs may help those who have no damage to the esophagus.

H2 blockers: H2 blockers, such as cimetidine (Tagamet HB), famotidine (Pepcid AC), nizatidine (Axid AR), and ranitidine (Zantac 75), impede acid production. They are available in prescription strength and over the counter. These drugs provide short-term relief, but over-the-counter H2 blockers should not be used for more than a few weeks at a time. They are effective for about half of those who have GERD symptoms. Many people benefit from taking H2 blockers at bedtime in combination with a proton pump inhibitor.

Proton pump inhibitors: Proton pump inhibitors include omeprazole (Prilosec), lansoprazole (Prevacid), pantoprazole (Protonix), rabeprazole (Aciphex), and esomeprazole (Nexium), which are all available by prescription. Proton pump inhibitors are more effective than H2 blockers and can relieve symptoms in almost everyone who has GERD.

Prokinetics: Another group of drugs, prokinetics, helps strengthen the sphincter and makes the stomach empty faster. This group includes bethanechol (Urecholine) and metoclopramide (Reglan).

Metoclopramide also improves muscle action in the digestive tract, but these drugs have frequent side effects that limit their usefulness. Erythromycin, an antibiotic, can also help your stomach empty faster.

Because drugs work in different ways, combinations of drugs may help control symptoms. People who get heartburn after eating may take both antacids and H2 blockers. The antacids work first to neutralize the acid in the stomach, while the H2 blockers act on acid production. By the time the antacid stops working, the H2 blocker will have stopped acid production. Your doctor is the best source of information on how to use medications for GERD.

What if Symptoms Persist?

If your heartburn does not improve with lifestyle changes or drugs, you may need additional tests.

- A *barium swallow radiograph* uses x rays to help spot abnormalities such as a hiatal hernia and severe inflammation of the esophagus. With this test, you drink a solution and then x rays are taken. Mild irritation will not appear on this test, although narrowing of the esophagus—called strictures—ulcers, hiatal hernia, and other problems will.

- *Upper endoscopy* is more accurate than a barium swallow radiograph and may be performed in a hospital or a doctor's office. The doctor will spray your throat to numb it and slide down a thin, flexible plastic tube called an endoscope. A tiny camera in the endoscope allows the doctor to see the surface of the esophagus and to search for abnormalities. If you have had moderate to severe symptoms and this procedure reveals injury to the esophagus, usually no other tests are needed to confirm GERD.

  The doctor may use tiny tweezers (forceps) in the endoscope to remove a small piece of tissue for biopsy. A biopsy viewed under a microscope can reveal damage caused by acid reflux and rule out other problems if no infecting organisms or abnormal growths are found.

- In an *ambulatory pH monitoring examination*, the doctor puts a tiny tube into the esophagus that will stay there for 24 hours. While you go about your normal activities, it measures the amount of and when acid comes up into your esophagus. This test is useful in people with GERD symptoms but no esophageal damage. The procedure is also helpful in detecting whether respiratory symptoms, including wheezing and coughing, are triggered by reflux.

Surgery

Surgery is an option when medicine and lifestyle changes do not work. Surgery may also be a reasonable alternative to a lifetime of drugs and discomfort.

Fundoplication, usually a specific variation called Nissen fundoplication, is the standard surgical treatment for GERD. The upper part of the stomach is wrapped around the LES to strengthen the sphincter and prevent acid reflux and to repair a hiatal hernia.

This fundoplication procedure may be done using a laparoscope and requires only tiny incisions in the abdomen. To perform the fundoplication, surgeons use small instruments that hold a tiny camera. Laparoscopic fundoplication has been used safely and effectively in people of all ages, even babies. When performed by experienced surgeons, the procedure is reported to be as good as standard fundoplication. Furthermore, people can leave the hospital in 1 to 3 days and return to work in 1 to 2 weeks.

In 2000, the U.S. Food and Drug Administration (FDA) approved two endoscopic devices to treat chronic heartburn. The Bard EndoCinch system puts stitches in the LES to create little pleats that help strengthen the muscle. The Stretta system uses electrodes to create tiny cuts on the LES. When the cuts heal, the scar tissue helps toughen the muscle. The long-term effects of these two procedures are unknown.

What Are the Long-Term Complications of GERD?

Sometimes GERD can cause serious complications. Inflammation of the esophagus from stomach acid causes bleeding or ulcers. In addition, scars from tissue damage can narrow the esophagus and make swallowing difficult. Some people develop Barrett's esophagus, where cells in the esophageal lining take on an abnormal shape and color, which over time can lead to cancer.

Also, studies have shown that asthma, chronic cough, and pulmonary fibrosis may be aggravated or even caused by GERD.

Points to Remember

- Heartburn, also called acid indigestion, is the most common symptom of GERD. Anyone experiencing heartburn twice a week or more may have GERD.

- You can have GERD without having heartburn. Your symptoms could be excessive clearing of the throat, problems swallowing, the feeling that food is stuck in your throat, burning in the mouth, or pain in the chest.

- In infants and children, GERD may cause repeated vomiting, coughing, and other respiratory problems. Most babies grow out of GERD by their first birthday.

- If you have been using antacids for more than 2 weeks, it is time to see a doctor. Most doctors can treat GERD. Or you may want to visit an internist—a doctor who specializes in internal medicine—or a gastroenterologist—a doctor who treats diseases of the stomach and intestines.

- Doctors usually recommend lifestyle and dietary changes to relieve heartburn. Many people with GERD also need medication or surgery.

Hope Through Research

No one knows why some people who have heartburn develop GERD. Several factors may be involved, and research is under way on many levels. Risk factors—what makes some people get GERD but not others—are being explored, as is GERD's role in other conditions such as asthma and bronchitis.

The role of hiatal hernia in GERD continues to be debated and explored. It is a complex topic because some people have a hiatal hernia without having reflux, while others have reflux without having a hernia.

Much research is needed into the role of the bacterium *Helicobacter pylori*. Our ability to eliminate *H. pylori* has been responsible for reduced rates of peptic ulcer disease and some gastric cancers. At the same time, GERD, Barrett's esophagus, and cancers of the esophagus have increased. Researchers wonder whether having *H. pylori* helps prevent GERD and other diseases. Future treatment will be greatly affected by the results of this research.

For More Information

Information about GERD is available from these organizations:

American College of Gastroenterology (ACG)
4900-B South 31st Street
Arlington, VA 22206-1656
Phone: (703) 820-7400
Fax: (703) 931-4520
Website: www.acg.gi.org

American Gastroenterological Association (AGA)
National Office
7910 Woodmont Avenue
Suite 700
Bethesda, MD 20814
Phone: (301) 654-2055
Fax: (301) 654-5920
E-mail: members@gastro.org
Website: www.gastro.org

Pediatric/Adolescent Gastroesophageal Reflux Association Inc. (PAGER)
P.O. Box 1153
Germantown, MD 20875-1153
Phone: (301) 601-9541 (East Coast) or (760) 747-5001 (West Coast)
E-mail: GERGROUP@aol.com
Website: www.reflux.org

Note: The U.S. Government does not endorse or favor any specific commercial product or company. Trade, proprietary, or company names appearing in this document are used only because they are considered necessary in the context of the information provided. If a product is not mentioned, this does not mean or imply that the product is unsatisfactory.

National Digestive Diseases Information Clearinghouse

National Digestive Diseases Information Clearinghouse
2 Information Way
Bethesda, MD 20892-3570
E-mail: nddic@info.niddk.nih.gov

The National Digestive Diseases Information Clearinghouse (NDDIC) is a service of the National Institute of Diabetes and Digestive and Kidney Diseases (NIDDK). The NIDDK is part of the National Institutes of Health under the U.S. Department of Health and Human Services. Established in 1980, the clearinghouse provides information about digestive diseases to people with digestive disorders and to their families, health care professionals, and the public. NDDIC answers inquiries, develops and distributes publications, and works closely with professional and patient organizations and Government agencies to coordinate resources about digestive diseases.

Publications produced by the clearinghouse are carefully reviewed by both NIDDK scientists and outside experts. This text was reviewed by G. Richard Locke, M.D., Mayo Clinic, and Joel Richter, M.D., Cleveland Clinic Foundation.

Chapter 23

Interstitial Cystitis

What Is Interstitial Cystitis?

Interstitial cystitis (IC), one of the chronic pelvic pain disorders, is a condition resulting in recurring discomfort or pain in the bladder and the surrounding pelvic region. The symptoms of IC vary from case to case and even in the same individual. People may experience mild discomfort, pressure, tenderness, or intense pain in the bladder and surrounding pelvic area. Symptoms may include an urgent need to urinate (urgency), frequent need to urinate (frequency), or a combination of these symptoms. Pain may change in intensity as the bladder fills with urine or as it empties. Women's symptoms often get worse during menstruation.

In IC, the bladder wall may be irritated and become scarred or stiff. Glomerulations (pinpoint bleeding caused by recurrent irritation) may appear on the bladder wall. Some people with IC find that their bladders cannot hold much urine, which increases the frequency of urination. Frequency, however, is not always specifically related to bladder size; many people with severe frequency have normal bladder capacity. People with severe cases of IC may urinate as many as 60 times a day.

Also, people with IC often experience pain during sexual intercourse. IC is far more common in women than in men. Of the more than 700,000 Americans estimated to have IC, 90 percent are women.

National Institute of Diabetes and Digestive and Kidney Diseases (NIDDK), National Institutes of Health (NIH), NIH Pub. No. 99-3220, August 1999, e-text last updated: February 2000.

Are There Different Types of IC?

Because IC varies so much in symptoms and severity, most researchers believe that it is not one, but several, diseases. In the past, cases were mainly categorized as ulcerative IC or nonulcerative IC, based on whether ulcers had formed on the bladder wall. But many researchers and clinicians have questioned the usefulness of this classification, since the vast majority of cases do not involve ulcers, and their presence or absence does not influence treatment options as much as other factors do.

How Is IC Diagnosed?

Because symptoms are similar to those of other disorders of the urinary system and because there is no definitive test to identify IC, doctors must rule out other conditions before considering a diagnosis of IC. Among these disorders are urinary tract or vaginal infections, bladder cancer, bladder inflammation or infection caused by radiation to the pelvic area, eosinophilic and tuberculous cystitis, kidney stones, endometriosis, neurological disorders, sexually transmitted

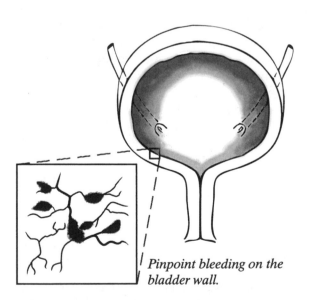

Pinpoint bleeding on the bladder wall.

Figure 23.1. Pinpoint bleeding on the bladder wall.

diseases, low-count bacteria in the urine and, in men, chronic bacterial and nonbacterial prostatitis.

The diagnosis of IC in the general population is based on:

- Presence of urgency, frequency, or pelvic/bladder pain.

- Cystoscopic evidence (under anesthesia) of bladder wall inflammation, including glomerulations or Hunner's ulcers present in 90 percent of patients with IC.

- Absence of other diseases that could cause the symptoms.

Diagnostic tests that help identify other conditions include urinalysis, urine culture, cystoscopy, biopsy of the bladder wall, urine cytology, and, in men, laboratory examination of prostate secretions. The most important test to confirm IC is a cystoscopy under anesthesia.

Cystoscopy under Anesthesia with Bladder Distention

During cystoscopy, the doctor uses a cystoscope—an instrument made of a hollow tube about the diameter of a drinking straw with several lenses and a light—to see inside the bladder and urethra. The doctor will also distend or stretch the bladder to its capacity by filling it with a liquid or gas. Because bladder distention is painful in patients with IC, they must be given either regional or general anesthesia before the doctor inserts the cystoscope. These tests can detect bladder wall inflammation; a thick, stiff bladder wall; and Hunner's ulcers. Glomerulations are usually seen only after the bladder has been stretched to capacity.

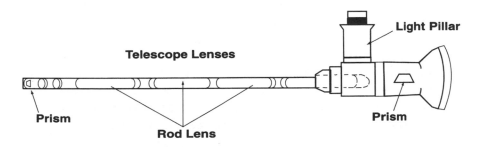

Figure 23.2. Cystoscope.

The doctor may also test the patient's maximum bladder capacity— the amount of liquid or gas the bladder can hold under anesthesia. Without anesthesia, capacity is limited by either pain or a severe urge to urinate. Many people with IC have normal or large maximum bladder capacities under anesthesia. However, a small bladder capacity under anesthesia helps support the diagnosis of IC.

What Are the Treatments for IC?

Because the causes of IC are unknown, treatments are aimed at relieving symptoms. Most people are helped for variable periods by one or a combination of treatments. As researchers learn more about IC, the list of potential treatments will change, so patients should discuss their options with a doctor.

- *Bladder distention:* Researchers are not sure why distention helps, but some believe that it may increase capacity and interfere with pain signals transmitted by nerves in the bladder. Symptoms may temporarily worsen 24 to 48 hours after distention, but should return to predistention levels or improve after 2 to 4 weeks.

- *Bladder instillation:* During a bladder instillation, also called a bladder wash or bath, the bladder is filled with a solution that is held for varying periods of time, averaging 10 to 15 minutes, before being emptied.

- *Oral drugs:* Pentosan polysulfate sodium (Elmiron), the first oral drug developed for IC, was approved by the FDA in 1996. Doctors do not know exactly how it works, but one theory is that it may repair defects that might have developed in the lining of the bladder.

- *Other oral medications:* Aspirin and ibuprofen are easy to obtain and may be a first line of defense against mild discomfort. Doctors may recommend other drugs to relieve pain. Some patients have experienced improvement in their urinary symptoms by taking antidepressants or antihistamines. Antidepressants help reduce pain and may also help patients deal with the psychological stress that accompanies living with chronic pain. In patients with severe pain, narcotic analgesics such as Tylenol with codeine or longer acting narcotics may be necessary.

- *Transcutaneous Electrical Nerve Stimulation (TENS):* With transcutaneous electrical nerve stimulation (TENS), mild electric pulses enter the body for minutes to hours two or more times a day either through wires placed on the lower back or just above the pubic area, between the navel and the pubic hair, or through special devices inserted into the vagina in women or into the rectum in men. Although scientists do not know exactly how TENS works, it has been suggested that the electric pulses may increase blood flow to the bladder, strengthen pelvic muscles that help control the bladder, or trigger the release of substances that block pain.

- *Diet:* There is no scientific evidence linking diet to IC, but many doctors and patients find that alcohol, tomatoes, spices, chocolate, caffeinated and citrus beverages, and high-acid foods may contribute to bladder irritation and inflammation. Some patients also note that their symptoms worsen after eating or drinking products containing artificial sweeteners. Patients may try eliminating various products from their diet and reintroducing them one at a time to determine which, if any, affect symptoms. It is important, however, to maintain a varied, well-balanced diet.

- *Smoking:* Many patients feel that smoking makes their symptoms worse. Because smoking is the major known cause of bladder cancer, one of the best things smokers can do for their bladder is to quit.

- *Exercise:* Many patients feel that gentle stretching exercises help relieve IC symptoms.

- *Bladder training:* People who have found adequate relief from pain may be able to reduce frequency by using bladder training techniques. Methods vary, but basically patients decide to void (that is, empty their bladder) at designated times and use relaxation techniques and distractions to keep to the schedule. Gradually, patients try to lengthen the time between scheduled voids. A diary that records voiding times is usually helpful in keeping track of progress.

Surgery for IC

Many approaches and techniques are used, each of which has its own advantages and complications that should be discussed with a surgeon. Surgery should be considered only if all available treatments have failed and the pain is disabling. Most doctors are reluctant to operate because the outcome is unpredictable—some people still have symptoms after surgery.

Those considering surgery should discuss the potential risks and benefits, side effects, and long- and short-term complications with a surgeon and with their family, as well as with people who have already had the procedure. Surgery requires anesthesia, hospitalization, and weeks or months of recovery, and as the complexity of the procedure increases, so do the chances for complications and failure.

To locate a surgeon experienced in performing specific procedures, check with your doctor.

Two procedures—*fulguration* and *resection* of ulcers—can be done with instruments inserted through the urethra. Fulguration involves burning Hunner's ulcers with electricity or a laser. When the area heals, the dead tissue and the ulcer fall off, leaving new, healthy tissue behind. Resection involves cutting around and removing the ulcers. Both treatments are done under anesthesia and use special instruments inserted into the bladder through a cystoscope. Laser surgery in the urinary tract should be reserved for patients with Hunner's ulcers and should be done only by doctors who have had special training and have the expertise needed to perform the procedure.

Another surgical treatment is augmentation, which makes the bladder larger. In most procedures, scarred, ulcerated, and inflamed sections of the patient's bladder are removed, leaving only the base of the bladder and healthy tissue. A piece of the patient's bowel (large intestine) is then removed, reshaped, and attached to what remains of the bladder. After the incisions heal, the patient may void less frequently. The effect on pain varies greatly; IC can sometimes recur on the segment of bowel used to enlarge the bladder.

Even in carefully selected patients—those with small, contracted bladders—pain, frequency, and urgency may remain or return after surgery, and the patient may have additional problems with infections in the new bladder and difficulty absorbing nutrients from the shortened intestine. Some patients are incontinent, while others cannot void at all and must insert a catheter into the urethra to empty the bladder.

Bladder removal, called a cystectomy, is another surgical option. Once the bladder has been removed, different methods can be used to reroute urine. In most cases, ureters are attached to a piece of bowel that opens onto the skin of the abdomen; this procedure is called a urostomy, and the opening is called a stoma. Urine empties through the stoma into a bag outside the body. Some urologists are using a second technique that also requires a stoma but allows urine to be stored in a pouch inside the abdomen. At intervals throughout the day, the patient puts a catheter into the stoma and empties the pouch. Patients with either type of urostomy must be very careful to keep the area in and around the stoma clean to prevent infection. Serious potential complications may include kidney infection and small bowel obstruction.

A third method to reroute urine involves making a new bladder from a piece of the patient's bowel and attaching it to the urethra. After healing, the patient may be able to empty the newly formed bladder by voiding at scheduled times or by inserting a catheter into the urethra. Few surgeons have the special training and expertise needed to perform this procedure.

Even after total bladder removal, some patients still experience variable IC symptoms in the form of phantom pain. Therefore, the decision to undergo a cystectomy should be undertaken only after testing all alternative methods and after seriously considering the potential outcome.

For More Information

National Institute of Diabetes and Digestive and Kidney Diseases
3 Information Way
Bethesda, MD 20892-3580
Phone: 800-891-5390
Website: http://www.niddk.nih.gov

Chapter 24

Kidney Stones

Overview

Kidney stones, one of the most painful of the urologic disorders, are not a product of modern life. Scientists have found evidence of kidney stones in a 7,000-year-old Egyptian mummy. Unfortunately, kidney stones are one of the most common disorders of the urinary tract; more than 1 million cases were diagnosed in 1996. An estimated 10 percent of people in the United States will have a kidney stone at some point in their lives. Men tend to be affected more frequently than women.

Most kidney stones pass out of the body without any intervention by a physician. Stones that cause lasting symptoms or other complications may be treated by various techniques, most of which do not involve major surgery. Also, research advances have led to a better understanding of the many factors that promote stone formation.

Introduction to the Urinary Tract

The urinary tract, or system, consists of the kidneys, ureters, bladder, and urethra. The kidneys are two bean-shaped organs located below the ribs toward the middle of the back. The kidneys remove extra water and wastes from the blood, converting it to urine. They

"Kidney Stones in Adults," National Institute of Diabetes and Digestive and Kidney Diseases (NIDDK), NIH Pub. No. 00-2495, February 2000, updated October 2000.

also keep a stable balance of salts and other substances in the blood. The kidneys produce hormones that help build strong bones and help form red blood cells.

Narrow tubes called ureters carry urine from the kidneys to the bladder, a triangle-shaped chamber in the lower abdomen. Like a balloon, the bladder's elastic walls stretch and expand to store urine. They flatten together when urine is emptied through the urethra to outside the body.

What Is a Kidney Stone?

A kidney stone is a hard mass developed from crystals that separate from the urine and build up on the inner surfaces of the kidney. Normally, urine contains chemicals that prevent the crystals from forming. These inhibitors do not seem to work for everyone, however,

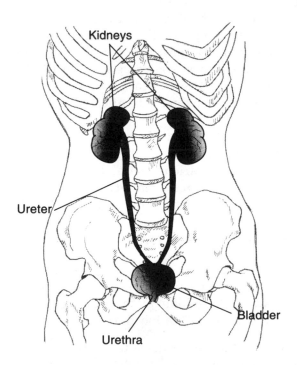

Figure 24.1. *The Urinary Tract.*

so some people form stones. If the crystals remain tiny enough, they will travel through the urinary tract and pass out of the body in the urine without being noticed.

Kidney stones may contain various combinations of chemicals. The most common type of stone contains calcium in combination with either oxalate or phosphate. These chemicals are part of a person's normal diet and make up important parts of the body, such as bones and muscles.

A less common type of stone is caused by infection in the urinary tract. This type of stone is called a struvite or infection stone. Much less common are the uric acid stone and the rare cystine stone.

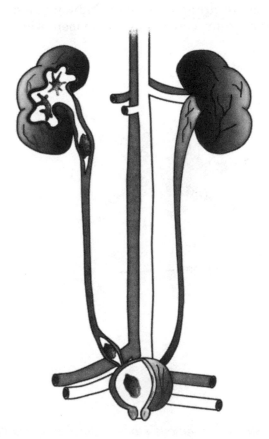

Figure 24.2. *Kidney stones in kidney, ureter, and bladder.*

Urolithiasis is the medical term used to describe stones occurring in the urinary tract. Other frequently used terms are urinary tract stone disease and nephrolithiasis. Doctors also use terms that describe the location of the stone in the urinary tract. For example, a ureteral stone (or ureterolithiasis) is a kidney stone found in the ureter. To keep things simple, however, the term "kidney stones" is used throughout this chapter.

Gallstones and kidney stones are not related. They form in different areas of the body. If you have a gallstone, you are not necessarily more likely to develop kidney stones.

Who Gets Kidney Stones?

For unknown reasons, the number of people in the United States with kidney stones has been increasing over the past 20 years. White Americans are more prone to develop kidney stones than African Americans. Stones occur more frequently in men. Kidney stones strike

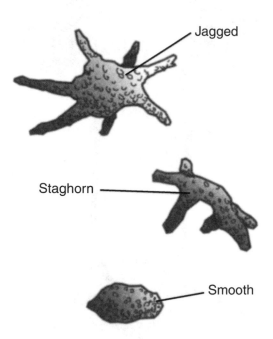

Figure 24.3. *Shapes of various stones. Sizes are usually smaller than shown here.*

most typically between the ages of 20 and 40. Once a person gets more than one stone, others are likely to develop.

What Causes Kidney Stones?

Doctors do not always know what causes a stone to form. While certain foods may promote stone formation in people who are susceptible, scientists do not believe that eating any specific food causes stones to form in people who are not susceptible.

A person with a family history of kidney stones may be more likely to develop stones. Urinary tract infections, kidney disorders such as cystic kidney diseases, and metabolic disorders such as hyperparathyroidism are also linked to stone formation.

In addition, more than 70 percent of people with a rare hereditary disease called renal tubular acidosis develop kidney stones.

Cystinuria and hyperoxaluria are two other rare, inherited metabolic disorders that often cause kidney stones. In cystinuria, too much of the amino acid cystine, which does not dissolve in urine, is voided. This can lead to the formation of stones made of cystine. In patients with hyperoxaluria, the body produces too much of the salt oxalate. When there is more oxalate than can be dissolved in the urine, the crystals settle out and form stones.

Absorptive hypercalciuria occurs when the body absorbs too much calcium from food and empties the extra calcium into the urine. This high level of calcium in the urine causes crystals of calcium oxalate or calcium phosphate to form in the kidneys or urinary tract.

Other causes of kidney stones are hyperuricosuria (a disorder of uric acid metabolism), gout, excess intake of vitamin D, and blockage of the urinary tract. Certain diuretics (water pills) or calcium-based antacids may increase the risk of forming kidney stones by increasing the amount of calcium in the urine.

Calcium oxalate stones may also form in people who have a chronic inflammation of the bowel or who have had an intestinal bypass operation, or ostomy surgery. As mentioned above, struvite stones can form in people who have had a urinary tract infection. People who take the protease inhibitor indinavir, a drug used to treat HIV infection and AIDS, are at risk of developing kidney stones.

What Are the Symptoms?

Usually, the first symptom of a kidney stone is extreme pain. The pain often begins suddenly when a stone moves in the urinary tract, causing irritation or blockage. Typically, a person feels a sharp, cramping pain in the back and side in the area of the kidney or in the lower abdomen. Sometimes nausea and vomiting occur. Later, pain may spread to the groin.

If the stone is too large to pass easily, pain continues as the muscles in the wall of the tiny ureter try to squeeze the stone along into the bladder. As a stone grows or moves, blood may appear in the urine. As the stone moves down the ureter closer to the bladder, you may feel the need to urinate more often or feel a burning sensation during urination.

If fever and chills accompany any of these symptoms, an infection may be present. In this case, you should contact a doctor immediately.

How Are Kidney Stones Diagnosed?

Sometimes "silent" stones—those that do not cause symptoms—are found on x-rays taken during a general health exam. These stones would likely pass unnoticed.

More often, kidney stones are found on an x-ray or sonogram taken on someone who complains of blood in the urine or sudden pain. These diagnostic images give the doctor valuable information about the stone's size and location. Blood and urine tests help detect any abnormal substance that might promote stone formation.

The doctor may decide to scan the urinary system using a special x-ray test called an IVP (intravenous pyelogram). The results of all these tests help determine the proper treatment.

How Are Kidney Stones Treated?

Fortunately, surgery is not usually necessary. Most kidney stones can pass through the urinary system with plenty of water (2 to 3 quarts a day) to help move the stone along. Often, you can stay home during this process, drinking fluids and taking pain medication as needed. The doctor usually asks you to save the passed stone(s) for testing. (You can catch it in a cup or tea strainer used only for this purpose.)

The First Step: Prevention

If you've had more than one kidney stone, you are likely to form another; so prevention is very important. To prevent stones from forming, your doctor must determine their cause. He or she will order laboratory tests, including urine and blood tests. Your doctor will also ask about your medical history, occupation, and eating habits. If a stone has been removed, or if you've passed a stone and saved it, the laboratory can analyze it to determine its composition.

You may be asked to collect your urine for 24 hours after a stone has passed or been removed. The sample is used to measure urine volume and levels of acidity, calcium, sodium, uric acid, oxalate, citrate, and creatinine (a product of muscle metabolism). Your doctor will use this information to determine the cause of the stone. A second 24-hour urine collection may be needed to determine whether the prescribed treatment is working.

Lifestyle Changes

A simple and most important lifestyle change to prevent stones is to drink more liquids—water is best. If you tend to form stones, you should try to drink enough liquids throughout the day to produce at least 2 quarts of urine in every 24-hour period.

People who form calcium stones used to be told to avoid dairy products and other foods with high calcium content. But recent studies have shown that foods high in calcium, including dairy foods, help prevent calcium stones. Taking calcium in pill form, however, may increase the risk of developing stones.

You may be told to avoid food with added vitamin D and certain types of antacids that have a calcium base. If you have very acidic urine, you may need to eat less meat, fish, and poultry. These foods increase the amount of acid in the urine.

To prevent cystine stones, you should drink enough water each day to dilute the concentration of cystine that escapes into the urine, which may be difficult. More than a gallon of water may be needed every 24 hours, and a third of that must be drunk during the night.

Medical Therapy

The doctor may prescribe certain medications to prevent calcium and uric acid stones. These drugs control the amount of acid or alkali in the urine, key factors in crystal formation. The drug allopurinol may also be useful in some cases of hypercalciuria and hyperuricosuria.

Another way a doctor may try to control hypercalciuria, and thus prevent calcium stones, is by prescribing certain diuretics, such as hydrochlorothiazide. These drugs decrease the amount of calcium released by the kidneys into the urine.

Some patients with absorptive hypercalciuria may be given the drug sodium cellulose phosphate, which binds calcium in the intestines and prevents it from leaking into the urine.

If cystine stones cannot be controlled by drinking more fluids, your doctor may prescribe the drug Thiola, which helps reduce the amount of cystine in the urine.

For struvite stones that have been totally removed, the first line of prevention is to keep the urine free of bacteria that can cause infection. Your urine will be tested regularly to be sure that no bacteria are present.

If struvite stones cannot be removed, your doctor may prescribe a drug called acetohydroxamic acid (AHA). AHA is used with long-term antibiotic drugs to prevent the infection that leads to stone growth.

People with hyperparathyroidism sometimes develop calcium stones. Treatment in these cases is usually surgery to remove the parathyroid glands (located in the neck). In most cases, only one of the glands is enlarged. Removing the glands cures the patient's problem with hyperparathyroidism and with kidney stones as well.

Surgical Treatment

Surgery should be reserved as an option for cases where other approaches have failed or shouldn't be tried. Surgery may be needed to remove a kidney stone if it

- Does not pass after a reasonable period of time and causes constant pain
- Is too large to pass on its own or is caught in a difficult place
- Blocks the flow of urine
- Causes ongoing urinary tract infection
- Damages kidney tissue or causes constant bleeding
- Has grown larger (as seen on followup x-ray studies).

Until recently, surgery to remove a stone was very painful and required a lengthy recovery time (4 to 6 weeks). Today, treatment for these stones is greatly improved, and many options do not require major surgery.

Extracorporeal Shockwave Lithotripsy

Extracorporeal shockwave lithotripsy (ESWL) is the most frequently used procedure for the treatment of kidney stones. In ESWL, shock waves that are created outside of the body travel through the skin and body tissues until they hit the dense stones. The stones break down into sand-like particles and are easily passed through the urinary tract in the urine.

There are several types of ESWL devices. In one device, the patient reclines in a water bath while the shock waves are transmitted. Other devices have a soft cushion on which the patient lies. Most devices use either x-rays or ultrasound to help the surgeon pinpoint the stone during treatment. For most types of ESWL procedures, anesthesia is needed.

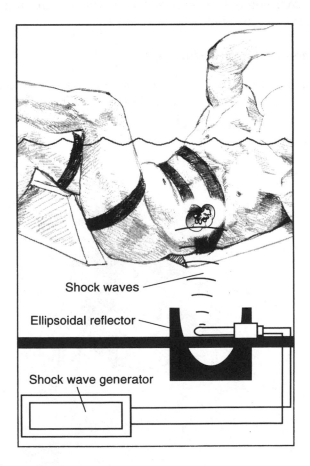

Figure 24.4. Extracorporeal shockwave lithotripsy.

In some cases, ESWL may be done on an outpatient basis. Recovery time is short, and most people can resume normal activities in a few days.

Complications may occur with ESWL. Most patients have blood in their urine for a few days after treatment. Bruising and minor discomfort of the back or abdomen from the shock waves are also common. To reduce the risk of complications, doctors usually tell patients to avoid taking aspirin and other drugs that affect blood clotting for several weeks before treatment.

Another complication may occur if the shattered stone particles cause discomfort as they pass through the urinary tract. In some cases, the doctor will insert a small tube called a stent through the bladder into the ureter to help the fragments pass. Sometimes the stone is not completely shattered with one treatment, and additional treatments may be needed.

Percutaneous Nephrolithotomy

Sometimes a procedure called percutaneous nephrolithotomy is recommended to remove a stone. This treatment is often used when

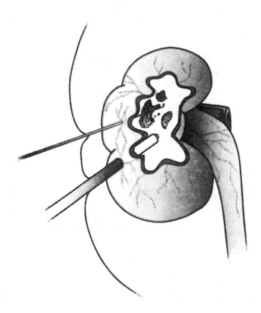

Figure 24.5. Percutaneous nephrolithotomy.

the stone is quite large or in a location that does not allow effective use of ESWL.

In this procedure, the surgeon makes a tiny incision in the back and creates a tunnel directly into the kidney. Using an instrument called a nephroscope, the surgeon locates and removes the stone. For large stones, some type of energy probe (ultrasonic or electrohydraulic) may be needed to break the stone into small pieces. Generally, patients stay in the hospital for several days and may have a small tube called a nephrostomy tube left in the kidney during the healing process.

One advantage of percutaneous nephrolithotomy over ESWL is that the surgeon removes the stone fragments instead of relying on their natural passage from the kidney.

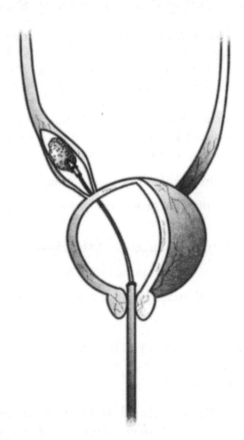

Figure 24.6. Ureteroscopic stone removal.

Ureteroscopic Stone Removal

Although some kidney stones in the ureters can be treated with ESWL, ureteroscopy may be needed for mid- and lower-ureter stones. No incision is made in this procedure. Instead, the surgeon passes a small fiberoptic instrument called a ureteroscope through the urethra and bladder into the ureter. The surgeon then locates the stone and either removes it with a cage-like device or shatters it with a special instrument that produces a form of shock wave. A small tube or stent may be left in the ureter for a few days to help the lining of the ureter heal. Before fiber optics made ureteroscopy possible, physicians used a similar "blind basket" extraction method. But this outdated technique should not be used because it may damage the ureters.

Is Any Research Being Done on Kidney Stones?

The Division of Kidney, Urologic, and Hematologic Diseases of the National Institute of Diabetes and Digestive and Kidney Diseases (NIDDK) funds research on the causes, treatments, and prevention of kidney stones. NIDDK is part of the Federal Government's National Institutes of Health in Bethesda, Maryland.

New drugs and the growing field of lithotripsy have greatly improved the treatment of kidney stones. Still, NIDDK researchers and grantees seek to answer questions such as

- Why do some people continue to have painful stones?

- How can doctors predict, or screen, those at risk for getting stones?

- What are the long-term effects of lithotripsy?

- Do genes play a role in stone formation?

- What is the natural substance(s) found in urine that blocks stone formation?

Researchers are also working on new drugs with fewer side effects.

Additional Reading

Coe, F. L., Parks, J. H., & Asplin, J. R. (1992). The pathogenesis and treatment of kidney stones. *New England Journal of Medicine,* 327(16), 1141-1152.

Curhan, G. C., Willet, W. C., Rimm, E. B., & Stampfer, M. J. (1993). A prospective study of dietary calcium and other nutrients and the risk of symptomatic kidney stones. *New England Journal of Medicine*, 328(12), 833-838.

Curhan, G. C., Willet, W. C., Speizer, F. E., Spiegelman, D., & Stampfer, M. J. (1997). Comparison of dietary calcium with supplemental calcium and other nutrients as factors affecting the risk for kidney stones in women. *Annals of Internal Medicine*, 126(7), 497-504.

Savitz, G., & Leslie, S. W. (1999). *Kidney stones handbook: A patient's guide to hope, cure, and prevention* (2nd ed.). Roseville, CA: Four Geez Press. (800) 2-KIDNEYS.

Understanding kidney stones . . . Management for a lifetime. (1995). San Bruno, CA: Krames Communication. (800) 333-3032.

Prevention Points to Remember

- If you have a family history of stones or have had more than one stone, you are likely to develop more stones.

- A good first step to prevent the formation of any type of stone is to drink plenty of liquids—water is best.

- If you are at risk for developing stones, your doctor may perform certain blood and urine tests to determine which factors can best be altered to reduce that risk.

- Some people will need medicines to prevent stones from forming.

- People with chronic urinary tract infections and stones will often need the stone removed if the doctor determines that the infection results from the stone's presence. Patients must receive careful followup to be sure that the infection has cleared.

Foods and Drinks Containing Oxalate

People prone to forming calcium oxalate stones may be asked by their doctor to cut back on certain foods on this list:

- Beets
- Cola
- Spinach
- Wheat bran
- Chocolate
- Nuts
- Strawberries
- Coffee
- Rhubarb
- Tea

People should not give up or avoid eating these foods without talking to their doctor first. In most cases, these foods can be eaten in limited amounts.

Other Resources

American Foundation for Urologic Disease
1128 North Charles Street
Baltimore, MD 21201
Phone: (800) 242-2383 or (410) 468-1800
email: admin@afud.org
website: www.afud.org

National Kidney Foundation
30 East 33rd Street
New York, NY 10016
Phone: (800) 622-9010 or (212) 889-2210

Oxalosis and Hyperoxaluria Foundation
12 Pleasant Street
Maynard, MA 01754
Phone: (888) 712-2432, PIN# 5392 or (508) 461-0614

For information about hyperparathyroidism:

National Institute of Diabetes and Digestive and Kidney Diseases
Building 31, Room 9A04
31 Center Drive MSC-2560
Bethesda, MD 20892
Phone: (301) 496-3583

For information about gout:

National Institute of Arthritis and Musculoskeletal and Skin Diseases Information Clearinghouse
1 AMS Circle
Bethesda, MD 20892-3675
Phone: (301) 495-4484
TTY: (301) 565-2966
Fax: (301) 718-6366
email: namsic@mail.nih.gov
website: www.nih.gov/niams/

National Kidney and Urologic Diseases Information Clearinghouse

National Kidney and Urologic Diseases Information Clearinghouse
3 Information Way
Bethesda, MD 20892-3580
email: nkudic@info.niddk.nih.gov

The National Kidney and Urologic Diseases Information Clearinghouse (NKUDIC) is a service of the National Institute of Diabetes and Digestive and Kidney Diseases (NIDDK). NIDDK is part of the National Institutes of Health under the U.S. Department of Health and Human Services. Established in 1987, the clearinghouse provides information about diseases of the kidneys and urologic system to people with kidney and urologic disorders and to their families, health care professionals, and the public. NKUDIC answers inquiries; develops, reviews, and distributes publications; and works closely with professional and patient organizations and Government agencies to coordinate resources about kidney and urologic diseases.

Publications produced by the clearinghouse are carefully reviewed for scientific accuracy, content, and readability.

Note

The U.S. Government does not endorse or favor any specific commercial product or company. Brand names appearing in this publication are used only because they are considered essential in the context of the information provided herein.

Chapter 25

Myofascial Pain Syndrome

Myofascial Pain—The Symptoms and Causes

Myofascial pain syndrome is a chronic local or regional musculoskeletal pain disorder that may involve either a single muscle or a muscle group. The pain may be of a burning, stabbing, aching or nagging quality. Importantly, where the patient experiences the pain may not be where the myofascial pain generator is located. This is known as referred pain. The pathophysiology of myofascial pain remains somewhat of a mystery due to limited clinical research; however, based on case reports and medical observation, investigators think it may develop from a muscle lesion or excessive strain on a particular muscle or muscle group, ligament or tendon. It is thought that the lesion or the strain prompts the development of a "trigger point" that, in turn, causes pain.

In addition to the local or regional pain, people with myofascial pain syndrome also can suffer from depression, fatigue and behavioral disturbances, as with all chronic pain conditions.

How to Diagnose and Treat Myofascial Pain Syndrome

Recognition of this syndrome is difficult and requires the physician to have a precise understanding of the body's anatomy. Trigger

"Myofascial Pain Syndrome," Department of Pain Medicine and Palliative Care at Beth Israel Medical Center, online at www.stoppain.org. © 2000 Continuum Health Partners, Inc.; reprinted with permission.

points can be identified by pain produced upon digital palpation (applying pressure with one to three fingers and the thumb). In diagnosing myofascial pain syndrome, four types of trigger points can be distinguished:

- active trigger point: an area of exquisite tenderness that is usually located in a skeletal muscle and is associated with local or regional pain;

- latent trigger point: a dormant area that can potentially behave like an active trigger point;

- secondary trigger point: a hyperirritable spot in a muscle that becomes active as a result of a trigger point and muscular overload in another muscle;

- satellite myofascial point: a hyperirritable spot in a muscle that becomes active because the muscle is located within the region of another trigger point.

The best treatments for myofascial pain syndrome are active and passive physical therapy methods. There is also the "stretch and spray" technique, in which the muscle with the trigger point is sprayed along its length with a coolant such as fluorimethane, and then stretched slowly.

Trigger point injection, whereby local anesthesia is injected directly into the trigger point, also is used. At times, corticosteroids and botulinum toxin can be injected. Massage therapy also can be of significant benefit in some patients. Often a combination of physical therapy, trigger point injections and massage are needed in refractory chronic cases.

Chapter 26

Neck Pain

Pain or discomfort in the neck is a common reason for patients to seek medical care. Most cases are not serious. A muscle spasm, brought on by poor posture, sleeping position or stress, is the most frequent causes of neck pain. But an aching neck can be a symptom of a more serious problem. Disk degeneration, narrowing of the spinal canal, arthritis and even cancer can cause neck pain. For serious neck problems a primary care physician and often a specialist, such as a neurosurgeon, should be consulted.

When to See a Physician

A doctor should be consulted if neck pain occurs after an injury or blow to the head. Also see a doctor if a fever or headache accompanies the neck pain, if a stiff neck prevents you from touching your chin to your chest, if pain shoots down one arm, if there is a tingling in your hands or if pain does not decrease after a week.

You can take a number of steps on your own to alleviate neck pain caused by strain or spasm of the neck muscles. Improve your posture and change the way you sleep. Take rest breaks at work instead of sitting or standing in the same position. Do exercises to stretch the neck and shoulder muscles. Use hot showers, hot compresses or a heating pad to relax tense muscles. Take aspirin or ibuprofen.

Reprinted with permission from Neurosurgery://On-CALL® at www.neurosurgery.org. Copyright © 2001 American Association of Neurological Surgeons/Congress of Neurological Surgeons.

Understanding the Neck

The neck is part of a long flexible column of bones and other tissue, often referred to as the spinal column or backbone, that extends through most of the body. The neck region of the spinal column is called the cervical spine, which consists of seven bones or vertebrae that are shaped like building blocks.

Intervertebral disks separate the vertebrae from one another. These disks allow the spine to move freely and act as shock absorbers when a person moves.

The back of each vertebra forms a tube-like canal of bone that runs down the back. This space is called the spinal canal, through which the spinal cord and nerves travel. The spinal cord is surrounded by cerebrospinal fluid and three protective membranes called the dura, the pia and the arachnoid.

A pair of spinal nerves exit each vertebra through small openings called foramina (one to the left and one to the right). These nerves connect to the muscles, skin and tissues of the body, providing sensation and movement to all parts of the body. The delicate spinal cord and nerves are further supported by strong muscles and ligaments that are attached to the vertebrae. The cervical spine needs to be strong because it also holds up the head, which can weigh 10 pounds or more.

Common Disorders of the Cervical Spine

Cervical Disk Disorders

The disks in the neck can wear out in the course of aging or can be damaged by sudden movement (whiplash), poor posture or diseases such as arthritis. Neck pain occurs when the herniated disk pinches the nerve or when arthritis progresses to the point where it involves the joints of the spine. Arthritis can lead to degeneration of the disk as well as abnormal bone growths (spurs) next to the joints. These spurs are the result of repetitive movement and can irritate the adjacent nerve and cause pain.

Cervical disk disorders are typically marked by intermittent neck pain, followed by severe neck and sometimes arm pain. The pain is sufficient to awaken a person from sleep. Irritated nerves also can lead to numbness or weakness in the arm or forearm, tingling in the fingers and coordination problems. Severe nerve impairment or even paralysis can develop if the disorder is left untreated.

Pressure on the spinal cord from a herniated disk or bone spur in the neck can also be a very serious problem. Virtually all of the nerves of the body have to pass through the neck to reach their final destination (arms, chest, abdomen, legs).

Cervical Stenosis

Cervical stenosis is a narrowing of the spinal canal that can pinch the spinal cord. The normal aging process is usually the cause. The disks dehydrate over time, causing them to lose their ability to act as shock absorbers. At the same time, degenerative changes in the vertebrae can lead to the growth of bone spurs that compress the nerve roots. The bones and ligaments that make up the spine gradually thicken and become less pliable. These changes cause the spinal canal to narrow.

Symptoms of cervical stenosis are neck pain, numbness and weakness in the hands, inability to walk at a quick pace, deterioration of fine motor skills and muscle spasms in the legs.

Osteoarthritis

The joints in the neck deteriorate as people age, sometimes leading to osteoarthritis. The symptoms of osteoarthritis are pain radiating to the shoulder or between the shoulder blades and pain that is worse at the start of the day, improves during the day and gets worse again at the close of the day. This pain usually diminishes with rest. Patients with a previous history of a whiplash injury are six times more likely to develop this condition.

Injury

Whiplash is one of the most common injuries to the neck and commonly occurs after a rear-end automobile crash. Whiplash symptoms include neck stiffness, shoulder or arm pain, headache, facial pain and vertigo. Pain from a whiplash injury can be caused by tears and bleeding in the muscles that support the neck, ligament rupture, or a disk tearing away from a vertebra.

Diagnosing Neck Problems

A physician investigates a neck problem through a medical history, physical exam and diagnostic tests. The physical examination includes an assessment of sensation, strength and reflexes in various parts of the body to help pinpoint which nerves or parts of the spinal cord are affected. The doctor may then order various diagnostic studies to determine more precisely the nature and extent of the disorder. These studies may include:

X-rays: An x-ray shows the bones of the neck and determines if there is significant wear and tear or disease of the bone. It also shows whether the bones are aligned (lined-up) properly.

Computed Tomography (CT): A CT (also known as a CAT scan) produces an image of the neck based on x-rays but displayed in slices. It helps clarify the relationship of the disk or bone spurs to the spinal cord and nerves. The CT may be done in conjunction with a myelogram of the neck to provide additional information.

Magnetic Resonance Imaging (MRI): The MRI uses a powerful magnetic field rather than x-rays to produce a detailed anatomical picture of the neck and the structures within it. An MRI is probably the best test to see herniated disks since they are soft tissues that are invisible to x-rays.

Myelogram: The myelogram is an x-ray with a special dye that highlights the spinal cord and nerves. The dye is usually injected into the fluid space around the spinal cord with a needle and then the x-rays are obtained. Myelograms have largely been replaced by CT and MRI scans.

Electromyogram and Nerve Conduction Studies (EMG/NCS): Unlike the other tests, which help a doctor determine anatomy and structure, these tests primarily study how the nerve and muscles are actually working together. They test for the impulse coming from the brain and/or spinal cord. If the impulse is blocked, it may be delayed or diminished enroute to its final destination (i.e., muscle, skin, toe, finger-tips). This information can assist in determining which nerves or muscles are functioning abnormally.

Discography: This is a special x-ray test that may help identify which disks are damaged and if they are a source of pain. It uses a contrast dye injected into the disk space to image the disk.

Treatment

Patients with neck pain are usually treated conservatively at first. Non-surgical treatments often can provide sufficient relief. Most cervical disk herniations, for example, heal with time and conservative treatment and do not require surgery.

Conservative treatment includes bed rest, reduction of physical activity, physical therapy and wearing a cervical collar, which provides support for the spine, reduces mobility and lessens pain and irritation. An injection of corticosteroids may be used to temporarily relieve pain. A cervical traction device may be used to further relieve the pressure on the nerves in the neck. This device attaches to the head and pulls up on the head using a pulley system and weights. It is usually applied a few times a day and can be used while sitting or lying in bed.

Mild cervical stenosis can be treated conservatively for extended periods of time as long as the symptoms are restricted to neck pain. Severe stenosis requires referral to a neurosurgeon.

Treatment of whiplash injuries consists of analgesics, non-steroidal anti-inflammatory drugs, muscle relaxants and aggressive physical therapy. Home cervical traction and manipulation are sometimes helpful. Approximately 65 percent of whiplash patients make a full recovery, 25 percent have minor residual symptoms and 5 to 10 percent develop chronic pain syndromes.

Conservative treatment options may continue for up to eight weeks. If there is severe muscle weakness or progressive symptoms, a more aggressive timetable may be warranted to avoid an irreversible wasting away of the muscles.

When Surgery Is Necessary

Surgery may be needed when conservative treatments for cervical disk problems do not provide relief. The choice of treatment and the decision as to when to perform the operation should be determined by a neurosurgeon, the medical specialist trained in the surgical treatment of disorders of the spine.

Surgery may be advisable if:

- You miss work because of pain.

- You are unable to join in family activities because of pain or muscle weakness.

- Your pain forces you to spend more time alone, away from friends and family.

- You feel frustrated or depressed because of your pain.

- You are otherwise in good health.

Factors in determining the type of surgical treatment include what type of disease (herniated disk or bone spurs), whether there is pressure on the spinal cord or spinal nerves and if the spine is dislocated in addition to pressure on the cord or nerves. Other factors include age, duration of disorder, other medical conditions and previous medical history.

Surgery has its limitations. It can't reverse all the effects of overuse or aging, and it carries risks. Yet it may be the only way to relieve pain, numbness and weakness.

Surgical Procedures

Anterior Cervical Discectomy

The most common surgical procedure on the neck relieves pressure on one or more nerve roots or on the spinal cord. The operation enlarges the nerve opening and removes the disk, as well as removing any attached bone spurs that could be compressing the spinal sac and nerve roots.

The surgeon makes an incision in the front (anterior) of the neck. The soft tissues within the neck are separated to allow the surgeon to reach the front of the spine, after which the disk and any bone spurs are removed. Sometimes the space between the vertebrae is refilled with a small piece of bone in a procedure called fusion. The bone may be the patient's, taken from the hipbone, or it may be taken from a donor bone bank. In addition to the bone, a metal plate at the fusion site may be attached to further strengthen the fusion. Over time, the vertebrae and bone fuse together, creating a more stable structure.

Anterior cervical discectomy typically involves few risks. These include infection, bleeding, stroke, injury to the recurrent laryngeal nerve (causing temporary or permanent hoarseness), and injury to the involved nerve root(s) or the spinal cord, both of which can cause paralysis. Overall, the risk is low and is much less than 5 percent for most healthy people.

Cervical Corpectomy

A more extensive version of the discectomy procedure, a cervical corpectomy involves removing vertebrae as well as disks. It is a more difficult surgery than a discectomy and the risks are slightly higher. These include nerve root and spinal cord damage, bleeding, infection, damage to the trachea or esophagus, graft dislodgement and continued pain. The most serious risk is complete or partial quadriplegia if the spinal cord is damaged.

Posterior Hemi-laminectomy

This operation is performed through a vertical incision in the back (posterior) of the neck, generally in the middle. The bone around the spinal cord or the bone around the nerve opening is removed, as are the attached ligaments exerting pressure on the spinal sac and nerve roots. Once the nerve is located, it is gently moved aside and an incision is made on the outside covering of the disk, through which the disk material is then removed.

Recovery after Surgery

A cervical collar or brace may be fitted around a patient's neck after surgery. Occasionally, a drainage tube may be used and is typically removed after a day or two. Intravenous (IV) fluids will be ordered during the early recovery period.

A patient who has had an anterior cervical discectomy or corpectomy may have a sore throat. If a piece of bone was taken from a hip for a graft, the area of incision is usually sore.

The length of the hospital stay is determined by the progress of recovery and by a patient's home situation. A patient is provided with instructions regarding his brace, incision care and physical activity when he leaves the hospital.

After Leaving the Hospital

Patients generally wear a brace for a few weeks and normally are not allowed to drive, lift heavy objects or engage in contact sports or vigorous physical activity for a while. Pain in the neck or arms may continue but will slowly lessen as the nerve heals. Medication may be necessary. Numbness or tingling sensations are often the last symptoms to fade away.

Patients need to adopt habits that reduce the risk of neck pain such as good posture and proper body mechanics when lifting and even during routine daily tasks.

Role of Neurosurgeons

Neurosurgeons are medical specialists trained to help patients suffering from neck pain. Neurosurgeons provide the operative and non-operative (prevention, diagnosis, evaluation, treatment, critical care and rehabilitation) care of neurological disorders. Neurosurgeons undergo six to eight years of specialized training following medical school, one of the longest training periods of any medical specialties. A major focus of neurosurgical training is management of disorders of the spine.

Chapter 27

Occipital Neuralgia

What Is Occipital Neuralgia?

Occipital neuralgia is a chronic pain disorder caused by irritation or injury to the occipital nerve located in the back of the scalp. Individuals with the disorder experience pain originating at the nape of the neck. The pain, often described as throbbing and migraine-like, spreads up and around the forehead and scalp. Occipital neuralgia can result from physical stress, trauma, or repeated contraction of the muscles of the neck.

Is There Any Treatment?

Treatment is generally symptomatic and includes massage and rest. In some cases, antidepressants may be used when the pain is particularly severe. Other treatments may include local nerve blocks and injections of steroids directly into the affected area.

What Is the Prognosis?

For most individuals with occipital neuralgia, the pain is eliminated or reduced with treatment and does not interfere with daily activities.

From "NINDS Occipital Neuralgia Information Page," National Institute of Neurological Disorders and Stroke (NINDS), at www.ninds.nih.gov. Reviewed July 2001.

What Research Is Being Done?

Within the NINDS research programs, occipital neuralgia is addressed primarily through studies on pain. NINDS vigorously pursues a research program that seeks to find new treatments for pain and nerve damage and to understand the underlying biological processes associated with pain.

Organizations

American Chronic Pain Association (ACPA)
P.O. Box 850
Rocklin, CA 95677-0850
Phone: (916) 632-0922
Fax: (916) 632-3208
Website: http://www.theacpa.org

National Chronic Pain Outreach Association (NCPOA)
P.O. Box 274
Millboro, VA 24460
Phone: (540) 862-9437
Fax: (540) 862-9485

National Headache Foundation
428 West St. James Place, 2nd Floor
Chicago, IL 60614-2750
Phone: (773) 388-6399
Toll Free: (888) NHF-5552 (888-643-5552)
Fax: (773) 525-7357
E-Mail: info@headaches.org
Website: http://www.headaches.org

Chapter 28

Paresthesia

What Is Paresthesia?

Paresthesia is a term that refers to an abnormal burning or prickling sensation which is generally felt in the hands, arms, legs, or feet, but may occur in any part of the body. The sensation, which arises spontaneously without apparent stimulus and is usually not painful, may also be described as tingling or numbness, skin crawling, buzzing, or itching. Most people have experienced transient (temporary) paresthesia at some time in their lives; it occurs whenever inadvertent pressure is placed on a nerve and causes what many describe as a "pins and needles" feeling. The feeling quickly goes away once the pressure is relieved. For some people, however, paresthesia can become a chronic condition caused by an underlying disorder. It more frequently occurs as a symptom of more widespread neurological disease or traumatic nerve damage. Paresthesia can be caused by disorders affecting the central nervous system, such as stroke, transient ischemic attack, multiple sclerosis, transverse myelitis, and encephalitis. A tumor or vascular lesion such as an arteriovenous malformation pressed up against the brain or spinal cord can also cause paresthesia. A wide range of conditions including diabetes, hypothyroidism, vitamin B_{12} deficiencies, alcoholism, heavy metal poisoning (lead, arsenic, and other metals), and nerve entrapment syndromes,

From "NINDS Paresthesia Information Page," National Institute of Neurological Disorders and Stroke (NINDS), at www.ninds.nih.gov. Reviewed July 2001.

such as carpal tunnel syndrome, can also damage peripheral nerves (peripheral neuropathy) and cause paresthesia. Connective tissue disorders such as rheumatoid arthritis or systemic lupus erythematosus also can cause peripheral neuropathy and lead to paresthesia. Paresthesia caused by peripheral neuropathy may be accompanied by pain. Diagnostic evaluation is largely based on determining the underlying condition causing the paresthetic sensations. An individual's medical history, physical examination, and laboratory tests are essential for the diagnosis. Physicians may order additional tests depending on the suspected cause of the paresthesia.

Is There Any Treatment?

The appropriate treatment for paresthesia depends on accurate diagnosis of the underlying cause.

What Is the Prognosis?

The prognosis for those with paresthesia depends on the severity of the sensations and the associated disorder(s).

What Research Is Being Done?

The National Institute of Neurological Disorders and Stroke (NINDS) supports research on disorders of the brain, spinal cord, and peripheral nerves that can cause paresthesia. The goals of this research are to increase scientific understanding of these disorders and to find ways to prevent, treat, and cure them.

Chapter 29

Pelvic Pain

Understanding the Principles of Chronic Pelvic Pain

Chronic Pelvic Pain: An Introduction

Chronic Pelvic Pain (CPP) is one of the most common medical problems affecting women today. Diagnosis and treatment of CPP accounts for 10% of all out-patient gynecologic visits, 20% of laparoscopies, and 12–16% of hysterectomies at a cost of as high as $2.8 billion annually.

The personal cost to those suffering from CPP is even greater, affecting all aspects of their lives. Pain puts about 25% of affected women in bed for much of the day for an average of 2.6 days a month; 58% must at least cut down on their usual activity one or more days a month. Emotionally, 56% noted significant changes; 47% felt "downhearted and blue" some of the time. Intercourse is compromised with pain in almost 90% of CPP patients.

Nearly 15% (1 in 7) of all American women ages 18–50 suffer from CPP. Yet of these 9.2 million sufferers, a surprising 61% still have no diagnosis. Why is this problem of epidemic proportions so poorly understood? Why have treatments until recently often proved so unsuccessful? How can you know if the problem you have truly is chronic pelvic pain versus another type of pain problem?

What Is Chronic Pelvic Pain?

The first step in solving this complex problem is to understand the definition of CPP and what factors must be present before this diagnosis can be made. Chronic Pelvic Pain is defined as any pelvic pain that lasts for more than six months.

Although acute pain may indicate specific active injury to some part of the body, chronic pain is very different. Often in CPP, the initial physical problem has lessened or even disappeared, but the pain continues because of changes in the nervous system, muscles, or other tissues.

This teaches us an important distinction:

- In acute pain, the pain is often a symptom of underlying tissue damage;

- In chronic pain, *the pain itself has become the disease.* Chronic pelvic pain is itself the diagnosis.

As this long-term, unrelenting pain process continues, even the strongest person's defenses may break down. This can result in associated emotional and behavioral changes. This symptom complex is termed "chronic pelvic pain syndrome."

There are six features common to all patients with chronic pelvic pain syndrome:

1. The pain has been present for six months or more;

2. Conventional treatments have yielded little relief;

3. The degree of pain perceived seems out of proportion to the degree of tissue damage detected by conventional means;

4. Physical appearance of depression is present (e.g., sleep disturbance, constipation, diminished appetite, "slow motion" body movements and reactions);

5. Physical activity has become increasingly limited; and

6. Emotional roles in the family are altered; the patient is displaced from her accustomed role (e.g., wife, mother, employee).

Thus, having associated psychological and behavioral symptoms with CPP is part of the typical expected evolution of chronic pelvic pain syndrome. Therefore, contrary to misguided beliefs, CPP is never "all in your head"; it is always a dynamic interaction of the *combined influences* of the mind, nervous system, and the body.

Can CPP Start One Place and End Up Somewhere Else?

Not only do emotional changes occur with the long-term tension of CPP, but also other organ systems beside that system where the pain originates become involved. For instance, we all can feel our muscles tense when we have pain—this tension can in turn cause changes in bowel and bladder function. It is therefore easy to imagine that long-term pain can cause more profound persistent problems in the muscles of the pelvis and adjacent areas, the urinary tract (bladder, urethra), the bowel, and even the overlying connective tissue and skin of the pelvic area. Often these secondary processes become the predominant problem, overshadowing the original disease process which may no longer even be detected.

Important principles:

1. By the time pain becomes chronic, multiple systems rather than a single problem is involved in the pain process. We must look for all the causes of CPP, not a single simple cause.

2. In searching for these causes, look *at*, then *beyond the female pelvic organs*.

How Is Pain Perceived?

The older theory of pain ("Cartesian Theory") is still the basic concept that many doctors and patients alike use to explain pain perception. This theory stated that specific nerve fibers ("neurons") act almost like a simple electric-wire connection carrying pain signals from damaged areas through the spinal cord directly to the cortex of the brain where pain is perceived. We now know that this concept is an oversimplification.

A newer theory called the "Gate Control Theory" likely is somewhat closer to the actual manner in which pain is perceived. Uncomfortable signals arise from injured or adversely stimulated tissues and travel through specialized nerve cells to the spinal cord. Here, these signals can be intensified, reduced, or even blocked. The spinal cord acts as a functional "gate", letting through, blocking, or at least changing the nature of pain signals before allowing their transmission to the brain.

The gate itself is influenced by local factors (other nerve inputs in the spinal cord), and by descending signals from the higher brain centers. Thus, other internal influences through the spinal cord and brain (besides the pain itself), and mood and external environmental factors from the brain all affect the nature of the pain's impulse transmission, and therefore pain perception. If the gates are damaged by chronic pain, they may remain open even after tissue damage is controlled, the pain will remain despite treating the originating cause; this type of pain is termed "neuropathic" pain.

What Are the Basic Elements of CPP? How Do They Apply to Pain Therapy?

To understand how to approach the treatment of chronic pelvic pain, three basic elements to chronic pain should be considered:

Pathology at the Site of Origin. Obviously, if the original source of tissue injury remains, pain will continue. This is called *pathology at the site of origin* (e.g., endometriosis, adhesions, infection, etc.).

Referred (Antidromic) Pain. The *Referred (Antidromic) Pain Concept* is of critical importance. Two types of nerves exist: *visceral nerves* carry impulses from intra-abdominal and thoracic structures into the spinal cord, while *somatic nerves* innervate superficial tissues, muscle, and skin. Visceral nerves and somatic nerves may synapse (meet) with the same nerve cell in the spinal cord and in this way have an influence on each other. When visceral nerves are chronically stimulated with unrelenting pain, the impulse will spill over in a reverse manner into the somatic nerve, which will carry the pain impulse in reverse fashion to areas of the abdominal wall, pelvic muscles, and superficial tissues. Specific areas of tenderness develop at those sites termed "trigger points", or referred pain. Although the trigger points may begin as a superficial expression of internal (visceral) pain, they may evolve into the patient's main source of pain. In some cases treatment of the trigger points may significantly reduce pain. In other cases, the visceral tissue injury must also be treated (surgical removal of endometriosis, adhesions, etc.).

Central Modulation by the Brain. The brain influences emotions and behavior and interacts with the spinal cord, modifying the perception of the visceral and referred pain. For instance, depression will allow more pain signals through to the brain. This is called central modulation by the brain. Central influences must also be treated with a variety of methods, including various psychological, physical, and pharmacologic (drug) therapies. *The simultaneous treatment of all levels of the pain process must be accomplished if there is to be any hope of success.*

How Do I Find Out if I Have CPP?

The history and physical examination (H&P) may tell us more about the reasons for your pain than any laboratory test or procedure. The H&P will also tell us which tests are appropriate for you specifically, and eliminate unnecessary testing.

History

Your ability to convey accurate, detailed, comprehensive information is directly related to how effective diagnostic evaluation and subsequent therapies may be.

In a single prolonged office visit, such a complex relaying of information may prove impossible and impose excessive stress on both you and your physician. Often, several shorter visits are more effective and productive.

To facilitate a "partnership in healing" between you and your physician, most pain practices first ask you to take the lead by conveying important information to the doctor's office *prior* to your first visit. This includes:

1. Obtaining all medical records of prior office, clinic, or hospital evaluations, and laboratory, radiological, psychological, and surgical testing. Any records of surgical treatments (including videotapes) are critical.

2. Carefully filling out a very detailed questionnaire concerning not only your pain problem, but also your entire medical, surgical, and family history. This will allow the physician to "know you well", even before you actually meet. It will not only speed the process of diagnosis and treatment, but will demonstrate how motivated you are in taking an active role in furthering your own care.

Completing the pain questionnaire also allows you the time to reflect and recall details otherwise missed during an interview and may allow you to more easily convey certain highly personal information that could be difficult for you to actually talk about. Lastly, this preliminary information frees the physician to immediately focus on those details you have already indicated are of the greatest significance.

Of great importance is an understanding of the past and present status of your pain and the chronology and how it developed. How and when did it begin? What actions or activities make it better or worse? Does it vary based on time of day, week, or menstrual cycle? Does it affect your sleep? Has it spread beyond where it was first noted? Is it associated with abnormal skin sensations, muscle or joint pain, or back pain? Is there any urinary pain or problems, constipation, diarrhea, or other bowel complaints? Has it affected your daily routine at home and at work? Has it led to emotional changes such as anxiety or depression? What have you personally done to attempt to alleviate the pain? What has your physician done? Have these been successful to any degree? What medications have you used in the past? What medications are you currently using? What do you think is causing your pain? What concerns you the most about your pain? All questions on the pain questionnaire were designed to elicit information that will be valuable in diagnosis and treatment of your pain condition.

Physical Examination

The physical examination for chronic pelvic pain will differ from a standard gynecologic exam since it is designed to provide information far beyond the condition of the female genital structures (e.g., cervix, uterus, tubes, and ovaries). Since the pelvis serves as the critical supporting structure for the upper body and is the connection to the lower body, the condition of upper and lower body structures may affect the pelvis, and vice-versa. Observations are made concerning your posture, gait, back and abdomen, thighs, and upper legs. Considerable detail is sometimes necessary regarding the musculoskeletal system, such as looking for problems that could increase general pelvic floor muscle tension or affect specific muscles. Changes in skin sensation, numbness, or tenderness can give clues to the specific pelvic nerves involved.

The abdomen and pelvis will be thoroughly checked for trigger points. The examination often proceeds in a precise grid-like pattern. You may be asked to tense your abdominal muscles by lifting your head to allow the doctor to distinguish internal pain from external abdominal wall pain. Hernias will be noted.

Not only will the vulva be examined, but also the entire areas surrounding the vagina and rectum will be carefully evaluated. The area of the glands on the inside of the minor lips of the vulva (the *vestibule*) are often a source of the pain (*vestibulitis*) and will be evaluated by lightly touching different sections of this area with a Q-tip.

Next, the vaginal area will be examined comprehensively, initially using only one examining finger rather than two (as in a standard exam) in order to obtain more precise information. Areas of tenderness may relate to problems with specific muscles, nerves, urinary tract structures, or cervical and paracervical problems. Following this, the bimanual exam will be done adding the abdominal hand's pressure into the pelvic region as needed to delineate conditions involving the uterus, cervix, tubes and ovaries, and to some extent the abdominal wall.

A rectovaginal examination is needed to further clarify findings, placing a finger in the rectum and one in the vagina. Characteristic areas of nodularity and tenderness in the area below the uterus (*cul-de-sac*) and uterosacral ligaments may be perceived most effectively in this manner and often suggests the presence of endometriosis.

You may be asked to tense and relax pelvic and abdominal muscles during the examination to clarify findings, and to reveal certain disorders of pelvic support (e.g., uterine prolapse).

The pelvic examination is completed by insertion of the speculum into the vagina to check for possible lesions of the vagina or cervix, infection, or other visible abnormalities.

During the course of the pelvic exam, you should inform the physician if anything being done causes you pain, and especially duplicates the specific pain that has been troubling you.

Diagnostic Testing

Diagnostic studies such as blood tests, x-rays, and ultrasound examinations may be necessary. Occasionally, more sophisticated imaging techniques such as CAT scans or MRI's may be required.

Most recently, pain mapping techniques that utilize a small diameter scope (*microlaparoscope*) may be done in a properly setup office setting or outpatient operating facility. While you are awake and conscious, you will be asked if touching certain areas inside the pelvis cause you pain, and if this duplicates components of the chronic pain you feel. Carefully noting these areas "maps" the location(s) of your pain for subsequent treatment.

Follow-up microlaparoscopic procedures ("second look") may be necessary to evaluate how effective lysis of adhesions has been, or to recut those adhesions that may have reformed.

Therapeutic Approaches

Several important common philosophies guide the clinician's therapeutic approaches to treating chronic pelvic pain:

1. Pain and its perception is located in the nervous system, which includes body and mind; therefore pain is not exclusively "all in your body", nor is it exclusively "all in your head." Therapies must be directed to both areas for effective treatment and reduction of pain.

2. Multiple interactive problems rather than a single problem are likely in CPP. The question is not what treatment is recommended, but what treatments.

3. The precise "percent" contribution of each pain factor to the total amount of your pain is difficult to assess. The initial factor that caused your pain, although important to locate and treat, may evolve into only a minor factor as pain becomes chronic, with secondary factors becoming more important. Therefore, all factors must be treated rather than just the ones you or prior physicians thought to be most important.

4. Improvement of your CPP may take considerable time, even though your physician is trying to give you relief as soon as possible. It took time for your pain to develop into the way it presents today. It may, therefore, take weeks to months for this stepwise progressive improvement to occur. Relaxation and emotional support techniques can be helpful during these periods to help preserve your patience and positive state of mind.

5. Pain medications (analgesics) may be used during the early stages of treatment since many therapies may take time to give relief. These medications are, however, not the cure for your pain, but merely a temporary supportive measure until other therapies "kick in" with their relieving effects. Remember that all medications have potential side effects, especially the narcotic analgesics with their strong dependency potential. Most clinicians choose to use non-narcotic analgesics as a first choice, and some avoid narcotic analgesics completely.

6. A combination of medications may prove more effective than a single type of medication. Analgesics may be more effective if

combined with different medications that have direct effects on mood and pain transmission, (e.g., certain antidepressants).

7. Pain medicines may not be given each time you complain of pain. This could reinforce your dependence on medication. A fixed time-schedule regimen of treatment called "time-contingent therapy" has proven far more effective in controlling pain than taking pain medicines whenever you feel the need. At each visit to the physician, you will be given prescriptions for a fixed amount of pain medication, and instructed to take a certain amount at regularly appointed time intervals. Should tolerance (decreased effectiveness to your current dose of medication) occur, it will be discussed at the next visit where changes in dose or particular medication can be made. As a rule, adjustments of pain medication will not be made by telephone. You must be seen with your clinic record in the office.

Particularly with narcotic analgesics, a written contract is frequently made to avoid their misuse. Lost or stolen prescriptions will not be replaced. It is your responsibility to be sure that your prescriptions are safe. Refills will not be given. If it is discovered that you have obtained additional narcotics from other physicians without permission, you may be discharged from the doctor's care.

Although these guidelines may seem severe, the potential damage from drug misuse is so dangerous that firm measures are mandatory to protect your health.

8. Physical Therapy is an integral part of therapy for recognition of many chronic pelvic pain conditions. Your musculoskeletal system will be evaluated by a physical therapist during a comprehensive examination. Your posture, gait, abdomen, pelvis, and lower extremities will be checked. You will also have an "internal" exam. Information concerning abnormalities, muscle strength, tenderness, length, and flexibility will be noted. Trigger points (exquisitely sensitive muscular points) will be mapped.

Therapy includes direct manipulative techniques externally and internally that will improve abnormal musculoskeletal physiology. Specific exercises to stretch or strengthen certain muscles or muscle groups may be advised and taught. Ancillary techniques may also be used, including the TENS (Transcutaneous Electrical Nerve Stimulation) unit, muscle stimulators, ultrasound, or various biofeedback modalities. Relaxation and breathing exercises may also be taught.

Effective treatment of trigger points may involve further consultation with the physician. A series of injections may be necessary to alleviate the source of pain.

9. Since it is often impossible to separate physical and emotional components of pain, adequate psychological evaluation and therapy is integral to successful pain reduction. Issues of anxiety, depression, work, family dynamics, sleep disturbances, sexual dysfunction, and sensitive issues of prior sexual or physical abuse are common factors in chronic pelvic pain syndrome.

    Through a variety of modalities, you will be better able to cope with your pain. This will improve your quality of life, reduce disabilities, and help you to overcome depression and anxiety. This is accomplished through changing behaviors that compound your pain.

10. Your chronic pain has affected not only you, but also your immediate family. The specifics of how your pain affects them and how their perceptions of your pain affects you must be understood. Educating your family as to the nature of problems found, treatments advised, and possible outcomes will help your recovery.

11. Surgical evaluation and treatment of certain CPP disorders are used. Laparoscopic exams are often critical in determining factors contributing to your pain as well as sometimes treating them. Classically, disorders such as pelvic adhesions and endometriosis are noted and treated with laparoscopy under general anesthesia in an outpatient setting, usually sending you home the very same day. The particular surgical procedure(s) used will depend on the conditions discovered.

12. During the course of evaluation and therapies, you must see your physician or therapist at regular preset intervals rather than just when the pain gets worse. You may begin with weekly or monthly visits with increasing or decreasing frequency as determined by your progress. Failure to keep your

appointments will prevent proper treatment. If you miss appointments and your pain level escalates, it will be more difficult to control the pain again.

Conclusion

You must at the very beginning of evaluation and therapy set realistic expectations for your treatment. Some chronic pelvic pain disorders cannot be completely resolved. Few patients are so resistant to a careful evaluation that significant pain reduction cannot be obtained. This may take time and often several modalities of therapy.

View successful management rather than elimination of your pain as your goal. Reduction of pain to low or barely noticeable levels which allows you to refocus your life away from pain and effectively resume your roles as wife, mother, and career woman is success.

Glossary

Acute Pain: pain that is episodic in nature, i.e., stubbing one's toe, having an accident, pain after surgery. Acute pain is temporary and centers on an injury.

Adhesions: fibrous structures that cause organs and structures which would not normally do so to adhere to each other.

Analgesics: a drug which eases pain without causing loss of consciousness.

Antidromic Pain: (see Referred Pain)

Cartesian Theory: an older theory of explaining pain which states that the nervous system is basically like electrical wires, carrying signals from the site of injury to the brain.

CAT Scan (computerized axial tomography): a diagnostic procedure more powerful than x-rays, but without the radiation.

Central Modulation by the Brain: the influence of emotion and behavior on your pain.

Chronic Pain: pain which lasts longer than 6 months.

Chronic Pelvic Pain: pelvic pain which lasts longer than 6 months. Chronic pelvic pain can appear without tissue injury, or remain after an original injury has healed. This is caused by changes in the nervous system, muscles, or other tissues. Chronic pelvic pain is itself a diagnosis.

Chronic Pelvic Pain Syndrome: a change in emotions and behaviors resulting from chronic pelvic pain.

Endometriosis: a condition in which tissue resembling the uterine lining occurs outside the uterus in various locations in the pelvic cavity.

Fibromyalgia: a chronic condition which causes widespread pain and profound fatigue along with other symptoms. Its effects are felt primarily in muscles, tendons, and ligaments throughout the body.

Fibroids: a benign tumor of smooth muscle and fibrous tissue occurring in the uterus and usually occurring in women in their 30's or 40's.

Gate Control Theory: a newer theory of pain which states that pain is transmitted through specialized nerve cells to the spinal cord, where the signals can be intensified, reduced, or even blocked. The spinal cord serves as a "gate" which can let pain signals through it, block them, or change them before transmission to the brain.

Laparoscope: a small instrument similar to a lighted telescope used for examining the pelvic area.

Levator: a muscle for elevating the organ or structure into which it is inserted.

Magnetic Resonance Imaging (MRI): produces internal images by generating powerful magnetic fields.

Microlaparoscope: a smaller version of the laparoscope.

Neurons: nerve fibers which perceive and transmit pain.

Neuropathic Pain: pain caused by changes in the spinal cord or nerve fibers which produce an abnormal signaling mechanism.

Pain Mapping: a procedure in which the physician attempts to duplicate the pain that a patient experiences in order to locate the exact source of the pain. The procedure is done while the patient is sedated, but conscious.

Pathology: the structural and functional ways a disease may present itself.

Pelvic Floor: muscles and soft tissues composing the support for the rectum, vagina, and bladder.

Referred (Antidromic) Pain: pain felt in superficial tissues, muscles, and skin and is caused by chronic internal organ (visceral) pain "spilling over" into these areas.

Somatic Nerves: nerves in the superficial tissues, muscles, and skin.

Synapse: the point at which a pain impulse is transmitted from one nerve to another.

Time-Contingent Therapy: medication taken on a strict timetable independent of pain level in order to maintain a constant blood level of the drug.

Transcutaneous Electrical Nerve Stimulation (TENS) Unit: battery-generated electrical impulses which can block pain by closing a gate of transmission.

Trigger Points: microscopic motor-neuron units that become exquisitely painful (see Gate Control Theory).

Uterosacral Ligaments: supporting ligaments which join the uterus and sacrum.

Vestibule: the entrance to the vagina.

Vestibulitis: exquisitely sensitive areas surrounding the entrance to the vagina which may produce pain on penetration.

Visceral Nerves: nerves which supply all internal organs, including uterus, tubes, ovaries, intestines, etc. A division of the autonomic (involuntary) nervous system.

About the International Pelvic Pain Society

The International Pelvic Pain Society was formed in 1996 for the purpose of educating health care professionals and women regarding the diagnosis and treatment of chronic pelvic pain in women.

Chronic pelvic pain is pelvic pain that occurs for at least six months. A few conditions that may cause this include: adhesions, endometriosis, vulvodynia, irritable bowel disease, interstitial cystitis and fibromyalgia. Over ten million women in the United States suffer with chronic pelvic pain. They are considered the medical "lepers" of the healthcare system. They face misdiagnosis, unnecessary surgeries, and prejudice as "drug seeker."

The Membership of the International Pelvic Pain Society is committed to an interdisciplinary approach to the treatment of chronic pelvic pain. Gynecologists, nurses, urologists, physical therapists, basic scientists, and other health care professionals are joining our membership. To join the IPPS, please go to our website. www.pelvic pain.org

Chapter 30

Phantom Pain

Any patient who undergoes an amputation, whether it be traumatic from an unexpected injury or from planned surgery, can develop phantom pain, stump pain, or both. Some studies suggest if a patient has pain in the area about to be amputated before the amputation, there is a greater likelihood of developing phantom pain.

Phantom Pain

Following an amputation, abnormal sensations can be felt from the amputated body part; that is, a patient may feel sensations in a limb (or any other amputated body part) which is no longer part of his/her body. In fact, these unusual phantom sensations occur in most people following amputation. The sensations can be changes in size or position, or actual feelings of heat, cold, or touch. In some patients, these abnormal sensations include pain. Because the pain is experienced in a part of the body that is no longer present, it is called phantom pain. Luckily, for most patients, both the phantom sensations and pain gradually resolve with time.

The actual cause of phantom pain is not known. Most authorities currently believe that both phantom pain and other phantom sensations are generated from the spinal cord and brain. It is believed that

"Phantom and Stump Pain," Department of Pain Medicine and Palliative Care at Beth Israel Medical Center, online at www.stoppain.org. © 2000 Continuum Health Partners, Inc.; reprinted with permission.

when a body part is amputated, the brain region responsible for perceiving sensation from that area begins to function abnormally, leading to the perception that the body part still exists.

Treatment of Phantom Pain

The treatment of phantom pain is difficult. No one treatment has shown to be effective in a majority of sufferers. Fortunately, there are treatment approaches that may be helpful in some patients.

Drug Therapy

Drugs used for phantom pain are:

- Antiseizure drugs (such as gabapentin, carbamazepine)
- Antidepressants (such as amitriptyline, nortriptyline)
- Local anesthetics (such as mexiletine)
- Alpha-2 adrenergic agonists (such as clonidine or tizanidine)
- Others, including calcitonin, badofen, dextromethorphan
- Opioids (such as morphine, oxycodone, methadone)

Other Therapies

Other approaches include:

- Nerve blocks
- Spinal cord stimulation
- Hypnosis, biofeedback, and other cognitive techniques (such as relaxation training and distraction)

Stump Pain

Stump pain is located at the end of an amputated limb's stump. Unlike phantom pain, it occurs in the body part that actually exists, in the stump that remains. It typically is described as a "sharp," "burning," "electric-like," or "skin-sensitive" pain.

Stump pain is due to a damaged nerve in the stump region. Nerves damaged in the amputation surgery try to heal and may form abnormally sensitive regions, called neuromas. A neuroma can cause pain and skin sensitivity.

Treatment of Stump Pain

No one treatment has been shown to be effective for stump pain. Because it is a pain due to an injured peripheral nerve, drugs used for nerve pain may be helpful. If the stump pain affects a limb, revision of the prosthesis is sometimes beneficial. Other approaches also are tried in selected cases, including:

- Nerve blocks

- Transcutaneous electrical nerve stimulation (TENS)

- Surgical revision of the stump or removal of the neuroma (This procedure may fail because the neuroma can grow back; some patients actually get worse after surgery.)

- Cognitive therapies

Chapter 31

Pinched Nerves

What Is Pinched Nerve?

The term pinched nerve describes one type of damage or injury to a nerve or set of nerves. The injury may result from compression, constriction, or stretching. Symptoms include numbness, "pins and needles" or burning sensations, and pain radiating outward from the injured area. One of the most common examples of a single compressed nerve is the feeling of having a foot or hand "fall asleep." Pinched nerves can sometimes lead to other conditions such as peripheral neuropathy, carpal tunnel syndrome, and tennis elbow. The extent of such injuries may vary from minor, temporary damage to a more permanent condition. Early diagnosis is important to prevent further damage or complications. Pinched nerve is a common cause of on-the-job injury.

Is There Any Treatment?

The most frequently recommended treatment for pinched nerve is rest for the affected area. Corticosteroids help alleviate pain. In some cases, surgery is recommended. Physical therapy may be recommended, and splints or collars may be used.

From "NINDS Pinched Nerve Information Page," National Institute of Neurological Disorders and Stroke (NINDS), at www.ninds.nih.gov. Reviewed July 2001.

What Is the Prognosis?

With treatment, most people recover from pinched nerve. However, in some cases, the damage is irreversible.

What Research Is Being Done?

Within the National Institute of Neurological Disorders and Stroke (NINDS) research programs, pinched nerves are addressed primarily through studies associated with pain research. NINDS vigorously pursues a research program seeking new treatments for pain and nerve damage with the ultimate goal of reversing debilitating conditions such as pinched nerves.

For More Information

National Rehabilitation Information Center (NARIC)
4200 Forbes Blvd., Suite 202
Lanham, MD 20706
Phone: (301) 459-5900
Fax: 301-562-2401
Website: http://www.naric.com

Chapter 32

Polymyalgia Rheumatica and Giant Cell Arteritis

What Are Polymyalgia Rheumatica and Giant Cell Arteritis?

Polymyalgia rheumatica is a rheumatic disorder that is associated with moderate to severe muscle pain and stiffness in the neck, shoulder, and hip area. Stiffness is most noticeable in the morning. This disorder may develop rapidly—in some patients, overnight. In other people, polymyalgia rheumatica develops more gradually. The cause of polymyalgia rheumatica is not known; however, possibilities include immune system abnormalities and genetic factors. The fact that polymyalgia rheumatica is rare in people under the age of 50 suggests it may be linked to the aging process.

Polymyalgia rheumatica may go away without treatment in one to several years. With treatment, the symptoms of polymyalgia rheumatica are quickly controlled, but relapse if treatment is stopped too early.

Giant cell arteritis, also known as temporal arteritis and cranial arteritis, is a disorder that results in swelling of arteries in the head (most often the temporal arteries, which are located on the temples on each side of the head), neck, and arms. This swelling causes the arteries to narrow, reducing blood flow. Early treatment is critical for good prognosis.

"Questions and Answers about Polymyalgia Rheumatica and Giant Cell Arteritis," National Institute of Arthritis and Musculoskeletal and Skin Diseases (NIAMS), February 2001.

How Are Polymyalgia Rheumatica and Giant Cell Arteritis Related?

It is unclear how or why polymyalgia rheumatica and giant cell arteritis are related, but an estimated 15 percent of people in the United States with polymyalgia rheumatica also develop giant cell arteritis. Patients can develop giant cell arteritis either at the same time as polymyalgia rheumatica or after the polymyalgia symptoms disappear. About half of the people affected by giant cell arteritis also have polymyalgia rheumatica.

When a person is diagnosed with polymyalgia rheumatica, the doctor also should look for symptoms of giant cell arteritis because of the risk of blindness. With proper treatment, the disease is not threatening. Untreated, however, giant cell arteritis can lead to serious complications including permanent vision loss and stroke. Patients must learn to recognize the signs of giant cell arteritis, because they can develop even after the symptoms of polymyalgia rheumatica disappear. Patients should report any symptoms to the doctor immediately.

Who Is at Risk?

White women over the age of 50 are most at risk of developing polymyalgia rheumatica and giant cell arteritis. Women are twice as likely as men to develop the conditions. Both conditions almost exclusively affect people over the age of 50. The average age at onset is 70 years. Polymyalgia rheumatica and giant cell arteritis are quite common. In the United States, it is estimated that 700 per 100,000 people in the general population over 50 years of age develop polymyalgia rheumatica. An estimated 200 per 100,000 people over the age of 50 develop giant cell arteritis.

What Are the Symptoms?

The primary symptoms of polymyalgia rheumatica are moderate to severe stiffness and muscle pain near the neck, shoulders, or hips. The stiffness is more severe upon waking or after a period of inactivity, and typically lasts longer than 30 minutes. People with this condition also may have flu-like symptoms, including fever, weakness, and weight loss.

Early symptoms of giant cell arteritis also may resemble the flu. People are likely to experience headaches, pain in the temples, and blurred or double vision. Pain may also affect the jaw and tongue.

How Are Polymyalgia Rheumatica and Giant Cell Arteritis Diagnosed?

No single test is available to definitively diagnose polymyalgia rheumatica. To diagnose the condition, a physician considers the patient's medical history, including symptoms that the patient reports, and results of laboratory tests that can rule out other possible diagnoses.

The most typical laboratory finding in people with polymyalgia rheumatica is an elevated erythrocyte sedimentation rate, commonly referred to as the sed rate. This test measures how quickly red blood cells fall to the bottom of a test tube of unclotted blood. Rapidly descending cells (an elevated sed rate) indicate inflammation in the body. While the sed rate measurement is a helpful diagnostic tool, it alone does not confirm polymyalgia rheumatica. An abnormal result indicates only that tissue is inflamed, which also is a symptom of many forms of arthritis and/or other rheumatic diseases. Before making a diagnosis of polymyalgia rheumatica, the doctor may perform additional tests to rule out other conditions, including rheumatoid arthritis, because symptoms of polymyalgia rheumatica and rheumatoid arthritis can be similar.

The doctor may recommend a test for rheumatoid factor (RF). RF is an antibody sometimes found in the blood. (An antibody is a special protein made by the immune system.) People with rheumatoid arthritis are likely to have RF in their blood, but most people with polymyalgia rheumatica do not. If the diagnosis still is unclear, a physician may conduct additional tests to rule out other disorders.

Doctors and patients both need to be aware of the risk of giant cell arteritis in people with polymyalgia rheumatica and should be on the lookout for symptoms of the disorder. Severe headaches, jaw pain, and vision problems are typical symptoms of giant cell arteritis. In addition, physical examination may reveal an abnormal temporal artery: tender to the touch, inflamed, and with reduced pulse. Because of the possibility of permanent blindness, a temporal artery biopsy is recommended if there is any suspicion of giant cell arteritis.

In a person with giant cell arteritis, the biopsy will show abnormal cells in the artery walls. Some patients showing symptoms of giant cell arteritis will have negative biopsy results. In such cases the doctor may suggest a second biopsy.

What Are the Treatments?

Polymyalgia rheumatica usually disappears without treatment in one to several years. With treatment, however, symptoms disappear quickly, usually in 24 to 48 hours. If there is no improvement, the doctor is likely to consider other possible diagnoses.

The treatment of choice is corticosteroid medication, usually prednisone. Polymyalgia rheumatica responds to a low daily dose of prednisone. The dose is increased as needed until symptoms disappear. Once symptoms disappear, the doctor may gradually reduce the dosage to determine the lowest amount needed to alleviate symptoms. The amount of time that treatment is needed is different for each patient. Most patients can discontinue medication after six months to two years. If symptoms recur, prednisone treatment is required again.

Nonsteroidal anti-inflammatory drugs (NSAIDs) such as aspirin and ibuprofen also may be used to treat polymyalgia rheumatica. The medication must be taken daily, and long-term use may cause stomach irritation. For most patients, NSAIDs alone are not enough to relieve symptoms.

Giant cell arteritis carries a small but definite risk of blindness. The blindness is permanent once it happens. A high dose of prednisone is needed to prevent blindness and should be started as soon as possible, perhaps even before the diagnosis is confirmed with a temporal artery biopsy. When treated, symptoms quickly disappear. Typically, people with giant cell arteritis must continue taking a high dose of prednisone for one month. Once symptoms disappear and the sed rate is normal and there is no longer a risk of blindness, the doctor can begin to gradually reduce the dose. When treated properly, giant cell arteritis rarely recurs.

People taking low doses of prednisone rarely experience side effects. Side effects are more common among people taking higher doses. But all patients should be aware of potential effects, which include:

- fluid retention and weight gain
- rounding of the face
- delayed wound healing
- bruising easily
- diabetes
- myopathy (muscle wasting)
- glaucoma
- increased blood pressure
- decreased calcium absorption in the bones, which can lead to osteoporosis

- irritation of the stomach

People taking corticosteroids may have some side effects or none at all. A patient should report any side effects to the doctor. When the medication is stopped, the side effects disappear. Because prednisone and other corticosteroid drugs change the body's natural production of corticosteroid hormones, the patient should not stop taking the medication unless instructed by the doctor. The patient and doctor must work together to gradually reduce the medication.

What Is the Outlook?

Most people with polymyalgia rheumatica and giant cell arteritis lead productive, active lives. The duration of drug treatment differs by patient. Once treatment is discontinued, polymyalgia may recur; but once again, symptoms respond rapidly to prednisone. When properly treated, giant cell arteritis rarely recurs.

What Research Is Being Conducted to Help People Who Have Polymyalgia Rheumatica and Giant Cell Arteritis?

Researchers studying possible causes of polymyalgia rheumatica and giant cell arteritis are investigating the role of genetic predisposition, immune system abnormalities, and environmental factors. Scientists also are looking for markers of the diseases, exploring treatments, and studying why the two disorders often occur together.

With funding from the National Eye Institute, a new mouse model of giant cell arteritis is being used to examine interactions between the immune system and blood vessels to explain tissue damage.

Where Can People Get More Information about Polymyalgia Rheumatica and Giant Cell Arteritis?

National Institute of Arthritis and Musculoskeletal and Skin Diseases Information Clearinghouse
NIAMS/National Institutes of Health
1 AMS Circle
Bethesda, MD 20892-3675
Phone: (301) 495-4484 or (877)-22-NIAMS (226-4267) (free of charge)
TTY: (301) 565-2966
Fax: (301) 718-6366
website: www.niams.nih.gov

National Eye Institute Information Clearinghouse
2020 Vision Place
Bethesda, MD 20892-3655
Phone: (301) 496-5248
Fax: (301) 402-1065
Website: www.nei.nih.gov

National Heart, Lung, and Blood Institute
31 Center Drive, MSC 2480
Bethesda, MD 20892-2480
Phone: (301) 496-4236
Fax: (301) 402-2405
Website: www.nhlbi.nih.gov

American College of Rheumatology
1800 Century Place, Suite 250
Atlanta, GA 30345
Phone: (404) 633-3777
Fax: (404) 633-1870
Website: www.rheumatology.org

Arthritis Foundation
1330 West Peachtree Street
Atlanta, GA 30309
Phone: (404) 872-7100 or (800) 283-7800 (free of charge) or call your
local chapter (listed in the telephone directory)
Website: www.arthritis.org

Acknowledgements

The NIAMS gratefully acknowledges the assistance of Gene G. Hunder, M.D., and Cornelia M. Weyland, M.D., of the Mayo Clinic, and Louis A. Healey, M.D. (retired), in the preparation and review of this text.

Chapter 33

Polyneuropathy

The Causes of Painful Polyneuropathy: Symptoms and Diagnosis

A "neuropathy" is a condition in which the peripheral nerves (the nerves in your body, aside from your spinal cord and brain) are damaged or not working correctly. There are hundreds of different types of neuropathies and many different ways to categorize them, including by the type of nerve damaged, the causes of the nerve damage, or the pattern of nerve damage.

A "polyneuropathy" is a neuropathy pattern, whereby the nerve damage initially starts in both feet and may progress to involve the feet, calves, and fingers/hands. Another word for this pattern is a "Stocking and Glove Neuropathy." Many patients with polyneuropathy may not even have any symptoms; in this case the diagnosis is made by a physical examination or a laboratory test (electromyography (EMG) and nerve conduction velocity test (NCV)). Some patients with polyneuropathy have only numbness, "tingling," and/or "pins and needles." Less often, some unlucky patients with polyneuropathy experience pain.

"Polyneuropathy—Diabetic Neuropathy, AIDS Neuropathy, and Others," Department of Pain Medicine and Palliative Care at Beth Israel Medical Center, online at www.stoppain.org. © 2000 Continuum Health Partners, Inc.; reprinted with permission.

The Causes of Painful Polyneuropathy

There are many causes of painful polyneuropathy. The most common cause is diabetes, both Type 1 and Type 2. Other causes include old age, certain drugs (such as some chemotherapy drugs), alcohol abuse, AIDS, environmental toxins, and inherited neurological neuropathies. However, in up to one-third of patients with painful polyneuropathy, no underlying cause can be found. Importantly, the chance of obtaining pain relief with proper treatment is the same for patients with or without a known etiology.

The actual injury to the nerves may result from several different problems. Possible injuries include:

- not enough blood supply to the nerves, resulting in loss of oxygen and other needed nutrients to the nerve and thus damage to the nerve, and

- abnormal function of the nerve itself, such that the nutrients within the nerve are not properly metabolized. In any individual patient, it is not possible to find out which type of problem exists. However, it does not matter which problem is present with regard to pain treatment.

Symptoms and Diagnosis

The symptoms of painful polyneuropathy start in the toes and feet (right and left). In some patients the symptoms gradually rise up the calves and into the knees. This is called a "stocking pattern." Then, in some the symptoms may also begin in the fingers and hands—causing a "stocking and glove pattern." It cannot be predicted how any one patient's symptoms will spread. In some patients, the pain does not spread beyond the toes or feet; in others, the progression to calves and hands occurs in months; and yet in others the spread is very gradual, over many years.

Patients who develop pain with polyneuropathy describe the pain using a variety of words, including "burning," "raw skin," "skin sensitivity," "sharp," "electric-like," "deep ache," "freezing cold," "like walking on ground glass," "itchy," and others. Some patients say they don't have pain but have unpleasant and irritating sensations, which may include "buzzing," "like bugs crawling," and "aching." Some patients have constant pains, day and night, whereas others only have noticeable pain at bedtime. Often, patients may complain that the pain interferes with their sleep.

Some patients with polyneuropathy may have difficulty feeling things with their feet or hands. Therefore, it is very important that these patients examine their affected skin areas regularly to make sure they haven't injured themselves (cuts, burns, infections, etc.). Also, some patients with neuropathy have trouble with their balance when walking; these patients should keep a nightlight on in their bedrooms and bathrooms, so they do not fall when they get up at night.

As with all chronic pain, patients with painful polyneuropathy may develop depression and sleep problems.

Diagnosing Polyneuropathy

Most often, a doctor should be able to diagnose painful polyneuropathy solely on a patient's description of his/her symptoms and a simple neurological examination. Sometimes, however, a doctor may order special nerve tests, electromyography (EMG) and nerve conduction testing (NCV); please note that EMG/NCV are painful tests: a doctor sticks a needle in the muscle and send electric shocks along the nerves to measure how well nerves are working. Another type of nerve test, quantitative sensory testing (QST), is less painful and measures how well the patient feels vibration and temperature changes. Importantly, in some painful polyneuropathy patients, the EMG/NCV tests may be completely normal.

Chapter 34

Reflex Sympathetic Dystrophy Syndrome

What Is Reflex Sympathetic Dystrophy Syndrome?

Reflex sympathetic dystrophy syndrome (RSDS)—also known as complex regional pain syndrome (see Chapter 17 for additional information)—is a chronic condition characterized by severe burning pain, pathological changes in bone and skin, excessive sweating, tissue swelling, and extreme sensitivity to touch. The syndrome, which is a variant of a condition known as causalgia, is a nerve disorder that occurs at the site of an injury (most often to the arms or legs). It occurs especially after injuries from high-velocity impacts such as those from bullets or shrapnel. However, it may occur without apparent injury.

Causalgia was first documented in the 19th century by physicians concerned about pain Civil War veterans continued to experience after their wounds had healed. Doctors often called it "hot pain," after its primary symptom. Over the years, the syndrome was classified as one of the peripheral neuropathies, and later, as a chronic pain syndrome. RSDS is currently classified as a variant of causalgia, not necessarily caused by trauma.

What Are the Symptoms of RSDS?

The symptoms of RSDS usually occur near the site of an injury, either major or minor, and include: burning pain, muscle spasms, local

"Reflex Sympathetic Dystrophy Syndrome," a fact sheet produced by the National Institute of Neurological Disorders and Stroke (NINDS), July 1, 2001.

swelling, increased sweating, softening of bones, joint tenderness or stiffness, restricted or painful movement, and changes in the nails and skin. One visible sign of RSDS near the site of injury is warm, shiny red skin that later becomes cool and bluish. The pain that patients report is out of proportion to the severity of the injury and gets worse, rather than better, over time. It is frequently characterized as a burning, aching, searing pain, which may initially be localized to the site of injury or the area covered by an injured nerve but spreads over time, often involving an entire limb. It can sometimes even involve the opposite extremity. Pain is continuous and may be heightened by emotional stress. Moving or touching the limb is often intolerable. Eventually the joints become stiff from disuse, and the skin, muscles, and bone atrophy.

The symptoms of RSDS vary in severity and duration. However, there are usually three stages associated with RSDS, and each stage is marked by progressive changes in the skin, nails, muscles, joints, ligaments, and bones.

Stage one lasts from 1 to 3 months and is characterized by severe, burning pain at the site of the injury. Muscle spasm, joint stiffness, restricted mobility, rapid hair and nail growth, and vasospasm (a constriction of the blood vessels) that affects color and temperature of the skin can also occur.

In stage two, which lasts from 3 to 6 months, the pain intensifies. Swelling spreads, hair growth diminishes, nails become cracked, brittle, grooved, and spotty, osteoporosis becomes severe and diffuse, joints thicken, and muscles atrophy.

As the patient reaches stage three, changes in the skin and bones become irreversible, and pain becomes unyielding and may now involve the entire limb. There is marked muscle atrophy, severely limited mobility of the affected area, and flexor tendon contractions (contractions of the muscles and tendons that flex the joints). Occasionally the limb is displaced from its normal position, and marked bone softening is more dispersed.

What Causes RSDS?

The cause of RSDS is unknown. The syndrome is thought to be the result of damaged nerves of the sympathetic nervous system—the part of the nervous system responsible for controlling the diameter of blood vessels. These damaged nerves send inappropriate signals to the brain, interfering with normal information about sensations, temperature, and blood flow.

Since RSDS is most often caused by trauma to the extremities, other conditions that can bring about RSDS include sprains, fractures, surgery, damage to blood vessels or nerves, and cerebral lesions. The disorder is unique in that it simultaneously affects the nerves, skin, muscles, blood vessels, and bones.

Who Gets It?

RSDS can strike at any age, but is more common between the ages of 40 and 60. It affects both men and women, but is most frequently seen in women. Although it can occur at any age, the number of RSDS cases among adolescents and young adults is increasing. Investigators estimate that two to five percent of those with peripheral nerve injury and 12 to 21 percent of those with hemiplegia (paralysis of one side of the body) will suffer from RSDS.

How Is RSDS Diagnosed?

RSDS is often misdiagnosed because it remains poorly understood. Diagnosis is complicated by the fact that some patients improve without treatment. A delay in diagnosis and/or treatment for this syndrome can result in severe physical and psychological problems. Early recognition and prompt treatment provide the greatest opportunity for recovery.

RSDS is diagnosed primarily through observation of the symptoms. However, some physicians use thermography—a diagnostic technique for measuring blood flow by determining the variations in heat emitted from the body—to detect changes in body temperature that are common in RSDS. A color-coded "thermogram" of a person in pain often shows an altered blood supply to the painful area, appearing as a different shade (abnormally pale or violet) than the surrounding areas of the corresponding part on the other side of the body. An abnormal thermogram in a patient who complains of pain may lead to a diagnosis of RSDS. X-rays may also show changes in the bone.

What Is the Prognosis?

Good progress can be made in treating RSDS if treatment is begun early, ideally within 3 months of the first symptoms. Early treatment often results in remission. If treatment is delayed, however, the disorder can quickly spread to the entire limb and changes in bone and muscle may become irreversible. In 50 percent of RSDS cases, pain persists longer than 6 months and sometimes for years.

What Is the Treatment?

Physicians use a variety of drugs to treat RSDS, including corticosteroids, vasodilators, and alpha- or beta-adrenergic-blocking compounds. Elevation of the extremity and physical therapy are also used to treat RSDS. Injection of a local anesthetic, such as lidocaine, is usually the first step in treatment. Injections are repeated as needed. TENS (transcutaneous electrical stimulation), a procedure in which brief pulses of electricity are applied to nerve endings under the skin, has helped some patients in relieving chronic pain.

In some cases, surgical or chemical sympathectomy—interruption of the affected portion of the sympathetic nervous system—is necessary to relieve pain. Surgical sympathectomy involves cutting the nerve or nerves, destroying the pain almost instantly. But surgery may also destroy other sensations as well.

Are There Any Other Disorders Like RSDS?

RSDS has many of the same features as causalgia, such as severe burning pain that is aggravated by physical or emotional stimuli. However, causalgia usually affects the lower limbs, the palm of the hand or the sole of the foot; RSDS may strike any part of the body.

RSDS also has characteristics similar to those of other disorders, such as shoulder-hand syndrome, which sometimes occurs after a heart attack and is marked by pain and stiffness in the arm and shoulder; Sudeck's syndrome, which is prevalent in older people and in women and is characterized by bone changes and muscular atrophy, but is not always associated with trauma; and Steinbrocker's syndrome, which affects both sexes but is slightly more prevalent in females, and includes such symptoms as gradual stiffness, discomfort, and weakness in the shoulder and hand.

What Research Is Being Done?

The National Institute of Neurological Disorders and Stroke (NINDS), a part of the National Institutes of Health (NIH), supports and conducts research on the brain and central nervous system, including research relevant to RSDS, through grants to major medical institutions across the country. NINDS-supported scientists are working to develop effective treatments for neurological conditions and, ultimately, to find ways of preventing them.

Investigators are studying new approaches to treat RSDS and intervene more aggressively after traumatic injury to lower the patient's chances of developing the disorder. In addition, NINDS-supported scientists are studying how signals of the sympathetic nervous system cause pain in RSDS patients. Using a technique called microneurography, these investigators are able to record and measure neural activity in single nerve fibers of affected patients. By testing various hypotheses, these researchers hope to discover the unique mechanism that causes the spontaneous pain of RSDS and that discovery may lead to new ways of blocking pain.

Other studies to overcome chronic pain syndromes are discussed in the pamphlet *"Chronic Pain: Hope Through Research,"* published by the NINDS.

Is Help Available?

The unrelenting pain from RSDS has caused many patients much physical and emotional misery. Family, friends, coworkers, and, regrettably, physicians themselves, may regard the patient as a complainer, thereby increasing the patient's distress. To meet the needs of individuals with RSDS and other conditions causing chronic pain, the following voluntary health agencies promote research, provide information, and may offer advice on coping. For information, write or call:

American Chronic Pain Association
P.O. Box 850
Rocklin, California 95677
Phone: (916) 632-0922
Website: www.theacpa.org

National Chronic Pain Outreach Association, Inc.
P.O. Box 274
Millboro, Virginia 24460
Phone: (540) 862-9437

RSDHope/ Maine RSDS Patient Advocacy Group
P.O. Box 875
Harrison, ME 04040-0875
Phone: (207) 583-4589
Website: www.rsdhope.org

RSDS Association
116 Haddon Avenue, Suite D
Haddonfield, New Jersey 08033
Phone: (856) 795-8845
Website: www.rsds.org

Chapter 35

Sciatica

If you suddenly start feeling pain in your lower back or hip that radiates down from your buttock to the back of one thigh and into your leg, your problem may be a protruding disk in your lower spinal column pressing on the roots to your sciatic nerve. Sciatica (lumbar radiculopathy) may feel like a bad leg cramp that lasts for weeks before it goes away. You may have pain, especially when you sit, sneeze or cough. You may also feel weakness, "pins and needles" numbness, or a burning or tingling sensation down your leg. See a doctor to have your condition diagnosed and start a course of treatment.

You're most likely to get sciatica when you're 30-50 years old. It may happen due to the effects of general wear and tear, plus any sudden pressure on the disks that cushion the vertebrae of your lower (lumbar) spine. The gel-like inside (nucleus) of a disk may protrude into or through the disk's outer lining (annulus). This herniated disk may press directly on nerve roots that become the sciatic nerve. The nerve may also get inflamed and irritated by chemicals from the disk's nucleus. About one in every 50 people experience a herniated disk. Of these, 10-25 percent have symptoms lasting more than six weeks. About 80-90 percent of people with sciatica get better, over time, without surgery.

Treatment

The condition usually heals itself if you give it enough time and rest. Tell your doctor how your pain started, where it travels and exactly what it feels like. A physical exam may help pinpoint the irritated nerve root. Your doctor may ask you to squat and rise, walk on your heels and toes or perform a straight leg raising test or other tests. Most cases of sciatica affect the L5 or S1 nerve roots. Later, X-rays and other specialized imaging tools such as MRI (magnetic resonance imaging) may confirm your doctor's diagnosis of which nerve roots are affected.

Treatment is aimed at helping you manage your pain without long-term use of medications. First, you'll probably need at least a few days of bed rest while the inflammation goes away. Nonsteroidal anti-inflammatory medications (NSAIDs) such as ibuprofen, aspirin or muscle relaxants may also help. You may find it soothing to put gentle heat or cold on your painful muscles. Find positions that are comfortable, but be as active as possible. Motion helps to reduce inflammation. Most of the time, your condition will get better within a few weeks. Sometimes, your doctor may inject your spine area with a cortisone-like drug. As soon as possible, start physical therapy with stretching exercises to help you resume your physical activities without sciatica pain. To start, your doctor may want you to take short walks.

You might need surgery only if after three months or more of treatment you still have disabling leg pain. A part of the herniated disk may be removed to stop it from pressing on your nerve. The surgery (laminotomy) may be done under local, spinal or general anesthesia. You have a 90 percent chance of successful surgery if most of your pain is in your leg. Avoid driving, excessive sitting, lifting or bending forward for at least a month after surgery. Your doctor may give you exercises to strengthen your back.

Following treatment for sciatica, you will probably be able to resume your normal lifestyle and keep your pain under control. However, it's always possible for your disk to rupture again. This happens to about five percent of people with sciatica.

Emergency Situation

In rare cases, a herniated disk may press on nerves that cause you to lose control of your bladder or bowel. If this happens, you may also have numbness or tingling in your groin or genital area. This is an emergency situation that requires surgery. Phone your doctor immediately.

Chapter 36

Sexual Pain (Dyspareunia)

Pain during sexual intercourse is not a normal condition, and it's not something you have to live with. Although you may think you are alone, a surprisingly large number of women experience this condition at some point in their lives.

What Is Dyspareunia?

The term dyspareunia (dis-pa-roon-ia) is the medical term for pain during sexual intercourse. Fear and embarrassment prevent many women from seeking help for dyspareunia. They may think they are abnormal. Or they may think nothing can be done. But that isn't true. Much can be done.

Thankfully, changing social attitudes have encouraged discussion of pain during sex. For more information about dyspareunia and its treatment, talk to your doctor or another healthcare professional.

What You Should Know about Dyspareunia

- Dyspareunia is quite common. Clinical studies show that approximately 10% of women experience pain during intercourse.

- Dyspareunia can be experienced during penetration or during deep thrusting. Women may experience either type or both.

- All kinds of women experience dyspareunia. It affects women regardless of marital status, income, age, race or childbearing history.

- Embarrassment prevents many women from seeking help and leads to unnecessary suffering and problems with their partner.

- Many effective treatments are available. These include medications, relaxation exercises and surgery.

Causes of Pain

Pain during sexual intercourse can occur for a variety of reasons such as an allergic reaction to a personal hygiene product or a physical problem. Sometimes, emotional issues play a role in the pain.

The causes of pain during sex include:

Infection: Bacterial or yeast infections are among the most common causes of pain during intercourse.

Lack of estrogen: During menopause, the vaginal walls thin, and the amount of vaginal lubrication decreases.

Vulvodynia: In this condition, the vulva is hypersensitive and extremely tender on touch.

Additional Causes of Pain

Pelvic floor muscle spasms: Involuntary muscle spasms can result in difficult and uncomfortable sex.

Drug side effects: Common drugs including those for allergy, high blood pressure or depression may affect the amount of vaginal lubrication, as well as the level of sexual arousal and desire.

Endometriosis: The tissue lining the uterus—the endometrium—may grow outside the uterus causing deep pain during sex.

Retroverted (tipped) uterus: If the uterus is retroverted or tipped backwards, the penis can hit the cervix or uterus during sexual intercourse causing deep and intense pain. This type of pain is called collision dyspareunia and may be more common than previously thought.

Other physical problems: Scar tissue from abdominal surgery or from delivering a baby can distort the anatomy and cause significant pain during sexual intercourse. A cyst on an ovary can also cause pain.

Emotional issues: Sometimes, past issues such as sexual abuse or communication problems in a relationship can translate into sexual difficulties.

Pain during sex may be caused by other reasons as well. Only consultation with your doctor or another healthcare professional will help you find out why you are experiencing pain and help you with a solution.

How Is Dyspareunia Diagnosed?

Basic Diagnostic Procedures

One of the easiest ways of diagnosing your problem is through a description of it. You can help by being open and candid. It may be helpful to think of the interview process as a heart to heart talk with a good friend.

Your doctor is aware that the subject is a sensitive one that involves private issues. He or she will be very supportive and will maintain confidentiality to protect your privacy Remember, your doctor is there to help you.

You may also want to write down any questions or concerns before your appointment.

During the appointment, your doctor will interview you about some of the following subjects:

- Characteristics of the pain such as its strength, how long it lasts and where it occurs
- When you feel the pain
- Other symptoms you may have such as headache, nausea or fatigue
- Past medical history
- Family history

A pelvic exam will help your doctor locate any areas of tenderness and identify other possible physical causes of your pain.

Additional Diagnostic Procedures

Depending on the results of your history and the pelvic exam, your physician may also use some of the following diagnostic tools:

- Lab tests: Cultures are used to check for infections.
- MRI and CT: Scans are used to check for physical problems.
- Ultrasound: This non-invasive procedure is used to check the ovaries and the uterus.
- Laparoscopy: A miniature camera is used to visualize your internal organs through small incisions made in your abdomen to check for physical problems.

Treatment Options

Depending on the results of your exam, your doctor will develop a personalized treatment plan that may include some of the following options:

Medications: In the case of an infection, treatment with medication often solves the problem.

Lubrication: Use of a cream or jelly can help make sexual intercourse more comfortable in cases when there is not enough natural lubrication.

Relaxation exercises: Relaxation exercises may help a woman regain control over vaginal muscles, thus reducing pain and making sexual intercourse more pleasurable.

Surgery: If diagnostic tests determine a physical problem is involved such as endometriosis or a tipped uterus, surgery may be recommended.

If You Need Surgery

If surgery is recommended, it may be performed using laparoscopic technique.

In laparoscopy, a small incision is made in the abdomen allowing the physician to insert a miniature camera or scope to visualize the internal organs. The physician then passes specialized surgical instruments through one or more additional small incisions to perform the procedure.

In most cases, recovery time is reduced, and patient comfort is improved compared to traditional surgery.

For example, deep pain related to a tipped uterus may be treated with a laparoscopic procedure known as the UPLIFT procedure. The UPLIFT procedure is one method of repositioning the uterus. In the UPLIFT procedure, the ligaments holding the uterus in place are shortened and strengthened to reposition the uterus in a more normal position. The procedure reduces the possibility of the penis hitting the cervix or uterus and causing pain during intercourse.

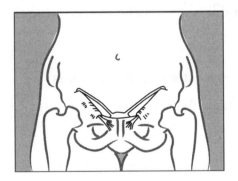

Figure 36.1. Tipped uterus

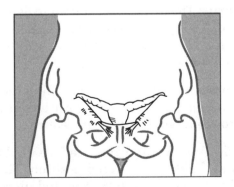

Figure 36.2. Uterus repositioned in normal position

Questions or Concerns

The following are questions or concerns you should discuss with your doctor or healthcare professional:

- Location of the pain (at entry, deep, etc.)

- Characteristics of the pain (dull, aching, sharp, etc.)

- When it happens (at entry, during intercourse, after intercourse, etc.)

- Methods used to cope with the pain (avoid intercourse, change positions, have intercourse only at certain times of the month, etc.)

- Reasons you think you may be experiencing the pain.

Glossary

Cervix: The narrow outer end of the uterus.

Collision dyspareunia: A type of dyspareunia caused by the penis hitting the cervix or uterus. The condition is associated with a retroverted or tipped uterus.

Dyspareunia: The medical term for pain during sexual intercourse.

Endometriosis: A condition in which the tissue lining the uterus begins to grow in other places causing pain and scar tissue.

Laparoscopy: A procedure in which a slender camera is inserted into a small incision in the abdomen to view the internal organs.

Retroverted uterus: The medical term used to describe a uterus that is tipped backward. A surgical procedure to reposition the uterus may be recommended if a woman with a retroverted uterus is experiencing collision dyspareunia.

UPLIFT procedure: A method of repositioning the uterus in which the ligaments holding the uterus in position are shortened and strengthened through a laparoscopic procedure.

Uterine repositioning: A surgical procedure used to reposition the uterus in a neutral/slightly anteverted position. The procedure may be recommended to women with a retroverted uterus who are experiencing collision dyspareunia.

Vaginitis: An inflammation of the vagina. Often caused by an infection.

Vulva: The outer area of a woman's genitals.

Vulvodynia: A chronic condition in which the vulva is hypersensitive to touch or pressure. Sexual intercourse is very painful. In some women, even a light touch associated with tampon use or tight clothing may provoke symptoms.

Additional Help and Information

Inlet Medical, Inc.
10180 Viking Drive
Eden Prairie, MN 55344
Phone: (612) 942-5034
Phone: (800) 969-0269
Fax: (612) 829-7112
Website: www.inletmedical.org
Website: www.inletmedical.com

Partners with gynecologists to design laparoscopic surgical instruments and kits to restore women's health.

The website is constantly updated with new information and resources. Visit http://www.inletmedical.org/html/new.htm for the most recent updates and content additions.

International Pelvic Pain Society
Phone: (800) 624-9676
Website: www.pelvicpain.org

A forum for professional and public education about the diagnosis and treatment of chronic pelvic pain.

Chapter 37

Shingles

In Italy, shingles is also called St. Anthony's fire, a fitting name for a disease that has bedeviled saints and sinners throughout the ages. Caused by the same varicella-zoster virus that causes chickenpox, shingles (also called herpes zoster) most commonly occurs in older people. Treatment was once limited to wet compresses and aspirin. Today's treatments provide a variety of ways to shorten the duration of a shingles outbreak and to control the associated pain. Sometimes, however, shingles leads to a chronic painful condition called post-herpetic neuralgia (PHN) that can be difficult to treat.

Initial Symptoms

After an attack of chickenpox, the varicella-zoster virus retreats to nerve cells in the body, where it may lie dormant for decades. But under certain conditions, usually related to aging or disease, the virus can reactivate and begin to reproduce. Once activated, the virus travels along the path of a nerve to the skin's surface, where it causes shingles.

Shingles' symptoms may be vague and nonspecific at first. People with shingles may experience numbness, tingling, itching, or pain before the classic rash appears. In the pre-eruption stage, diagnosis may be difficult, and the pain can be so severe that it may be mistaken for pleurisy, kidney stones, gallstones, appendicitis, or even a heart attack, depending on the location of the affected nerve.

"Shingles: An Unwelcome Encore," by Evelyn Zamula, *FDA Consumer*, U.S. Food and Drug Administration (FDA), May-June 2001.

The Outbreak

Pain may come first, but when the migrating virus finally reaches the skin—usually the second to the fifth day after the first symptoms—the rash tells all. The virus infects the skin cells and creates a painful, red rash that resembles chickenpox.

Doctors can distinguish shingles from chickenpox (or dermatitis or poison ivy) by the way the spots are distributed. Since shingles occurs in an area of the skin that is supplied by sensory fibers of a single nerve—called a dermatome—the rash usually appears in a well-defined band on one side of the body, typically the torso; or on one side of the face, around the nose and eyes. (Shingles' peculiar name derives from the Latin *cingulum*, which means girdle or belt.) If a diagnosis is in doubt, lab tests can confirm the presence of the virus.

The rash usually begins as clusters of small bumps that soon develop into fluid-filled blisters (vesicles). In turn, the blisters fill with pus (pustules), break open, and form crusty scabs. In about four or five weeks, the disease runs its course, the scabs drop off, the skin heals, and the pain fades. Most healthy individuals make an uneventful, if not particularly pleasant, recovery.

Not everyone sails through without incident, however. Although it's difficult to resist scratching the itchy rash, it's better to keep hands off, as the damaged skin may develop a bacterial infection requiring antibiotic treatment. After such an infection, the skin may be left with significant scarring, some of it serious enough to require plastic surgery.

Another complication called the Ramsay Hunt syndrome occurs when the varicella-zoster virus spreads to the facial nerve, causing intense ear pain. The rash can appear on the outer ear, inside the ear canal, on the soft palate (part of the roof of the mouth), around the mouth and on the face, neck and scalp. The hearing loss, vertigo and facial paralysis that may result are usually, but not always, temporary.

Occasionally, the rash will appear as a single spot or cluster of spots on the tip of the nose, called Hutchinson's sign. This is not good news. It means that the ophthalmic nerve is probably involved and the eye may become affected, possibly causing temporary or permanent blindness.

"My husband was undergoing chemotherapy treatment for prostate cancer," says Julia Hershfield, of Kensington, Md., "when he developed shingles in his right eye. The pain was so bad, that he lost all will to live. Shingles finished him." In people whose immune systems

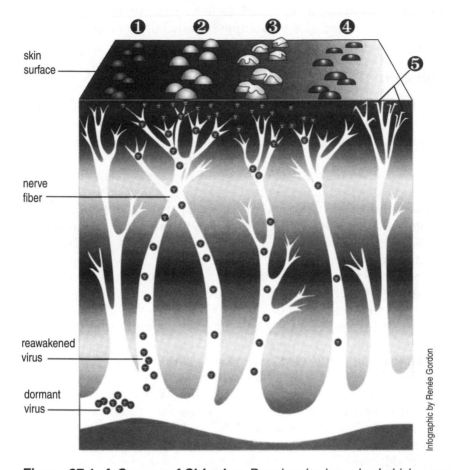

Figure 37.1. A Course of Shingles. *People who have had chickenpox (varicella zoster) in their youth can develop shingles (herpes zoster) in later years. During an acute attack of the chickenpox virus, most of the viral organisms are destroyed, but some survive, travel up nerve fibers along the spine, and lodge in nerve cells where they may lie dormant for many years. A decrease in the body's resistance can cause the virus to reawaken decades later. It then travels back down the nerve fibers to the skin's surface. The reawakened virus generally causes a vague burning sensation or tingling over an area of skin. A painful rash usually occurs two to five days after the first symptoms appear. A cluster of small bumps (1) turns into blisters (2) that resemble chickenpox lesions. The blisters fill with pus, break open (3), crust over (4), and finally disappear. This process takes four to five weeks. A painful condition called post-herpetic neuralgia can sometimes occur. This condition is thought to be caused by damage to the nerves (5), and can last from weeks to years after the rash disappears.*

are extremely weakened, the shingles virus can also spread to the internal organs and affect the lungs, central nervous system and the brain, sometimes causing death.

Chickenpox Redux

Like other members of the herpes family (such as the herpes simplex viruses that cause cold sores and genital herpes), the varicella-zoster virus that causes chickenpox never completely leaves the body. Most people don't get chickenpox a second time. However, anyone who has had chickenpox has the potential to develop shingles, because after recovery from chickenpox, the virus settles in the nerve roots.

Researchers are not sure exactly what triggers the virus to spontaneously start reproducing in nerve cells later in life and reappear as shingles. However, they do know the virus may reactivate when the immune system is weak.

Certain factors can cause the immune system to let down its guard. Age is one of them. Immunity declines with aging, so susceptibility to disease increases. The incidence of shingles and of resulting PHN rises with increasing age. More than 50 percent of cases occur in people over 60. Older people may also lack exposure to children with chickenpox, thereby losing an opportunity to boost immunity and prevent virus reactivation. Although most people have only one attack of shingles, about four percent will have further attacks.

People who have had chickenpox cannot "catch" shingles from someone who has it. However, people who've never had chickenpox can be infected with chickenpox if exposed to someone with an active case of shingles. The rash sheds the varicella-zoster virus and can be contagious. A caregiver or other person who lacks immunity developed from a prior case of chickenpox or the vaccine must avoid coming into contact with the rash or contaminated materials.

Also at risk for shingles are people with leukemia, lymphoma, or Hodgkin's disease, and those whose immune systems have been weakened because they are HIV-positive, or have undergone chemotherapy, radiation, transplant surgery with immunosuppression, or treatment with corticosteroids. Moreover, about five percent of people with shingles are found to have an underlying cancer, about twice the number of people in the population expected to have undiagnosed cancer.

It pays to be vigilant when unexplained symptoms occur. "New development of a rash or pain, especially when it occurs on only one side of the chest or face, should prompt a visit to the health-care provider," says Therese A. Cvetkovich, M.D., a medical officer in the Food and Drug Administration's Center for Drug Evaluation and Research (CDER).

Controlling the Outbreak

Although viral diseases can't be cured, doctors can prescribe oral antiviral medications, such as Zovirax (acyclovir), Famvir (famciclovir) and Valtrex (valacyclovir), that help control the infection by hindering reproduction of the virus in the nerve cells. "Antiviral therapy may shorten the course of an episode of shingles," says Cvetkovich. "However, therapy must be started as early as possible after symptoms develop—within 48 hours—in order to have an effect."

To relieve pain, the doctor may recommend over-the-counter analgesics (pain-relieving drugs), such as ibuprofen and naproxen, or prescription drugs, such as indomethacin, all members of a class of medications known as nonsteroidal anti-inflammatory drugs. Acetaminophen is also commonly used to relieve the pain. If pain is severe, doctors may add stronger analgesics, such as codeine or oxycodone.

When the Pain Persists

In some patients, the misery continues long after the rash has healed. Many of the 1 million people who develop shingles each year experience a complication called post-herpetic neuralgia (PHN). This term refers to pain that is present in the affected area for months, or even years, afterward. Although the acute pain of shingles and the chronic pain of PHN (called neuropathic pain) both originate in the nerve cells, their duration and the reaction to treatment is different.

Pain that occurs with the initial outbreak responds to treatment and is limited in duration. In contrast, PHN lasts longer, is difficult to treat and can be incapacitating. Furthermore, for unknown reasons, older people suffer more from this debilitating pain than younger people. In many individuals, the skin is so sensitive that clothing or even a passing breeze cannot be tolerated on the affected area. Described by PHN sufferers as agonizing, excruciating, and burning, the pain can result in an inability to perform daily tasks of living, and lead to loss of independence and, ultimately, depression and isolation.

"I would rather have ten babies than the pain I've endured for the past ten years," says 87-year-old Etta Watson Zukerman of Bethesda, Md., who has lost partial use of her right arm and hand due to nerve damage from PHN. "Nothing my doctor prescribed helped. I even went to a sports medicine specialist who recommended exercises. They didn't help either." Many PHN sufferers receive no relief at all, no matter what medications or therapies they use. And what works for one doesn't necessarily work for another.

Treating the Pain

Doctors use other methods to alleviate pain with varying degrees of success. "One of the relatively new medications that I'm enthusiastic about is the Lidoderm patch," says Veronica Mitchell, M.D., director of the pain management center and inpatient pain service at Georgetown University Hospital, Washington, D.C. "It's the transdermal form of lidocaine and it's been studied in the PHN population with very good results," adds Mitchell. "We prescribed the Lidoderm patch for a patient who had intolerable side effects with oral medications—and no relief—and she's had about a 50 percent-plus improvement in pain relief. It's one of my first-line therapies." The medication contained in this soft, pliable patch penetrates the skin, reaching the damaged nerves just under the skin without being absorbed significantly into the bloodstream. This means that the patch can be used for long periods of time without serious side effects.

Yet another method used to treat PHN is transcutaneous electrical nerve stimulation, or TENS. A device that generates low-level pulses of electrical current is applied to the skin's surface, causing tingling sensations and offering some people pain relief. One theory as to how TENS works is that the electrical current stimulates production of endorphins, the body's natural painkillers.

TENS is not for everyone. "TENS didn't help at all," says Einar Raysor of Rockville, Md. "I found there was a problem in fine-tuning the administration of the electrical current. Low doses of the electrical current didn't do anything for me. When the technician increased the current, it gave me a painful response. After this happened a couple of times, we dropped the treatment."

As a last resort, invasive procedures called nerve blocks may be used to provide temporary relief. These procedures usually entail the injection of a local anesthetic into the area of the affected nerves. "We have controversial results in the terms of the efficacy of nerve blocks," says Mitchell. "I do consider nerve blocks in treating PHN and I would perform them because there's some evidence that they work, but the real efficacy is to catch and treat the patient in the acute shingles phase. As PHN presents mostly in the elderly, and the older patient often is unable to tolerate some of the medications we use, I find nerve blocks useful in these cases."

Injection directly into the spine is another option for relief of pain that is not easily treated. A Japanese clinical study published in the *New England Journal of Medicine* found that an injection of the steroid methylprednisone combined with the anesthetic lidocaine reduced pain by more than 70 percent in one patient group compared with groups that received lidocaine alone or an inactive substance.

Prevention, Almost Perfect

Before the FDA approved the chickenpox vaccine in 1995, about 95 percent of the U.S. population developed chickenpox before age 18. Since then, more than 60 percent of American youngsters have been vaccinated against chickenpox.

"The vaccine is a live attenuated strain of the chickenpox virus," says Philip R. Krause, M.D., lead research investigator in the FDA's Center for Biologics Evaluation and Research. "However, it's a weaker form so it gives rise to a milder infection. But in the course of giving rise to this milder infection, it induces enough immunity to prevent people from getting the natural infection." It is estimated that the vaccine is between 75 and 85 percent effective in preventing chickenpox. "But the important thing," says Krause, "is that it is almost completely effective in preventing severe cases of chickenpox."

Now that we have a chickenpox vaccine, are shingles and PHN on their way out? Although the FDA hasn't evaluated the effects of the vaccine on shingles, Krause believes that "in the long term, if you can prevent enough people from getting the wild (natural) type of chickenpox, you're likely to see a beneficial effect on the incidence of shingles and post-herpetic neuralgia. But it may take several generations for this to happen."

Shingles Prevention Study

Since shingles can be very serious in older people, the Department of Veterans Affairs, the National Institute of Allergy and Infectious Diseases, and Merck & Co. Inc. are conducting a five-year clinical study at 22 sites nationwide to determine whether vaccination can prevent shingles in people ages 60 years and older who have had chickenpox.

As with the chickenpox vaccine now in use, the experimental vaccine is made from a weakened form of the chickenpox virus, but is much more potent than the existing vaccine.

"Immunity to the virus declines with advancing age, making older adults vulnerable to shingles," says Norberto Soto, M.D., principal investigator for the Shingles Prevention Study at the National Institutes of Health site in Bethesda, Md. "We believe that by boosting the body's immune response with this vaccine, shingles and its complications may be prevented."

The clinical trial hopes to recruit 37,200 volunteers. Besides the age requirement, the enrollees must be in good health and never have experienced shingles.

The study, which began in 1999, is a "double-blind" study, which means that neither the researchers nor the participants know who is receiving the experimental vaccine or an inactive substance (placebo).

If the vaccine is effective, it may help reduce illness and health-care costs among older people. For more information on the study, call 1-877-841-6251, or visit www.niaid.nih.gov/shingles.

— by Evelyn Zamula

Evelyn Zamula is a freelance writer in Potomac, Md.

Chapter 38

Shoulder Pain

This chapter first answers general questions about the shoulder and shoulder problems. It then answers questions about specific shoulder problems (dislocation, separation, tendinitis, bursitis, impingement syndrome, torn rotator cuff, frozen shoulder, and fracture) as well as shoulder pain caused by arthritis of the shoulder.

How common are shoulder problems?

According to the American Academy of Orthopaedic Surgeons, about 4 million people in the United States seek medical care each year for shoulder sprain, strain, dislocation, or other problems. Each year, shoulder problems account for about 1.5 million visits to orthopaedic surgeons—doctors who treat disorders of the bones, muscles, and related structures.

What are the structures of the shoulder and how does the shoulder function?

The shoulder joint is composed of three bones: the clavicle (collarbone), the scapula (shoulder blade), and the humerus (upper arm bone) (see Figure 38.1). Two joints facilitate shoulder movement. The acromioclavicular (AC) joint is located between the acromion (part of

"Questions and Answers about Shoulder Problems" National Institute of Arthritis and Musculoskeletal and Skin Diseases (NIAMS), NIH Pub. No. 01-4865, May 2001.

the scapula that forms the highest point of the shoulder) and the clavicle. The glenohumeral joint, commonly called the shoulder joint, is a ball-and-socket type joint that helps move the shoulder forward and backward and allows the arm to rotate in a circular fashion or hinge out and up away from the body. (The "ball" is the top, rounded portion of the upper arm bone or humerus; the "socket," or glenoid, is a dish-shaped part of the outer edge of the scapula into which the ball fits.) The capsule is a soft tissue envelope that encircles the glenohumeral joint. It is lined by a thin, smooth synovial membrane.

The bones of the shoulder are held in place by muscles, tendons, and ligaments. Tendons are tough cords of tissue that attach the shoulder muscles to bone and assist the muscles in moving the shoulder. Ligaments attach shoulder bones to each other, providing stability.

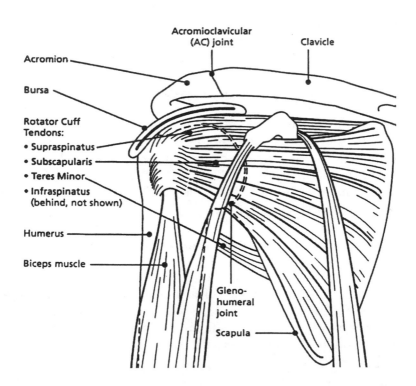

Figure 38.1. *Structure of shoulder*

For example, the front of the joint capsule is anchored by three gle-nohumeral ligaments.

The rotator cuff is a structure composed of tendons that, with as-sociated muscles, holds the ball at the top of the humerus in the gle-noid socket and provides mobility and strength to the shoulder joint.

Two filmy sac-like structures called bursae permit smooth gliding between bone, muscle, and tendon. They cushion and protect the ro-tator cuff from the bony arch of the acromion.

What are the origin and causes of shoulder problems?

The shoulder is the most movable joint in the body. However, it is an unstable joint because of the range of motion allowed. It is easily subject to injury because the ball of the upper arm is larger than the shoulder socket that holds it. To remain stable, the shoulder must be anchored by its muscles, tendons, and ligaments. Some shoulder prob-lems arise from the disruption of these soft tissues as a result of in-jury or from overuse or underuse of the shoulder. Other problems arise from a degenerative process in which tissues break down and no longer function well.

Shoulder pain may be localized or may be referred to areas around the shoulder or down the arm. Disease within the body (such as gall-bladder, liver, or heart disease, or disease of the cervical spine of the neck) also may generate pain that travels along nerves to the shoulder.

How are shoulder problems diagnosed?

Following are some of the ways doctors diagnose shoulder prob-lems:

- Medical history (the patient tells the doctor about an injury or other condition that might be causing the pain).

- Physical examination to feel for injury and discover the limits of movement, location of pain, and extent of joint instability.

- Tests to confirm the diagnosis of certain conditions. Some of these tests include:

  - x-ray

  - arthrogram—Diagnostic record that can be seen on an x-ray after injection of a contrast fluid into the shoulder joint to outline structures such as the rotator cuff. In disease or in-jury, this contrast fluid may either leak into an area where it does not belong, indicating a tear or opening, or be blocked from entering an area where there normally is an opening.

- MRI (magnetic resonance imaging)—A non-invasive procedure in which a machine produces a series of cross-sectional images of the shoulder.

- Other diagnostic tests, such as injection of an anesthetic into and around the shoulder joint, are discussed in specific sections of this chapter.

Dislocation

What is a shoulder dislocation?

The shoulder joint is the most frequently dislocated major joint of the body. In a typical case of a dislocated shoulder, a strong force that pulls the shoulder outward (abduction) or extreme rotation of the joint pops the ball of the humerus out of the shoulder socket. Dislocation commonly occurs when there is a backward pull on the arm that either catches the muscles unprepared to resist or overwhelms the muscles. When a shoulder dislocates frequently, the condition is referred to as shoulder instability. A partial dislocation where the upper arm bone is partially in and partially out of the socket is called a subluxation.

What are the signs of a dislocation and how is it diagnosed?

The shoulder can dislocate either forward, backward, or downward. Not only does the arm appear out of position when the shoulder dislocates, but the dislocation also produces pain. Muscle spasms may increase the intensity of pain. Swelling, numbness, weakness, and bruising are likely to develop. Problems seen with a dislocated shoulder are tearing of the ligaments or tendons reinforcing the joint capsule and, less commonly, nerve damage. Doctors usually diagnose a dislocation by a physical examination, and x-rays may be taken to confirm the diagnosis and to rule out a related fracture.

How is a dislocated shoulder treated?

Doctors treat a dislocation by putting the ball of the humerus back into the joint socket—a procedure called a reduction. The arm is then immobilized in a sling or a device called a shoulder immobilizer for several weeks. Usually the doctor recommends resting the shoulder and applying ice three or four times a day. After pain and swelling have been controlled, the patient enters a rehabilitation program that includes exercises to restore the range of motion of the shoulder and strengthen the muscles to prevent future dislocations. These exercises may progress from simple motion to the use of weights.

After treatment and recovery, a previously dislocated shoulder may remain more susceptible to reinjury, especially in young, active individuals. Ligaments may have been stretched or torn, and the shoulder may tend to dislocate again. A shoulder that dislocates severely or often, injuring surrounding tissues or nerves, usually requires surgical repair to tighten stretched ligaments or reattach torn ones.

Sometimes the doctor performs surgery through a tiny incision into which a small scope (arthroscope) is inserted to observe the inside of the joint. After this procedure, called arthroscopic surgery, the shoulder is generally immobilized for about six weeks and full recovery takes several months. Arthroscopic techniques involving the shoulder are relatively new and many surgeons prefer to repair a recurrent dislocating shoulder by the time-tested open surgery under direct vision. There are usually fewer repeat dislocations and improved movement following open surgery, but it may take a little longer to regain motion.

Separation

What is a shoulder separation?

A shoulder separation occurs where the collarbone (clavicle) meets the shoulder blade (scapula). When ligaments that hold the joint together are partially or completely torn, the outer end of the clavicle may slip out of place, preventing it from properly meeting the scapula. Most often the injury is caused by a blow to the shoulder or by falling on an outstretched hand.

What are the signs of a shoulder separation and how is it diagnosed?

Shoulder pain or tenderness and, occasionally, a bump in the middle of the top of the shoulder (over the AC joint) are signs that a separation may have occurred. Sometimes the severity of a separation can be detected by taking x-rays while the patient holds a light weight that pulls on the muscles, making a separation more pronounced.

How is a shoulder separation treated?

A shoulder separation is usually treated conservatively by rest and wearing a sling. Soon after injury, an ice bag may be applied to relieve pain and swelling. After a period of rest, a therapist helps the patient perform exercises that put the shoulder through its range of motion. Most shoulder separations heal within 2 or 3 months without further intervention. However, if ligaments are severely torn, surgical repair may be required to hold the clavicle in place. A doctor may wait to see if conservative treatment works before deciding whether surgery is required.

Tendinitis, Bursitis, and Impingement Syndrome

What are tendinitis, bursitis, and impingement syndrome of the shoulder?

These conditions are closely related and may occur alone or in combination. If the rotator cuff and bursa are irritated, inflamed, and swollen, they may become squeezed between the head of the humerus and the acromion. Repeated motion involving the arms, or the aging process involving shoulder motion over many years, may also irritate and wear down the tendons, muscles, and surrounding structures.

Tendinitis is inflammation (redness, soreness, and swelling) of a tendon. In tendinitis of the shoulder, the rotator cuff and/or biceps tendon become inflamed, usually as a result of being pinched by surrounding structures. The injury may vary from mild inflammation to involvement of most of the rotator cuff. When the rotator cuff tendon becomes inflamed and thickened, it may get trapped under the acromion. Squeezing of the rotator cuff is called impingement syndrome.

Tendinitis and impingement syndrome are often accompanied by inflammation of the bursa sacs that protect the shoulder. An inflamed bursa is called bursitis. Inflammation caused by a disease such as rheumatoid arthritis may cause rotator cuff tendinitis and bursitis. Sports involving overuse of the shoulder and occupations requiring frequent overhead reaching are other potential causes of irritation to the rotator cuff or bursa and may lead to inflammation and impingement.

What are the signs of tendinitis and bursitis?

Signs of these conditions include the slow onset of discomfort and pain in the upper shoulder or upper third of the arm and/or difficulty sleeping on the shoulder. Tendinitis and bursitis also cause pain when the arm is lifted away from the body or overhead. If tendinitis involves the biceps tendon (the tendon located in front of the shoulder that helps bend the elbow and turn the forearm), pain will occur in the front or side of the shoulder and may travel down to the elbow and forearm. Pain may also occur when the arm is forcefully pushed upward overhead.

How are these conditions diagnosed?

Diagnosis of tendinitis and bursitis begins with a medical history and physical examination. X-rays do not show tendons or the bursae but may be helpful in ruling out bony abnormalities or arthritis. The doctor may remove and test fluid from the inflamed area to rule out infection. Impingement syndrome may be confirmed when injection of a small amount of anesthetic (lidocaine hydrochloride) into the space under the acromion relieves pain.

How are tendinitis, bursitis, and impingement syndrome treated?

The first step in treating these conditions is to reduce pain and inflammation with rest, ice, and anti-inflammatory medicines such as aspirin, naproxen (Naprosyn), ibuprofen (Advil, Motrin, or Nuprin), or cox-2 inhibitors (Celebrex, or Vioxx). (Brand names included in this text are provided as examples only, and their inclusion does not mean that these products are endorsed by the National Institutes of Health or any other Government agency. Also, if a particular brand name is not mentioned, this does not mean or imply that the product is unsatisfactory.) In some cases the doctor or therapist will use ultrasound (gentle sound-wave vibrations) to warm deep tissues and improve blood flow. Gentle stretching and strengthening exercises are added gradually. These may be preceded or followed by use of an ice pack. If there is no improvement, the doctor may inject a corticosteroid medicine into the space under the acromion. While steroid injections are a common treatment, they must be used with caution because they may lead to tendon rupture. If there is still no improvement after 6 to 12 months, the doctor may perform either arthroscopic or open surgery to repair damage and relieve pressure on the tendons and bursae.

Torn Rotator Cuff

What is a torn rotator cuff?

One or more rotator cuff tendons may become inflamed from overuse, aging, a fall on an outstretched hand, or a collision. Sports requiring repeated overhead arm motion or occupations requiring heavy lifting also place a strain on rotator cuff tendons and muscles. Normally, tendons are strong, but a longstanding wearing down process may lead to a tear.

What are the signs of a torn rotator cuff?

Typically, a person with a rotator cuff injury feels pain over the deltoid muscle at the top and outer side of the shoulder, especially when the arm is raised or extended out from the side of the body. Motions like those involved in getting dressed can be painful. The shoulder may feel weak, especially when trying to lift the arm into a horizontal position. A person may also feel or hear a click or pop when the shoulder is moved.

How is a torn rotator cuff diagnosed?

Pain or weakness on outward or inward rotation of the arm may indicate a tear in a rotator cuff tendon. The patient also feels pain when lowering the arm to the side after the shoulder is moved backward and the arm is raised. A doctor may detect weakness but may not be able to determine from a physical examination where the tear is located. X-rays, if taken, may appear normal. An MRI can help detect a full tendon tear, but does not detect partial tears. If the pain disappears after the doctor injects a small amount of anesthetic into the area, impingement is likely to be present. If there is no response to treatment, the doctor may use an arthrogram, rather than an MRI, to inspect the injured area and confirm the diagnosis.

How is a torn rotator cuff treated?

Doctors usually recommend that patients with a rotator cuff injury rest the shoulder, apply heat or cold to the sore area, and take medicine to relieve pain and inflammation. Other treatments might be added, such as electrical stimulation of muscles and nerves, ultrasound, or a cortisone injection near the inflamed area of the rotator cuff. The patient may need to wear a sling for a few days. If surgery is not an immediate consideration, exercises are added to the treatment program to build flexibility and strength and restore the shoulder's function. If there is no improvement with these conservative treatments and functional impairment persists, the doctor may perform arthroscopic or open surgical repair of the torn rotator cuff.

Frozen Shoulder (Adhesive Capsulitis)

What is a frozen shoulder?

As the name implies, movement of the shoulder is severely restricted in people with a "frozen shoulder." This condition, which doctors call adhesive capsulitis, is frequently caused by injury that leads to lack of use due to pain. Rheumatic disease progression and recent shoulder surgery can also cause frozen shoulder. Intermittent periods of use may cause inflammation. Adhesions (abnormal bands of tissue) grow between the joint surfaces, restricting motion. There is also a lack of synovial fluid, which normally lubricates the gap between the arm bone and socket to help the shoulder joint move. It is this restricted space between the capsule and ball of the humerus that distinguishes adhesive capsulitis from a less complicated painful, stiff shoulder. People with diabetes, stroke, lung disease, rheumatoid arthritis, and heart disease, or who have been in an accident, are at a higher risk for frozen shoulder. The condition rarely appears in people under 40 years old.

What are the signs of a frozen shoulder and how is it diagnosed?

With a frozen shoulder, the joint becomes so tight and stiff that it is nearly impossible to carry out simple movements, such as raising the arm. People complain that the stiffness and discomfort worsen at night. A doctor may suspect the patient has a frozen shoulder if a physical examination reveals limited shoulder movement. An arthrogram may confirm the diagnosis.

How is a frozen shoulder treated?

Treatment of this disorder focuses on restoring joint movement and reducing shoulder pain. Usually, treatment begins with nonsteroidal anti-inflammatory drugs and the application of heat, followed by gentle stretching exercises. These stretching exercises, which may be performed in the home with the help of a therapist, are the treatment of choice. In some cases, transcutaneous electrical nerve stimulation (TENS) with a small battery-operated unit may be used to reduce pain by blocking nerve impulses. If these measures are unsuccessful, the doctor may recommend manipulation of the shoulder under general anesthesia. Surgery to cut the adhesions is only necessary in some cases.

Fracture

What happens when the shoulder is fractured?

A fracture involves a partial or total crack through a bone. The break in a bone usually occurs as a result of an impact injury, such as a fall or blow to the shoulder. A fracture usually involves the clavicle or the neck (area below the ball) of the humerus.

What are the signs of a shoulder fracture and how is it diagnosed?

A shoulder fracture that occurs after a major injury is usually accompanied by severe pain. Within a short time, there may be redness and bruising around the area. Sometimes a fracture is obvious because the bones appear out of position. Both diagnosis and severity can be confirmed by x-rays.

How is a shoulder fracture treated?

When a fracture occurs, the doctor tries to bring the bones into a position that will promote healing and restore arm movement. If the clavicle is fractured, the patient must at first wear a strap and sling around the chest to keep the clavicle in place. After removing the strap and sling, the doctor will prescribe exercises to strengthen the shoulder and restore movement. Surgery is occasionally needed for certain clavicle fractures.

Fracture of the neck of the humerus is usually treated with a sling or shoulder immobilizer. If the bones are out of position, surgery may be necessary to reset them. Exercises are also part of restoring shoulder strength and motion.

Arthritis of the Shoulder

What is arthritis of the shoulder?

Arthritis is a degenerative disease caused by either wear and tear of the cartilage (osteoarthritis) or an inflammation (rheumatoid arthritis) of one or more joints. Arthritis not only affects joints; it may also affect supporting structures such as muscles, tendons, and ligaments.

What are the signs of shoulder arthritis and how is it diagnosed?

The usual signs of arthritis of the shoulder are pain, particularly over the AC joint, and a decrease in shoulder motion. A doctor may suspect the patient has arthritis when there is both pain and swelling in the joint. The diagnosis may be confirmed by a physical examination and x-rays. Blood tests may be helpful for diagnosing rheumatoid arthritis, but other tests may be needed as well. Analysis of synovial fluid from the shoulder joint may be helpful in diagnosing some kinds of arthritis. Although arthroscopy permits direct visualization of damage to cartilage, tendons, and ligaments, and may confirm a diagnosis, it is usually done only if a repair procedure is to be performed.

How is arthritis of the shoulder treated?

Most often osteoarthritis of the shoulder is treated with nonsteroidal anti-inflammatory drugs, such as aspirin, ibuprofen, or cox-2 inhibitors. (Rheumatoid arthritis of the shoulder may require physical therapy and additional medicine, such as corticosteroids.) When non-operative treatment of arthritis of the shoulder fails to relieve pain or improve function, or when there is severe wear and tear of the joint causing parts to loosen and move out of place, shoulder joint replacement (arthroplasty) may provide better results. In this operation, a surgeon replaces the shoulder joint with an artificial ball for the top of the humerus and a cap (glenoid) for the scapula. Passive shoulder exercises (where someone else moves the arm to rotate the shoulder joint) are started soon after surgery. Patients begin exercising on their own about 3 to 6 weeks after surgery. Eventually, stretching and strengthening exercises become a major part of the rehabilitation program. The success of the operation often depends on the condition of rotator cuff muscles prior to surgery and the degree to which the patient follows the exercise program.

If you receive a shoulder injury, here's what you can do:

RICE = Rest, Ice, Compression, and Elevation

Rest—Reduce or stop using the injured area for 48 hours.

Ice—Put an ice pack on the injured area for 20 minutes at a time, 4 to 8 times per day. Use a cold pack, ice bag, or a plastic bag filled with crushed ice that has been wrapped in a towel.

Compression—Compression may help reduce the swelling. Compress the area with bandages, such as an elastic wrap, to help stabilize the shoulder.

Elevation—Keep the injured area elevated above the level of the heart. Use a pillow to help elevate the injury.

If pain and stiffness persist, see a doctor.

Additional Information

National Institute of Arthritis and Musculoskeletal and Skin Diseases Information Clearinghouse
National Institutes of Health
1 AMS Circle
Bethesda, MD 20892-3675
Phone: (301) 495-4484 or 877-22-NIAMS (226-4267) (free of charge)
TTY: (301) 565-2966
Fax: (301) 718-6366
Website: http://www.niams.nih.gov/

The clearinghouse provides information about various forms of arthritis and rheumatic disease and bone, muscle, and skin diseases. It distributes patient and professional education materials and refers people to other sources of information. Additional information and updates can also be found on the NIAMS website.

American Academy of Orthopaedic Surgeons
6300 North River Road
Rosemont, IL 60018-4262
Toll Free: 800-346-AAOS
Phone: 847-823-7186
Website: http://www.aaos.org

The academy publishes brochures on total joint replacement, arthritis, arthroscopy, and other subjects. Single copies of a brochure are available free of charge by sending a self-addressed, stamped (business-size) envelope to (name of brochure) at the address above.

American College of Rheumatology
1800 Century Place, Suite 250
Atlanta, GA 30345
Phone: (404) 633-3777

Fax: (404)-633-1870
Website: www.rheumatology.org

This national professional organization can provide referrals to rheumatologists and allied health specialists, such as physical therapists. One-page fact sheets are also available on various forms of arthritis. Lists of specialists by geographic area and fact sheets are also available on their website.

American Physical Therapy Association
1111 North Fairfax Street
Alexandria, VA 22314-1488
Phone: (703) 684-2782 or (800) 999-2782, ext. 3395 (free of charge)
Website: www.apta.org

This national professional organization represents physical therapists, allied personnel, and students. Its objectives are to improve research, public understanding, and education in the physical therapies. A free brochure titled "Taking Care of Your Shoulder: A Physical Therapist's Perspective" is available on the association's website or by sending a business-size, stamped, self-addressed envelope to the address above.

Arthritis Foundation
1330 West Peachtree Street
Atlanta, GA 30309
Phone: (404) 872-7100 or (800) 283-7800 (free of charge) or call your local chapter (listed in the telephone directory)
Website www.arthritis.org

This is the major voluntary organization devoted to arthritis. The foundation publishes pamphlets on arthritis, such as "Arthritis Answers," that may be obtained by calling the toll-free telephone number. The foundation also can provide physician and clinic referrals. Local chapters also provide information and organize exercise programs for people who have arthritis.

Acknowledgments

The NIAMS gratefully acknowledges the assistance of James Panagis, M.D., M.P.H., of the NIAMS; Frank A. Pettrone, M.D., of Arlington, Virginia; and Thomas J. Neviaser, M.D., of Fairfax, Virginia, in the preparation and review of this text.

Chapter 39

Temporomandibular Disorders (TMD)

You may have read articles in newspapers and magazines about "TMD" —temporomandibular (jaw) disorders, also called "TMJ syndrome." Perhaps you have even felt pain sometimes in your jaw area, or maybe your dentist or physician has told you that you have TMD.

If you have questions about TMD, you are not alone. Researchers, too, are looking for answers to what causes TMD, what are the best treatments, and how can we prevent these disorders. The National Institute of Dental Research has written this information to share with you what we have learned about TMD.

TMD is not just one disorder, but a group of conditions, often painful, that affect the jaw joint (temporomandibular joint, or TMJ) and the muscles that control chewing. Although we don't know how many people actually have TMD, the disorders appear to affect about twice as many women as men.

The good news is that for most people, pain in the area of the jaw joint or muscles is not a signal that a serious problem is developing. Generally, discomfort from TMD is occasional and temporary, often occurring in cycles. The pain eventually goes away with little or no treatment. Only a small percentage of people with TMD pain develop significant, long-term symptoms.

"Temporomandibular Disorders (TMD)," an undated pamphlet produced by the National Institute of Dental Research (NIDR), text available online at www.nidr.nih.gov; accessed October 2001.

What Is the Temporomandibular Joint?

The temporomandibular joint connects the lower jaw, called the mandible, to the temporal bone at the side of the head. If you place your fingers just in front of your ears and open your mouth, you can feel the joint on each side of your head. Because these joints are flexible, the jaw can move smoothly up and down and side to side, enabling us to talk, chew and yawn. Muscles attached to and surrounding the jaw joint control its position and movement.

When we open our mouths, the rounded ends of the lower jaw, called condyles, glide along the joint socket of the temporal bone. The condyles slide back to their original position when we close our mouths. To keep this motion smooth, a soft disc lies between the condyle and the temporal bone. This disc absorbs shocks to the TMJ from chewing and other movements.

What Are Temporomandibular Disorders?

Today, researchers generally agree that temporomandibular disorders fall into three main categories:

- **myofascial pain**, the most common form of TMD, which is discomfort or pain in the muscles that control jaw function and the neck and shoulder muscles;

- **internal derangement of the joint**, meaning a dislocated jaw or displaced disc, or injury to the condyle;

- **degenerative joint disease**, such as osteoarthritis or rheumatoid arthritis in the jaw joint.

A person may have one or more of these conditions at the same time.

What Causes TMD?

We know that severe injury to the jaw or temporomandibular joint can cause TMD. A heavy blow, for example, can fracture the bones of the joint or damage the disc, disrupting the smooth motion of the jaw and causing pain or locking. Arthritis in the jaw joint may also result from injury. Other causes of TMD are less clear. Some suggest, for example, that a bad bite (malocclusion) can trigger TMD, but recent research disputes that view. Orthodontic treatment, such as braces and the use of headgear, has also been blamed for some forms of TMD, but studies now show that this is unlikely.

And there is no scientific proof that gum chewing causes clicking sounds in the jaw joint, or that jaw clicking leads to serious TMJ problems. In fact, jaw clicking is fairly common in the general population. If there are no other symptoms, such as pain or locking, jaw clicking usually does not need treatment.

Researchers believe that most people with clicking or popping in the jaw joint likely have a displaced disc—the soft, shock-absorbing disc is not in a normal position. As long as the displaced disc causes no pain or problems with jaw movement, no treatment is needed.

Some experts suggest that stress, either mental or physical, may cause or aggravate TMD. People with TMD often clench or grind their teeth at night, which can tire the jaw muscles and lead to pain. It is not clear, however, whether stress is the cause of the clenching/grinding and subsequent jaw pain, or the result of dealing with chronic jaw pain or dysfunction. Scientists are exploring how behavioral, psychological and physical factors may combine to cause TMD.

TMD Signs and Symptoms

A variety of symptoms may be linked to TMD. Pain, particularly in the chewing muscles and/or jaw joint, is the most common symptom. Other likely symptoms include:

- limited movement or locking of the jaw,
- radiating pain in the face, neck or shoulders,
- painful clicking, popping or grating sounds in the jaw joint when opening or closing the mouth.
- a sudden, major change in the way the upper and lower teeth fit together.

Symptoms such as headaches, earaches, dizziness and hearing problems may sometimes be related to TMD. It is important to keep in mind, however, that occasional discomfort in the jaw joint or chewing muscles is quite common and is generally not a cause for concern. Researchers are working to clarify TMD symptoms, with the goal of developing easier and better methods of diagnosis and improved treatment.

Diagnosis

Because the exact causes and symptoms of TMD are not clear, diagnosing these disorders can be confusing. At present, there is no widely accepted, standard test to correctly identify TMD. In about 90 percent of cases, however, the patient's description of symptoms, combined with a simple physical examination of the face and jaw, provides information useful for diagnosing these disorders.

The examination includes feeling the jaw joints and chewing muscles for pain or tenderness; listening for clicking, popping or grating sounds during jaw movement; and examining for limited motion or locking of the jaw while opening or closing the mouth. Checking the patient's dental and medical history is very important. In most cases, this evaluation provides enough information to locate the pain or jaw problem, to make a diagnosis, and to start treatment to relieve pain or jaw locking.

Regular dental X-rays and TMJ x-rays (transcranial radiographs) are not generally useful in diagnosing TMD. Other x-ray techniques, such as arthrography (joint x-rays using dye); magnetic resonance imaging (MRI), which pictures the soft tissues; and tomography (a special type of x-ray), are usually needed only when the practitioner strongly suspects a condition such as arthritis or when significant pain persists over time and symptoms do not improve with treatment. Before undergoing any expensive diagnostic test, it is always wise to get another independent opinion.

One of the most important areas of TMD research is developing clear guidelines for diagnosing these disorders. Once scientists agree on what these guidelines should be, it will be easier for practitioners to correctly identify temporomandibular disorders and to decide what treatment, if any, is needed.

Treatment

The key words to keep in mind about TMD treatment are "conservative" and "reversible." Conservative treatments are as simple as possible and are used most often because most patients do not have severe, degenerative TMD. Conservative treatments do not invade the tissues of the face, jaw or joint. Reversible treatments do not cause permanent, or irreversible, changes in the structure or position of the jaw or teeth.

Because most TMD problems are temporary and do not get worse, simple treatment is all that is usually needed to relieve discomfort. Self-care practices, for example, eating soft foods, applying heat or ice packs, and avoiding extreme jaw movements (such as wide yawning, loud singing and gum chewing) are useful in easing TMD symptoms. Learning special techniques for relaxing and reducing stress may also help patients deal with pain that often comes with TMD problems.

Other conservative, reversible treatments include physical therapy you can do at home, which focuses on gentle muscle stretching and relaxing exercises, and short-term use of muscle-relaxing and anti-inflammatory drugs.

The health care provider may recommend an oral appliance, also called a splint or bite plate, which is a plastic guard that fits over the upper or lower teeth. The splint can help reduce clenching or grinding, which eases muscle tension. An oral splint should be used only for a short time and should not cause permanent changes in the bite. If a splint causes or increases pain, stop using it and see your practitioner.

The conservative, reversible treatments described are useful for temporary relief of pain and muscle spasm—they are not "cures" for TMD. If symptoms continue over time or come back often, check with your doctor.

There are other types of TMD treatment, such as surgery or injections, that invade the tissues. Some involve injecting pain relieving medications into painful muscle sites, often called "trigger points." Researchers are studying this type of treatment to see if these injections are helpful over time.

Surgical treatments are often irreversible and should be avoided where possible. When such treatment is necessary, be sure to have the doctor explain to you, in words you can understand, the reason for the treatment, the risks involved, and other types of treatment that may be available.

Scientists have learned that certain irreversible treatments, such as surgical replacement of jaw joints with artificial implants, may cause severe pain and permanent jaw damage. Some of these devices may fail to function properly or may break apart in the jaw over time. *Before undergoing any surgery on the jaw joint, it is very important to get other independent opinions.*

The Food and Drug Administration has recalled artificial jaw joint implants made by Vitek, Inc., which may break down and damage surrounding bone. If you have these implants, see your oral surgeon or dentist. If there are problems with your implants, the devices may need to be removed. Persons who have Vitek implants should call Medic Alert at 1-800-554-5297 for more information.

Other irreversible treatments that are of little value—and may make the problem worse—include orthodontics to change the bite; restorative dentistry, which uses crown and bridge work to balance the bite; and occlusal adjustment, grinding down teeth to bring the bite into balance.

Although more studies are needed on the safety and effectiveness of most TMD treatments, scientists strongly recommend using the most conservative, reversible treatments possible before considering invasive treatments. Even when the TMD problem has become chronic, most patients still do not need aggressive types of treatment.

If You Think You Have TMD...

Keep in mind that for most people, discomfort from TMD will eventually go away whether treated or not. Simple self-care practices are often effective in easing TMD symptoms. If more treatment is needed, it should be conservative and reversible. Avoid, if at all possible, treatments that cause permanent changes in the bite or jaw. If irreversible treatments are recommended, be sure to get a reliable second opinion.

Many practitioners, especially dentists, are familiar with the conservative treatment of TMD. Because TMD is usually painful, pain clinics in hospitals and universities are also a good source of advice and second opinions for these disorders. Specially trained facial pain experts can often be helpful in diagnosing and treating TMD.

Research

The National Institute of Dental Research supports an active research program on TMD. Developing reliable guidelines for diagnosing these disorders is a top priority. Studies are also under way on the causes, treatments, and prevention of TMD. Through continued research, pieces of the TMD puzzle are falling slowly but steadily into place.

Chapter 40

Thoracic Outlet Syndrome

What Is Thoracic Outlet Syndrome?

Thoracic outlet syndrome consists of symptoms caused by compression of the nerves in the brachial plexus (nerves that pass into the arms from the neck) or blood vessels. Patients may have pain in the shoulder, arm, or hand, or in all three locations. The hand pain is often most severe in the fourth and fifth fingers. The pain is aggravated by the use of the arm, and "fatigue" of the arm is often prominent.

Is There Any Treatment?

The goals of treatment are two-fold: to correct postural abnormalities that might contribute to the compression, and to establish an exercise program to strengthen the shoulder muscles. Most often a conservative course of treatment is followed. If vascular or major neurological impairment is present, surgical decompression may be considered. However, only a small number of patients require surgery.

What Is the Prognosis?

The prognosis for the majority of individuals who receive therapy for thoracic outlet syndrome is good.

From "NINDS Thoracic Outlet Syndrome Information Page," National Institute of Neurological Disorders and Stroke (NINDS), available at www.ninds.nih.gov. Reviewed July 2001.

What Research Is Being Done?

Within the National Institute of Neurological Disorders and Stroke (NINDS) research programs, thoracic outlet syndrome is addressed through research on pain. NINDS vigorously pursues a research program seeking new treatments for pain and nerve damage with the ultimate goal of reversing cumulative trauma disorders such as thoracic outlet syndrome.

Organizations

American Chronic Pain Association (ACPA)
P.O. Box 850
Rocklin, CA 95677-0850
Phone: (916) 632-0922
Fax: (916) 632-3208
Website: http://www.theacpa.org

National Rehabilitation Information Center (NARIC)
4200 Forbes Blvd., Suite 202
Lanham, MD 20706
Toll Free: (800) 346-2742
Phone: (301) 459-5900
Fax: (301) 562-2401
Website: http://www.naric.com

National Chronic Pain Outreach Association (NCPOA)
P.O. Box 274
Millboro, VA 24460
Phone: (540) 862-9437
Fax: (540) 862-9485

Chapter 41

Tooth Pain

Symptom:
Momentary sensitivity to hot or cold foods.

Possible problem: If the discomfort lasts only moments, sensitivity to hot and cold foods generally does not signal a problem. The sensitivity may be caused by a loose filling or by minimal gum recession which exposes small areas of the root surface.

What to do: Try using toothpastes made for sensitive teeth. Brush up and down with a soft brush; brushing sideways wears away exposed root surfaces. If this is unsuccessful, see your dentist.

Symptom:
Sensitivity to hot or cold foods after dental treatment.

Possible problem: Dental work may inflame the pulp, inside the tooth, causing temporary sensitivity.

What to do: Wait four to six weeks. If the pain persists or worsens, see your dentist.

Symptom:
Sharp pain when biting down on food.

Possible problem: There are several possible causes of this type of pain: decay, a loose filling, or a crack in the tooth. There may be damage to the pulp tissue inside the tooth.

What to do: See a dentist for evaluation. If the problem is a cracked tooth, your dentist may send you to an endodontist. Cracked tooth pain comes from damage to the inner soft tissue of the tooth, the pulp. Endodontists are dentists who specialize in pulp-related procedures. Endodontic treatment, also known as root canal treatment, can relieve that pain.

Symptom:
Lingering pain after eating hot or cold foods.

Possible problem: This probably means the pulp has been damaged by deep decay or physical trauma.

What to do: See your endodontist to save the tooth with root canal treatment.

Symptom:
Constant and severe pain and pressure, swelling of gum, and sensitivity to touch.

Possible problem: A tooth may have become abscessed, causing the surrounding bone to become infected.

What to do: See your endodontist for evaluation and treatment to relieve the pain and save the tooth. Take over-the-counter analgesics until you see the endodontist.

Symptom:
Dull ache and pressure in upper teeth and jaw.

Possible problem: The pain of a sinus headache is often felt in the face and teeth. Grinding of teeth, a condition known as bruxism, can also cause this type of ache.

What to do: For sinus headache, try over-the-counter analgesics or sinus medicine. For bruxism, consult your dentist. If pain is severe and chronic, see your physician or endodontist for evaluation.

Symptom:
Chronic pain in head, neck, or ear.

Possible problem: Sometimes pulp-damaged teeth cause pain in other parts of the head and neck, but other dental or medical problems may be responsible.

What to do: See your endodontist for evaluation. If the problem is not related to the tooth, your endodontist will refer you to an appropriate dental specialist or a physician.

For More Information

American Association of Endodontists
211 E. Chicago Ave., Suite 1100
Chicago, Illinois 60611-2691
Phone: (800) 872-3636 or (312) 266-7255
Fax: (312) 266-9867
Website: www.aae.org

Chapter 42

Trigeminal Neuralgia

What is trigeminal neuralgia?

Trigeminal neuralgia, also called tic douloureux, is a condition that affects the trigeminal nerve (the 5th cranial nerve), one of the largest nerves in the head. The trigeminal nerve is responsible for sending impulses of touch, pain, pressure, and temperature to the brain from the face, jaw, gums, forehead, and around the eyes. Trigeminal neuralgia is characterized by a sudden, severe, electric shock-like or stabbing pain typically felt on one side of the jaw or cheek. The disorder is more common in women than in men and rarely affects anyone younger than 50. The attacks of pain, which generally last several seconds and may be repeated one after the other, may be triggered by talking, brushing teeth, touching the face, chewing, or swallowing. The attacks may come and go throughout the day and last for days, weeks, or months at a time, and then disappear for months or years.

Is there any treatment?

Treatment for trigeminal neuralgia typically includes anticonvulsant medications such as carbamazepine or phenytoin. Baclofen, clonazepam, gabapentin, and valproic acid may also be effective and may be used in combination to achieve pain relief. If medication fails to relieve pain, surgical treatment may be recommended.

From "NINDS Trigeminal Neuralgia Information Page," National Institute of Neurological Disorders and Stroke (NINDS), available at www.ninds.nih.gov. Reviewed July 2001.

What is the prognosis?

The disorder is characterized by recurrences and remissions, and successive recurrences may incapacitate the patient. Due to the intensity of the pain, even the fear of an impending attack may prevent activity. Trigeminal neuralgia is not fatal.

What research is being done?

Within the National Institute of Neurological Disorders and Stroke (NINDS) research programs, trigeminal neuralgia is addressed primarily through studies associated with pain research. NINDS vigorously pursues a research program seeking new treatments for pain and nerve damage with the ultimate goal of reversing debilitating conditions such as trigeminal neuralgia. NINDS has notified research investigators that it is seeking grant applications both in basic and clinical pain research.

Selected References

Fields, H. Treatment of Trigeminal Neuralgia [Editorial] in *The New England Journal of Medicine*, 334:17; 1125-1126 (April 1996)

Kitt, C.A., et al. Trigeminal Neuralgia: Opportunities for Research and Treatment. *Pain*, 85:1-2; 3-7 (March 2000)

Loeser, J. *Cranial Neuralgias In The Management of Pain, vol. 1, 2nd edition*, Lea & Febiger, Philadelphia, pp. 676-686 (1990)

Maciewicz, R, and Scrivani, S. Trigeminal Neuralgia: Gamma Radiosurgery May Provide New Options for Treatment. *Neurology*, 48; 565-566 (March 1997)

Trigeminal Neuralgia. *Surgical Neurology*, 45:5; 818-825 (May 1996)

Weigel, G, and Casey, K.F. *Strike Back! The Trigeminal Neuralgia Handbook*, Gates Publishing, Co. (January 2000)

Organizations

American Chronic Pain Association (ACPA)
P.O. Box 850
Rocklin, CA 95677-0850
Phone: (916) 632-0922

Fax: (916) 632-3208
Website: http://www.theacpa.org

National Chronic Pain Outreach Association (NCPOA)
P.O. Box 274
Millboro, VA 24460
Phone: (540) 862-9437
Fax: (540) 862-9485

Trigeminal Neuralgia Association
2801 SW Archer Rd., Suite C
Gainsville, FL 32608
Phone: (352) 376-9955
Fax: (352) 376-8688
Website: http://www.tna-support.org
E-Mail: tnanational@tna-support.org

Related NINDS Publications and Information

Chronic Pain: Hope Through Research: Chronic pain information booklet compiled by NINDS, the National Institute of Neurological Disorders and Stroke.

Headache: Hope Through Research: Information booklet about headaches, including migraines.

Trigeminal Neuralgia: Opportunities for Research and Treatment: Summary of a workshop, "Trigeminal Neuralgia: Opportunities for Research and Treatment," September 1999.

Chapter 43

Vulvar Pain (Vulvodynia)

The word "vulvodynia" simply means vulvar pain. The root "vulv" refers to the vulva and "odynia" is derived from the Greek word for pain. Scrotodynia is the analogous condition in the male. (One must be careful to use the word vulvodynia, rather than vulvadynia, when doing a literature or Internet search.) Vulvodynia is a symptom which may have multiple causes. There is no prevalence data available at the present time, so one can only guess at its magnitude. A rough estimation is that 7% of the female population experiences painful sexual intercourse of a chronic nature, with 2-3% of these women suffering from vulvodynia. The chronicity of the problem differentiates this entity from acute causes of vulvar pain such as bacterial or fungal infections.

Physical Examination

The patient often presents with intermittent or constant burning of the vulva, sometimes described as rawness or irritation. The first diagnostic step is a thorough physical and comprehensive history. While taking a patient's history, I specifically listen for the nature, location, and duration of the symptoms. Here we must differentiate

From "Classification and Treatment of Vulvodynia" by Stanley Marinoff, M.D., Center for Vulvovaginal Disorders, Washington D.C. This article was originally published in the Summer 1998 issue of the newsletter of the National Vulvodynia Association. © 1998 National Vulvodynia Association. Reprinted with permission.

vulvodynia from pruritus (itching) and determine the chronicity of the problem. The results of previous treatments and medications must be evaluated. It is not unusual for a patient to bring to the appointment a large assortment of medications that have been prescribed. It is important to take the time to review these medications and the positive or negative results they have produced. The patient's sexual history, especially changes in sexual practices or contraceptive methods, must be explored. Hygienic patterns also must be assessed. Many women feel "unclean" in this area and respond by excessive washing and douching, which may lead to a vicious cycle of irritation and burning.

A pertinent medical history of trauma or metabolic disorders, such as diabetes mellitus, may be the clue to the origin of vulvar pain. Additionally, there is a high incidence of relationship between vulvar pain and other disorders such as interstitial cystitis, fibromyalgia, and irritable bowel syndrome. The cause of this commonality is not yet known.

In the physical examination, the entire vulva must be carefully inspected. Adequate lighting and magnification are essential. A colposcope (magnifying instrument) helps to identify genital warts and lesions that may be cancerous. Abnormal-looking tissue should be biopsied. However, biopsies are not generally indicated for areas that show only erythema (redness), because the finding will most likely be chronic inflammation.

In particular, the vestibule (tissue immediately surrounding the entrance to the vagina) must be evaluated. To localize specific areas of tenderness in the vestibule, I use a moistened cotton-tipped applicator stick. Vaginitis must be ruled out so appropriate cultures are obtained and wet mounts with both saline and potassium hydroxide are inspected.

Categorizing Vulvar Pain

Because vulvar pain conditions are not all the same, I use the objective findings shown in Table 43.1 to develop a treatment strategy.

Table 43.1. Vulvodynia

Lesions on cutaneous and mucosal surfaces:	Erosive Vulvovaginitis
Tender red spots in vestibule only:	Vulvar Vestibulitis Syndrome
No visible lesions or only mild erythema:	Essential Vulvodynia or Pudendal Neuralgia

Dermatoses

The first category consists of dermatologic problems such as inflammatory dermatoses, which typically present as itching. These are grouped as the "lichens," an unfortunate term since it brings to mind a picture of the plant form. The three types are lichen sclerosus, lichen planus, and lichen simplex chronicus. One must be able to recognize these entities and refer the patient to a dermatologist or vulvologist for appropriate treatment. These are treatable dermatological diseases.

Vulvar Vestibulitis Syndrome

The second subset is vulvar vestibulitis syndrome (VVS), a chronic condition with three diagnostic criteria:

1. Severe pain on vestibular touch or attempted vaginal entry.

2. Tenderness to pressure localized within the vulvar vestibule.

3. Physical findings confined to vestibular erythema of various degrees.

The *sine qua non* of VVS is introital dyspaurenia, pain in the vestibule upon pressure or penetration. Initial therapy consists of various conservative measures such as removal of irritants, and treatment of concomitant infections and dermatoses. Rehabilitation of the pelvic floor muscles with biofeedback has been helpful in some patients. Interlesional alpha-interferon injections into the vestibule also have been somewhat successful; 30-40% of patients who receive these injections exhibit improvement in sexual function. If all non-surgical methods fail to provide relief, surgery may be recommended. Outcome research on surgery patients has found that surgery leads to marked improvement in the ability to engage in sexual relations in 65-85% of cases. The key to this success is careful patient selection, i.e., patients with pure vulvar vestibulitis syndrome, rather than dysesthetic vulvodynia, experience the best results.

Essential Vulvodynia

Essential vulvodynia and pudendal neuralgia comprise the third category of vulvar pain syndromes. The difference between these two entities is ill-defined, but I separate them on the basis of whether definitive neurological findings can be demonstrated. In these cases, I prefer the term pudendal neuralgia. These individuals usually report a constant or intermittent burning in a diffuse pattern over the entire vulvar area. With pudendal neuralgia, the pain follows the distribution of the pudendal nerve, so the localization of the pain may include a combination of any of these areas: clitoris, vestibule, urethra, labia minora with or without labia majora, perineum with or without the peri-rectal area, the mons, upper thighs, and even the posterior thighs and legs. The symptoms become worse as the day progresses, especially when there are long periods of sitting.

Because the vulva is an area with many sensory nerves, Reid (1995) first suggested that nerve sensitization might be involved in chronic vulvar irritation. To understand the neurological theory of vulvodynia pain, we must review the basic physiology of the burning sensation. The experience of burning pain involves nerves, mediators, and perception. Pain receptors known as nociceptors are activated when there is tissue damage. These receptors normally transmit "pain" and "touch" sensations along unmyelinated C fibers (peripheral nerve fibers). Inflamed tissue contains biochemical mediators which activate the nociceptors, causing prolonged firing of the nerve fibers. (This sensitization of the nerve fibers explains why a sensation remains even after the original stimulus has been removed.) The prolonged firing of the C fibers sensitizes neurons (nerve cells) in the dorsal horn, a part of the spinal cord. From the dorsal horn, neurons transmit the impulse to the brain stem and thalamus, where it is perceived as pain. In summary, the neurological theory says that sensitized peripheral nerves cause the brain to react similarly to "touch" and "pain" impulses, such that stimulation of either type will be perceived as pain.

The initiating factor of vulvodynia can be any event that causes irritation. Possible causal factors may be: chronic yeast infections or the many topical medications used in their treatment; herpes virus infection, resulting in a pseudo post-herpetic neuralgia syndrome; accidental trauma; prolonged stretching of the pudendal nerve due to childbirth; chemical or laser destruction of subclinical human papilloma virus (HPV); or certain metabolites in the urine.

Causes of pudendal neuralgia may include trauma, neoplasms (new benign or malignant growths) of the spinal cord, infection, neurologic disorders, and muscle spasm. Unfortunately, a specific initiating factor is not discovered in most cases, and the cause is termed idiopathic.

Treatment

The main treatment of both essential vulvodynia and pudendal neuralgia is the use of tricyclic antidepressants such as amitriptyline or desipramine. These norepinephrine re-uptake inhibitors previously have been shown to be effective in the management of neuropathic pain conditions such as post-herpes zoster neuralgia and diabetic neuropathy. I start by prescribing the smallest dose and increase the dosage until improvement is noted or the patient complains of significant side effects. These drugs should not be discontinued abruptly as severe reactions can occur. The pure serotonin re-uptake inhibitors such as Prozac have not been found to be as useful in the treatment of neuropathic pain, although some clinical pain specialists report some success with Effexor.

Other types of medications that are used to manage essential vulvodynia and pudendal neuralgia are anticonvulsants such as Neurontin and Trileptal, a modified version of Tegretol. These drugs are especially helpful in patients who experience shooting pains in addition to constant burning pain. Their method of action is to raise the threshold at which nerve transmission occurs. Obtaining a detailed history of other medications being taken by the patient is important, as drug interactions with anticonvulsants are common. Prophylaxis with acyclovir, 400 mg. twice a day, should be reserved for patients who have active herpes lesions associated with flare-ups of their symptoms. In these situations, acyclovir is given in addition to the tricyclic antidepressant or anticonvulsant.

In conjunction with medication, measures that reduce irritation of the sensitive vulvar mucosa (inner lining of the labia minora) are indicated. Loose fitting clothes, white cotton underwear, hypo-allergenic soaps, cold soaks, and the elimination of bubble bath and feminine deodorant sprays are helpful. I also recommend that a protective layer of an emollient—like plain petroleum or Crisco vegetable shortening be applied to the mucosa.

It should be noted that no single therapy works all the time in every patient. As mentioned earlier, **surgical procedures should primarily be limited to patients with vulvar vestibulitis syndrome**. On the other hand, medication is the treatment of choice for essential vulvodynia, but not for vulvar vestibulitis. Recent articles have suggested that pelvic floor adjustment with physical therapy and biofeedback has helped some vulvar pain patients. Many alternative therapies have been tried with some success in some patients; for example, acupuncture and transepidermal nerve stimulation (TENS) have been used with varying results.

Psychological Support

Even though vulvar pain is a physical disorder, psychological support often is necessary to enable the patient to cope with what can be a severely disabling condition. In addition to its newsletter, the National Vulvodynia Association has organized a support network throughout the United States and Canada, as well as five other countries.

Some patients also may benefit from professional counseling to deal with depression and interpersonal/sexual issues. Any patient with chronic pain that interferes with normal functioning for more than three months is by definition depressed. I am always asked which came first, the chicken or the egg! A few psychological studies have shown that, in general, these patients do not differ significantly from control patients with regard to many psychological parameters. Given my personal experience with vulvar pain patients, once the diagnosis has been made they are no different from other patients. One factor that contributes to the frustration and depression initially exhibited by these patients is that they have been shifted from one physician to another, repeatedly mis-diagnosed and treated for yeast infections which do not get any better.

Summary

In conclusion, the key to vulvodynia treatment is early diagnosis! Potential therapies include:

1. Vigorously treating the initiating event.

2. Stabilizing the dorsal horn with tricyclic antidepressants and/ or anticonvulsants.

3. Interrupting the mucosal pain loop with symptomatic treatment and removal of all irritants.

4. Breaking the deeper "pain loop" with biofeedback or physical therapy.

5. Providing emotional support and encouraging psychological counseling as needed.

—by Stanley Marinoff, M.D

Dr. Marinoff is the director of the Center for Vulvovaginal Disorders and clinical professor of OB/GYN at George Washington University School of Medicine, Washington, D.C. He also serves on the NVA medical advisory board and is a fellow of the International Society for the Study of Vulvovaginal Disease.

Part Three

Pain Management

Chapter 44

Principles of Pain Management

The Management of Acute, Chronic and Cancer Pain

For thousands of years, doctors have been helping to relieve their patients' pain with a variety of medications and treatments. Like other areas of medicine, a new subset of doctors have become specialists in treating pain. They are focused on managing all types of pain—studying what causes it, how the body reacts to it, how different medications dull or eliminate the pain, and how other treatments can be used to relieve many painful conditions.

Doctors Who Specialize in Treating Pain

Doctors who manage pain are frequently anesthesiologists. Anesthesiologists are doctors of medicine (M.D.) or osteopathy (D.O.) who make sure that you are safe, pain-free and comfortable during and following surgery. They also provide their services in other areas of the hospital—especially in the labor and delivery area—or in doctors' offices where painful medical tests or procedures are performed.

But not everyone realizes that decades of research and work done by anesthesiologists have led to the development of newer, more effective treatments for patients who have pain unrelated to surgery. Many techniques used to make surgery and childbirth virtually painless are now being used to relieve other types of pain. In fact, the work pioneered by anesthesiologists that led to these new medications and treatments also has created a new category of medicine called pain medicine.

Frequently the anesthesiologist heads a team of other specialists and doctors who work together to help you manage your pain. The anesthesiologist or other pain medicine doctors (such as neurologists, oncologists, orthopedists, physiatrists and psychiatrists) and non-physician specialists (such as nurses, nurse practitioners, physician assistants, physical or rehabilitation therapists and psychologists) all work together to evaluate your condition. Then this "team" of specialists will develop a treatment plan designed just for you.

What type of training does a pain medicine doctor have?

Like other physicians, anesthesiologists earned a college degree and then completed four years of medical school. They spent four more years learning the medical specialty of anesthesiology and pain medicine during residency training. Many anesthesiologists who specialize in pain medicine receive an additional year of fellowship training to become a "subspecialist," or an expert in treating pain. Some also have done research, and many have special certification in pain medicine through the American Board of Anesthesiology (ABA). The ABA is the only organization recognized by the American Board of Medical Specialties to offer special credentials in pain medicine.

When would I need to see a pain medicine doctor?

People develop pain for many reasons. Pain from a recent surgery, injury or medical illness is called acute pain. In many cases, this pain can be managed immediately and will usually get better in just a short time. For more serious pain, however, your primary care doctor may ask a pain medicine doctor to help manage your pain while you are healing.

If your pain persists after the healing process should be over, you might have what is called chronic pain. If the current treatment you are receiving stops working or your pain begins to get worse over time, your primary care doctor may suggest that you see a pain medicine doctor.

Cancer pain is another condition that can be managed by a pain medicine doctor while the patient continues to receive treatment for various types of cancer. The pain can be due to cancer surgery or treatment procedures, including radiation therapy and chemotherapy, or the tumor itself.

What does a pain medicine doctor do? Can these doctors find out why I hurt?

Pain medicine doctors are experts at diagnosing why you are having pain as well as treating the pain itself. Some of the more common pain problems they manage include: arthritis, back and neck pain, cancer pain, nerve pain, migraine headaches, shingles, phantom limb pain for amputees and pain caused by AIDS.

They also manage acute pain caused by surgery, a debilitating illness or a serious injury. Examples include: pain after a knee-joint replacement, pain during recovery from a car accident, pain following stomach or chest surgery, or pain associated with sickle cell disease. You may be treated in the hospital or in an outpatient clinic.

- The pain medicine doctor will work closely with your primary care doctor.

- Pain medicine doctors will review your medical records and X-rays as needed.

- They will ask you to describe your pain in detail, such as where it hurts, for how long, what makes the pain worse or what makes it feel better.

- They may ask you to fill out a detailed questionnaire that helps them to assess the impact that your pain is having on your lifestyle and if it is interfering with your daily activities.

- They also will do a complete physical examination on you.

- They may need to order other tests and will then review all of their findings to determine what is causing your pain and how the problem can be corrected.

Medications for Managing Pain

Due to rapid advances in medicine, a wide variety of medications and treatments are available for acute, chronic and cancer pain. Patients often will be prescribed medications before receiving other forms of therapy. In addition, your pain medicine doctor may conclude that a combination of medication and treatments may be right for you. Your therapy plan will be tailored to your specific needs and circumstances.

Your pain medicine doctor may suggest that you use certain over-the-counter pain relievers or may prescribe stronger medicine for your condition. **Do not mix pain prescription drugs with over-the-counter**

pain relievers without consulting your doctor. Advise your doctor if you are taking any herbal medicines or dietary supplements.

Common pain relievers: Nonaspirin pain relievers such as acetaminophen (Tylenol®) can relieve headaches and minor pain but do not reduce swelling. They are sometimes used in combination with other drugs to provide greater pain relief.

Anti-inflammatory drugs: Aspirin (Anacin®, Bayer®), coated or buffered aspirin (Ascripton®, Bufferin®) and aspirin with acetaminophen (Excedrin®) may be used to reduce swelling and irritation as well as to relieve pain. There also are non-steroidal anti-inflammatory drugs (NSAIDs, commonly called "N-sayeds") such as ibuprofen (Advil®, Motrin®) and naproxen (Aleve®). Anti-inflammatory drugs are used to relieve pain, inflammation and fever. There also are steroidal drugs (like cortisol and prednisone), available only by prescription, that are used to treat more serious inflammatory conditions such as chronic arthritis.

Opioid pain medications: Morphine-like drugs called opioids are prescribed to treat acute pain or cancer pain. They are occasionally used for certain chronic, noncancer pain as well.

Anti-depressants: These drugs were originally used only to treat depression. Studies now show, however, that they also can relieve certain pain. Available only by prescription, they often are used to help you sleep better at night.

Anti-seizure medicines: These medications are used to relieve what some patients describe as "shooting" pain by decreasing abnormal painful sensations caused by damaged nerves.

Other medicines: The doctor may also prescribe other types of medication that will be helpful for your specific pain problems. In addition, medications that counteract the side effects of opioids or treat the anxiety and depression associated with pain may also be prescribed.

Treatments for Managing Pain

Medication alone may not be enough to manage certain kinds of pain. Some medicines are more effective in fighting pain when they are combined with other methods of treatment. In some cases, the patient's pain condition may respond to treatment instead of medication. In fact, for some patients, certain therapies may eventually replace the need for taking any pain medicine, or less of it, over time. Here are just some of the available treatments being used successfully to treat pain patients.

Injection treatments: Local anesthetics (such as Novocain®), with or without cortisone-like medicines, can be injected around nerve roots and into muscles or joints. These medicines reduce swelling, irritation, muscle spasms and abnormal nerve activity that can cause pain.

Nerve blocks: Often a group of nerves, called a plexus or ganglion, that causes pain to a specific organ or body region can be blocked with local anesthetics. If successful, another solution that numbs the nerves can then be injected.

Physical and aquatic therapy: The physiatrist or physical therapist may suggest an exercise program tailored for you that will increase your daily functioning and decrease your pain. Other treatments may include whirlpool therapy, ultrasound and deep-muscle massage.

Electrical stimulation: Transcutaneous electrical nerve stimulation (TENS) is the most common form of electrical stimulation used in pain management. It is not painful and does not require needles or medicine. TENS consists of a small, battery-operated device that can diminish pain by stimulating nerve fibers through the skin.

Acupuncture: This ancient Chinese practice uses very thin needles at very specific points on the skin to treat disease and pain. Practitioners of acupuncture undergo specialized training in these techniques and may offer this treatment for certain painful conditions.

Psychological support: Many patients who are in pain feel the emotional effects of suffering along with the physical aspects of pain. These may include feelings of anger, sadness, hopelessness or despair. In addition, pain can alter one's personality, disrupt sleep, interfere with work and relationships and often have a profound effect on family members. Support and counseling from a psychiatrist or psychologist, combined with a comprehensive pain treatment program, may be needed to help you manage your condition. These trained professionals also can teach you additional self-help therapies such as relaxation training or biofeedback to relieve pain, lessen muscle spasms and reduce stress.

Surgery: When necessary, surgical treatment may be recommended. In rare instances when severe pain has not responded to other treatments and procedures, surgery on certain nerves can be done to give the patient some relief and allow them to resume near-normal activities. Usually all other avenues of treatment are tried before surgery is considered.

Pain Treatment Centers

Because this is a highly specialized field of medicine that is still growing, not every community has a pain treatment center yet. These centers are called by many different names, including: pain clinic, pain management center, pain center, pain unit or pain service. These facilities may be in a wing of your local hospital or medical center, in a separate medical-professional building or in a doctor's office. Some are affiliated with medical schools and large health care centers.

Where can I find a pain treatment center, and how do I decide if it's the right one for me?

There are many different forms of pain treatment and therapy, and one center may offer a service or specific kind of specialist that another center does not have. Some have pain medicine doctors on staff, and others may offer only nonmedical treatments such as acupuncture and massage therapy. Thus before consenting to treatment, it is best to find out what types of pain therapies are offered, what the specialists' credentials are and if they have successfully helped others with your type of pain.

To find a pain medicine doctor or pain specialist, generally your regular doctor should be able to refer you to an individual or group who offers services that are best for helping your specific pain problem. If your doctor is not able to refer you, try the sources below:

1. Call your local hospital or medical center and ask if they have a pain treatment center there or if they are affiliated with a pain treatment center or clinic nearby.

2. If your area does not have a specialized pain treatment center, ask the hospital to connect you to the Department of Anesthesiology. They may have doctors on staff who can provide treatment or who can refer you to another hospital.

3. If your local hospital does not have information on a pain treatment center, contact the nearest school of medicine, which is usually affiliated with a private college or state university. (Medical school listings are available at the public library.) Ask them if they offer pain treatment or if they have research programs that study pain.

4. If you have access to the internet, you can obtain information through the American Society of Anesthesiologists (ASA) at www.ASAhq.org. While ASA does not maintain a list of pain centers nationwide, we may be able to assist you with some additional information in your area.

Throughout the generations, pain has been a unique, often misunderstood condition that affects every age, gender, ethnic and social group all over the world. It can occur for many reasons, and there is no one "silver bullet" that can cure pain. Yet great progress in pain medicine has been made in recent years and is expected to advance further as doctors learn more about the causes of pain.

Anesthesiologists, through ASA, will continue to support research, medical training and patient education to help those who suffer from pain—whether it is acute, chronic or cancer pain—so these patients can live comfortably and be productive members of their families and communities.

Certain product names used in this chapter are included as a point of reference for patients and should not be considered all inclusive or construed as an endorsement by the American Society of Anesthesiologists (ASA), its committees or its members.

Patients should consult their physicians for recommendation or prescription of an appropriate course of treatment.

Chapter 45

Answers for Pain Patients

Who practices pain management?

Healthcare professionals with experience and/or special training in pain management who continue to obtain knowledge on a regular basis.

When should I seek a pain management practitioner?

When pain does not respond to the usual and customary treatments within a reasonable period of time.

My physician says I am in pain because my body is "deconditioned" and has referred me to physical therapy. The therapists where I live don't seem to understand complicated pain and I always get worse with the exercise programs. How can I improve my ability for movement without "flaring" up my pain?

Movement is a better word to use than exercise. People with complicated pain need to start with gentle and specific stretching of trigger points in muscles, all body joints, and the spine; under the guidance of their therapist.

How do I choose a pain management facility?

1. Call the State Board of Examiners to be sure you are seeing licensed health care professionals.

2. Call the facility and ask to have the case manager speak to you about becoming a patient.

3. Call your insurance company to review your benefits.

4. Interview the case manager and others about their experience with complicated pain and discuss any possible limitations or exclusions of your insurance and payment plans for services.

5. Ask about policy and procedures for patient rights and responsibilities, informed consent, billing procedures, and credential of practitioners.

How can I find professionals in pain management?

Look first for a type of practitioner and their current state licensure. Many state boards can confirm the status as well as any prior disciplinary problems. In addition, look for membership in professional organizations at the state or national level that indicate a higher level of commitment to practice. Finally, look for specialized training focused on pain issues such as membership or diplomat status with the American Academy of Pain Management.

Why should I bother seeking out an accredited pain program?

Pain Program Accreditation speaks to several issues. First, it shows that your treating professionals are committed to the best possible organized care for you and the best way to address the issues you bring. Second, accreditation shows that your treating professionals meet peer review standards for treating your problem. Finally, accreditation means that your treating professionals wish to compare their treatment outcomes to others in the field. This means that the program's treatment can constantly get better. The bottom line is that accreditation means you get a program that has met peer based standards, can be cost effective, and reflects a belief in the patient as a health team member with rights about treatment.

My doctor says I should have some biofeedback. Is he trying to dump me since my pain isn't responding too well right now?

Absolutely not! Your doctor is trying to be sure you have the comprehensive care you need. Pain is not just a physical issue, but effects all aspects of your physical and mental health. Despite centuries of trying to separate mind and body, treatment of chronic pain forces us to admit this can't be done. We will never say your pain is in your head but thoughts and emotion are related to pain. We call this the pain/stress/depression cycle. Biofeedback can give us the opportunity to interfere throughout this cycle. The more places and ways we can interfere with the pain- stress cycle, the more likely we are able to be of lasting help.

How does the pain professional interact with patients to make sure they understand condition, goals, treatment and outcome?

1. The client making clear their desired outcome at intake.

2. Use of a pain analog scale before and after treatment.

3. Each patient has a chance to review their progress on a regular basis.

4. All goals are measurable.

5. Clients are asked about treatment satisfaction.

6. Interaction and dialogue is central to the program.

What are the concerns of pain practitioners who prescribe narcotics for the management of chronic pain?

Licensing issues, peer review, state disciplinary action, protection from legal prosecution for over-prescribing (under-prescribing) of controlled substances, etc.

I've been to my family doctor and several specialists and no one can tell me what is wrong. What should I do?

Schedule time to speak with your health care professional. Ask for clarification. Ask for a referral to a good pain program where you can get information. Ask to see your file and request an explanation of the reports.

My doctor says there is no objective basis for my pain, why isn't there any?

Laboratory and imaging tests for your condition may be negative, but that doesn't mean your pain doesn't exist. Your doctor should also consider your subjective pain complaints. You know your body best, sometimes a condition does not show up on a test until later. You may request a visit with a pain management counselor to help clarify your situation.

Why hasn't my doctor referred me to a pain clinic sooner?

Conservative measures are usually tried before you are seen by a pain consultant. However, if your pain has not resolved within a reasonable period of time ask for a referral to a pain clinic.

Are there risks to injections?

There are potential risks any time the skin is broken. All treatment should be explained prior to being performed. You should have the opportunity to ask questions and sign a consent form.

Are opioids for everyone?

Nothing is for everyone! Opioids may relieve certain types of pain. If pain limits function, opioids may help improve function. There is debate even among pain specialists about the need for opioids for chronic pain. There is an increasing trend to use opioids for painful conditions. Always speak to your doctor about recommended medications. Be clear why you are taking medications, how to take your medications and any potential adverse risk from taking the medication.

Is pain management covered by health insurance?

Policies differ. It depends on your coverage and the type of intervention. Please check with your health care provider or insurance company to see if you qualify for specific benefits.

Chapter 46

Managing Pain in Palliative Care

All patients with medical illness should be made as comfortable as possible by relieving pain and other distressing symptoms. This is a fundamental goal of palliative care.

Pain

Many serious diseases, such as cancer and AIDS, cause pain. Pain can be intermittent or constant, and can vary in severity from mild to severe. It can have many different qualities, such as burning, shooting, aching, piercing or pinching. Many factors influence the perception of pain, including mood, activity level, stress, and the availability of pain-relieving therapies.

Pain can be caused by:

- The activation of pain receptors by something that injures pain-sensitive tissues (nociceptive pain). Tissue damage from a mass (like a tumor) or from inflammation, for example, can cause this type of pain

- Nerve damage (neuropathic pain) from a virus, chemotherapy, trauma or a disease such as multiple sclerosis

---

Excerpted from "Management of Pain and Other Symptoms," Department of Pain Medicine and Palliative Care at Beth Israel Medical Center, online at www.stoppain.org. © 2000 Continuum Health Partners, Inc.; reprinted with permission.

Treating pain is important. Unrelieved pain can cause patients to:

- Experience depression
- Experience disruptions in activity, appetite and sleep
- Feel helpless and anxious
- Give up hope
- Reject treatment programs
- Stop participating in life to the fullest extent possible

Pain usually can be controlled. There are many treatment options. To offer the best approaches for pain, doctors must recognize that pain is different in every person. All patients who experience pain deserve a detailed evaluation of the pain, the effect of the pain, and the diseases that may be causing the pain.

Pain in Cancer Patients

Many people with cancer experience pain. Thirty to 40 percent of patients in active cancer therapy and 70 to 90 percent of patients with advanced cancer report pain.

Cancer pain can be caused by:

- Tumors pressing on organs, nerves or bone
- Treatment such as surgery, chemotherapy or radiation
- Other conditions related to the cancer, such as stiffness from inactivity, muscle spasms, constipation and bedsores
- Conditions unrelated to the cancer, such as arthritis or migraine

In most cases, cancer pain can be controlled through relatively simple means. Doctors usually use medications, which are prescribed according to a plan that was first described by the World Health Organization and is called the Analgesic Ladder approach to cancer pain management.

Other ways to alleviate cancer pain include:

- Surgery, radiation or chemotherapy to shrink tumors causing pain
- Antibiotic therapy or drainage for pain caused by infection

- Psychological therapies, and social and spiritual support, to influence the perception of pain

- Other pain treatments

World Health Organization's Analgesic Ladder Approach for Relief of Cancer Pain

Step 1. Patients with mild to moderate pain should receive:

- A nonopioid analgesic, such as acetaminophen or a nonsteroidal anti-inflammatory drug (NSAID)

- Adjuvant drugs if a specific indication exists

Step 2. Patients with moderate to severe pain (or who have failed to achieve adequate relief with Step 1) should receive:

- An opioid conventionally used for moderate pain (usually codeine, hydrocodone, dihydrocodeine, oxycodone, propoxyphene, or tramadol)

- A nonopioid analgesic, such as acetaminophen or an NSAID

- An adjuvant drug in some cases

Step 3. Patients with severe pain (or who have failed to achieve adequate relief with Step 2) should receive:

- An opioid conventionally used for severe pain, such as morphine, oxycodone, hydromorphone, methadone, levorphanol or fentanyl

- A nonopioid analgesic in some cases

- Adjuvant drugs in some cases

Pain in AIDS Patients

Pain is just as common in AIDS as it is in cancer. Like cancer pain, AIDS-related pain can be caused by the disease itself and from therapies.

AIDS patients commonly experience:

- Pain due to nerve damage, such as peripheral neuropathy and postherpetic neuralgia

341

- Headaches from meningitis
- Abdominal pain from gastrointestinal disease
- Chest pain from pneumonia
- Muscle pains

To find an appropriate treatment, a doctor should perform a detailed assessment.

Treatment of Pain

Treatments that can successfully control pain include:

Pharmacological Therapies (Medication)

- Non-opioid pain relievers
- Opioids
- Adjuvant medications (drugs whose primary purpose is not for pain but rather for other conditions)
- Topical treatments (drugs are applied directly to the skin, as a patch, gel, or cream)

Because the effects of a medication can vary widely from person to person, treatment of pain needs to be tailored to fit each individual. Some patients may need to try many different kinds of treatments before they find the right balance between pain relief and side effects.

Patients should be sure their doctors are aware of all medications they are taking, even for conditions unrelated to their pain or over-the-counter drugs such as aspirin. Many medications should not be taken together because they increase or decrease each other's effects or produce new adverse reactions. Of course, the doctor should also be informed if the patient is pregnant or breast feeding.

Non-pharmacological Treatments

Non-pharmacological treatments (treatments that do not rely primarily on medication to achieve their effect) offer a variety of approaches to pain relief. Most are non-invasive.

Simple, relatively safe non-pharmacological approaches include:

- Physiatric Approaches

- Non-invasive Stimulatory Approaches

- Psychological Approaches

- Complementary/Alternative Approaches

In most cases, these techniques should be used in addition to, not instead of, other approaches to pain relief.

More invasive non-pharmacological treatments include:

- Anesthesiologic Approaches

- Invasive Stimulatory Approaches

- Surgical Approaches

Physiatric Approaches

Therapeutic Exercise. Exercising is important because it can:

- Strengthen weak muscles

- Mobilize stiff joints

- Help restore coordination and balance

- Promote a sense of well-being

- Decrease anxiety and stress

- Keep the heart healthy

- Help maintain an appropriate weight

A physical therapist, exercise physiologist or certified athletic trainer can help patients get started safely and learn exercises designed specifically to target problem areas. Even bedridden patients can benefit from range-of-motion exercises.

Heat Therapy. Heat therapy can reduce pain, especially the pain of muscle tension or spasm. Sometimes patients with other types of pain benefit.

Heat therapy acts to:

- Increase the blood flow to the skin

- Dilate blood vessels, increasing oxygen and nutrient delivery to local tissues

- Decrease joint stiffness by increasing muscle elasticity

Heat should be applied for 20 minutes. Patients can use hot packs, hot water bottles, hot and moist compresses, electric heating pads, or chemical and gel packs carefully wrapped to avoid burns. Patients can also submerge themselves or the painful part in warm water.

Heat therapy is not recommended on tissue that has received radiation treatment. Pregnant women should avoid using hot tubs or any method that subjects the developing baby to prolonged heat.

Deep heat delivered to underlying tissue by short wave diathermy, microwave diathermy or ultrasound is also sometimes used to relieve pain. Deep heat should be used with caution by patients with active cancer and should not be applied directly over a cancer site.

Cold Therapy. Cold therapy, which constricts blood vessels near the skin, sometimes can relieve the pain of muscle tension or spasm. Other types of pain also benefit in some cases. It can also reduce swelling if applied soon after an injury.

Ice packs, towels soaked in ice water or commercially prepared chemical gel packs should be applied for 15 minutes. Cold sources should be sealed to prevent dripping, flexible to conform to the body, and adequately wrapped to prevent irritation or damage to the skin.

Non-Invasive Stimulatory Approaches

Transcutaneous Electrical Nerve Stimulation (TENS). Transcutaneous electrical nerve stimulation (TENS) is a method of applying a gentle electric current to the skin to relieve pain. Studies have shown that it can be effective in certain cases of chronic pain.

A small box-shaped device, which patients can put in their pocket or hang on their belt, transmits electrical impulses through wires to electrodes taped to the skin in the painful area. Patients describe the sensation of TENS as buzzing, tingling or tapping.

The patient should experiment with the placement of the electrodes and the timing, intensity, amplitude and frequency of the electrical current to find the most effective setting. Pain relief usually lasts beyond the period when current is applied. TENS can become less effective at relieving pain over time.

TENS is usually safe and well tolerated. However, it is not recommended on inflamed, infected or otherwise unhealthy skin, over a pregnant uterus (except for obstetric pain relief), or in the presence of a cardiac pacemaker.

Psychoeducational Approaches

Cognitive Behavioral Techniques. Cognitive behavioral techniques are used to reduce the body's unproductive responses to stress, helping to relieve pain or improve the ability to tolerate it.

Some techniques are:

- *Deep breathing.* In this simple technique, the patient focuses his or her attention on breathing deeply. This may shift attention away from the source of pain.

- *Progressive muscle relaxation.* In this technique, developed in the 1930s, patients contract, then relax, muscles throughout the body, group by group. Progressive muscle relaxation can help patients learn about the tension in their body and the contrast between tense and relaxed muscles.

- *Imagery.* In this technique, patients focus on pleasant thoughts, for example waves gently hitting a sandy beach. One variation is to think of an image that represents the pain (such as a hot, blazing concrete sidewalk), then imagine it changing into an image representing a pain-free state (a pretty, snow-covered forest).

- *Meditation.* In this technique, practiced routinely in Asia, the individual aims to empty his or her mind of thoughts, focusing instead on the sensation of breathing and the rhythms of his or her body.

- *Biofeedback Therapy.* Biofeedback is a method in which people learn to reduce their body's unproductive responses to stress, and thus decrease their sensitivity to pain. Children are particularly quick to learn from biofeedback.

  In biofeedback, electrodes are placed at various points on the patient's skin to measure:

  - Muscle tension. As a muscle contracts, electrical activity increases

  - Temperature. The stress response is related to blood flow in the hands or feet, and blood flow determines temperature

  - Heart beat

  - Sweating

  Patients watch the monitor and listen to the tones measuring their stress indicators. They use these as a guide in learning to release tension throughout their body.

- *Distraction*. Distraction is a pain management technique in which patients focus their attention on something other than their pain and negative emotions. To distract themselves, patients can:

  - Sing

  - Count

  - Listen to music

  - Watch TV

  - Listen to the radio

  - Talk to friends or family

  - Read

  - Listen to stories being read

- *Reframing*. Reframing is a pain and stress management technique that teaches patients to monitor negative thoughts and images and replace them with positive ones.

  Patients can learn to have a more positive outlook by recognizing some counterproductive thought patterns, such as:

  - Blaming, in which the individual avoids taking responsibility. Thoughts such as "It's my boss's fault I have this headache" can be replaced with "I'm going to focus on what I can do to feel better."

  - "Should" or "must" statements, which imply that someone has failed to live up to an arbitrary standard. Statements such as "I should have been more careful" can be counteracted with "I do not have to be perfect" or "I made the best decision I could have at the time."

  - Polarized thinking, in which everything is black or white, with no shades of gray. Statements such as "I'm still in pain, so this program is useless" can be counteracted with "I wish I could be free of pain, but I have made some progress. Sometimes small improvements add up."

  - Catastrophizing, in which the person images the worst possible scenario then acts as if it will surely come true. Statements such as "This pain must mean I am going downhill" can be counteracted with "I am jumping to conclusions" or "I'll find a way to cope with whatever happens."

- Control fallacy, in which the person sees him or herself as completely controlled by others (or controlling everything). Thoughts such as "My spouse doesn't think I need to see a counselor, so I can't go" can be counteracted with "I am not a helpless victim" (or thoughts such as "My family will fall apart without me" can be counteracted with "Members of my family are not helpless").

- Emotional reasoning, in which the individual believes that what he or she feels must be true. Statements such as "I'm so frightened the pain will never stop, I know it never will" can be counteracted with "I'm scared, but that does not give me an accurate view of the situation" or "When I calm down, I will think about what this means."

- Filtering, in which people focus on one thing (such as pain) to the exclusion of any other experience or point of view. Statements such as "I can't take it'" can be replaced with "I have coped before and can cope again."

- Entitlement fallacy, in which individuals believe they have the right to what they want. Statements such as "Life is so unfair" or "I have been cheated" can be counteracted with "No one promised me a rose garden. I will focus on finding ways to make things better."

Psychotherapy and Social Support. Psychotherapy and social support can help a patient cope with pain.

- Psychotherapy may be useful for anyone whose pain is difficult to manage, who has developed clinical depression or anxiety or who has a history of psychiatric illness.

  Among the goals of psychotherapy are the following:

  - Emphasize the patient's past strengths
  - Support the patient's use of previously successful coping strategies
  - Teach new coping skills
  - Establish a bond to decrease a patient's sense of isolation
  - Foster a sense of self-worth

- Psychological Approaches

- Group Approaches: Peer groups, in which a patient meets with others with the same condition, can help by:

  - Providing support

  - Showing the patient how others have coped effectively

  - Helping the patient maintain a social identity

  - Providing access to information and material aid

- Spiritual leaders are another potential source of support for patients.

Complementary / Alternative Approaches

Acupuncture. Acupuncture is an ancient method for relieving pain and controlling disease, used in China for thousands of years. It appears to be effective for some patients with chronic pain.

Thin gold or metal needles, gently twirled for ten to twenty minutes, can be used to stimulate acupuncture points, which relieve pain in specific parts of the body (for example, a point on the leg targets stomach pain). Patients usually feel a tingling, warm sensation, similar to that of transcutaneous electrical nerve stimulation. Acupuncture points can also be stimulated with deep massage (acupressure), electric currents (electroacupuncture), or lasers.

The risk of side effects is low. Side effects can include post-needling pain, bleeding, bruising, dizziness, fainting, and local skin reactions. Rarely, organ damage can occur with deep needling techniques. Infection because of inadequately sterilized needles is a hazard: disposable needles are recommended.

Acupuncture is not recommended for patients with serious blood clotting problems. Acupuncture, should be used with caution by pregnant women.

Massage. Massage can be a useful addition to a pain management program, especially for patients who are bedridden.

Massage can:

- Stimulate blood flow

- Relax muscles that are tight or in spasm

- Promote a feeling of well-being

Muscles can be stroked, kneaded or rubbed in a circular motion. A lotion can reduce friction on the skin.

Massage is not recommended in cases of swollen tissue. It should be used in addition to, and not instead of, exercise by patients who can walk.

Anesthesiologic Approaches

For patients with pain who fail conservative therapies, simple to complex interventional therapies such as nerve blocks, epidural steroid injections, intraspinal drug administration, or trigger point injections may be helpful. These therapies are typically provided by anesthesiologists with advanced training in pain management.

Nerve Blocks and Epidural Steroid Injections. Nerve blocks can relieve pain by inhibiting the impulses that travel along specific nerves in the body. To achieve a block, the doctor usually injects a local anesthetic along the course of a nerve or nerves. Although this is called a "temporary" block, in the best outcome, pain relief lasts for a long time. In very selected cases, the doctor can inject a solution that damages the nerve and produces a more permanent block.

Sympathetic nerve blocks inhibit the nerves of the sympathetic nervous system, which are responsible for increasing heart rate, constricting blood vessels and raising blood pressure in response to stress. Sympathetic nerve blocks can be useful in treating some pains due to nerve damage, such as some types of complex regional pain syndrome (also called reflex sympathetic dystrophy or causalgia).

Blocks of somatic nerves can be targeted to any area of the body. In some cases, nerve blocks fail to provide pain relief, or provide only a brief respite.

Epidural steroids, administered through injection, can help to interrupt the passage of painful impulses through nerves.

Spinal Infusion. Intraspinal drug administration involves the delivery of low doses of analgesic drugs, such as morphine or clonidine, through a catheter inserted directly into the spine. This approach is used often to manage cancer pain.

Triggerpoint Injections. This approach may be helpful.

Invasive Stimulatory Approaches

Invasive Nerve Stimulation. Invasive nerve stimulation can provide pain relief for some patients who have not responded to other therapies. In this technique, electrodes are implanted in the patient's

349

body to send a gentle electrical current to nerves in the spinal column or the brain.

Spinal cord stimulation has been used for chronic back and/or leg pain following lumbar surgery, pain due to nerve damage (complex regional pain syndrome and postherpetic neuralgia) and intractable angina. Few controlled studies of this method exist.

Deep brain stimulation may help as many as half of patients with central pain, a challenging condition that can develop as a result of damage to the central nervous system from stroke.

Disadvantages of this therapy include its high cost, risks of an invasive treatment (such as infection), and difficulty predicting before a trial which patients will benefit.

Surgical Approaches

Surgery to treat pain (rather than the underlying disease) is only appropriate in cases where more conservative approaches have failed and where trained neurosurgeons and follow-up care are available.

A surgeon can cut a nerve close to the spinal cord (rhizotomy) or bundles of nerves in the spinal cord (cordotomy) to interrupt the pathways that send pain signals to the brain. In the best possible outcome, surgery relieves pain and the need for most or all pain medication.

However, surgery carries the risk of:

- Stopping the pain only briefly

- Creating new pain from nerve damage at the site of the operation

- Limiting the patient's ability to feel pressure and temperature in the region, putting him or her at risk for injury

Chapter 47

Pain Treatments: An Overview

How to Prescribe

When using a drug to treat pain, it is very important to use it as prescribed by the physician. Many drugs used for pain must be started at a low dose, then slowly increased—a method called titration. Because not every patient is the same with regard to his or her pain and body chemistry, every patient responds differently to each drug. Patients with the same pain syndrome may or may not experience pain relief or side effects from any particular drug and, additionally, the best dose often varies from patient to patient.

Over-the-Counter (OTC) Pain Relievers (Non-Prescription Drugs)

Over-the-counter (OTC) pain relievers are among the most widely used drugs. Most people self-medicate their usual aches and pains with medications such as acetaminophen and nonsteroidal anti-inflammatory agents (aspirin, ibuprofen, naproxen, and ketoprofen). Acetaminophen, the active ingredient in Tylenol®, has few side effects. However, long-term regular use of high dose acetaminophen can cause serious liver damage.

"General Treatments," Department of Pain Medicine and Palliative Care at Beth Israel Medical Center, online at www.stoppain.org. © 2000 Continuum Health Partners, Inc.; reprinted with permission.

Nonsteroidal Anti-Inflammatory Drugs (NSAIDs)

Nonsteroidal anti-inflammatory drugs (NSAIDs) are commonly used as OTC pain relievers and are also prescribed by doctors in larger doses ("prescription strength"). NSAIDs reduce the production or release of prostaglandins, chemicals in the body responsible for inflammatory pain. Most NSAIDs are taken orally. There are many drugs, and the best drug varies from person to person. NSAIDs are nonspecific analgesics but are most commonly used to treat musculoskeletal pains and headache. The most important side effect is peptic ulcer disease.

Adjuvant Medications

By definition, adjuvant analgesics are drugs whose initial use was not for pain but rather for other conditions. They are a diverse group of drugs that includes antidepressants, anticonvulsants (antiseizure drugs), and others.

Antidepressants

The best studied adjuvant analgesics are the tricyclic antidepressants (TCAs), such as amitriptyline (Elavil®), and desipramine. There is overwhelming evidence that this class of drugs can be effective for migraine headache, tension-type headache, postherpetic neuralgia, painful diabetic neuropathy, arthritis, low back pain, and other painful conditions. These drugs have been shown to relieve pain independent of their effects on depression; that is, patients who are not depressed may experience pain relief. Once the correct dose is found for the individual patient, favorable results are usually seen within a week; however, side effects, including weight gain, dry mouth, blurred vision and constipation, are possible.

There are many newer antidepressants, such as the selective serotonin reuptake inhibitors (like fluoxetine [Prozac®], paroxetine [Paxil®], sertraline [Zoloft®]), and others (like venlafaxine [Effexor®] and nefazadone [Serzone®]. Most of these antidepressant drugs have not been shown to be effective pain relievers in clinical studies, but some have, and many pain specialists believe that most, if not all, can potentially relieve pain. They are usually better tolerated than the TCA's.

Anticonvulsants

Drugs that are primarily used to treat epilepsy (seizures) have been used to treat nerve pain conditions and migraine headache for several decades. Many anticonvulsant drugs have been shown in clinical studies to be effective.

Gabapentin (Neurontin®) has become a first-line drug for neuropathic conditions due to its proven effectiveness and its low incidence of side effects. Other anticonvulsant drugs may be useful, including carbamazepine [Tegretol®], phenytoin [Dilantin®], valproate [Depakote®], clonazepam [Klonopin®], topiramate [Topamax®], and lamotrigine [Lamictal®]. The most common use of these drugs is for nerve pains, such as trigeminal neuralgia, postherpetic neuralgia, painful diabetic neuropathy, and migraine headache.

Alpha-2-Adrenergic Agonists

Currently, there are two alpha-2-adrenergic agonists that have some evidence as pain relievers: tizanidine (Zanaflex®) and clonidine (Catapres®). There are some studies showing that tizanidine can be effective for tension-type headache, back pain, neuropathic pain, and myofascial pains. Clonidine has been used to treat refractory neuropathic pain. Tizanidine tends to be better tolerated than clonidine and, unlike clonidine, rarely decreases blood pressure.

Local Anesthetics

Mexiletine is a drug that was first approved to treat irregular heart rhythms. However, several scientific studies have shown this drug to be effective in chronic nerve pain syndromes. Other oral local anesthetics are also used. Intravenous infusion of a local anesthetic is a special technique that may be used by pain specialists.

Steroids

Corticosteroids can be used as an effective analgesic for treating some cancer pain syndromes. Also, corticosteroids given as short-term tapers can be effective in treating migraine headache and complex regional pain syndrome (reflex sympathetic dystrophy).

Other Adjuvant Analgesics

Baclofen is on the market as a muscle relaxant and is used to treat nerve pain syndromes. There is very good evidence that it works in trigeminal neuralgia.

Drugs that block a specific receptor involved in the experience of pain, the N-methyl-D-aspartate (NMDA) receptor, may also be analgesic in nerve pain. These include dextromethorphan (the cough suppressant, but at higher doses than those needed to block cough), ketamine (an anesthetic), and amantadine.

There are many drugs that are called "muscle relaxants" and are used to treat minor musculoskeletal pains. These include carisoprodol (Soma®), cyclobenzaprine (Flexeril®), metaxolone (Skelaxin®), and others. These drugs do not actually relax skeletal muscle, but they can relieve pain, and they are commonly used.

Topical Drugs

Topical drugs are applied directly to the skin, as a patch, gel, or cream and have their pharmacologic activity directly under the skin site without any significant amount of drug entering the blood stream. Thus, true topical drugs should not produce any systemic side effects, that is, side effects caused by the drug's effects throughout the body. Currently, only one topical drug has an FDA approved indication for pain treatment—a topical lidocaine patch (Lidoderm®)—for the treatment of postherpetic neuralgia. This patch can be tried for many types of nerve pain.

A widely used topical pain reliever is capsaicin, which is available as an over-the-counter cream. There have been some studies that show pain relief with capsaicin and others that do not. This drug is being used to treat nerve pain and arthritis pain.

Interventional Approaches

For patients with chronic pain who fail conservative therapies, an interventional therapy might be helpful. The simpler of these approaches include trigger point injections (injecting local anesthetic and/or steroid into myofascial trigger points), epidural steroid injections and joint injections. The more complex include nerve blocks, spinal cord stimulation, and intraspinal drug administration. These more sophisticated procedures are typically provided by anesthesiologists with advanced training in pain management.

Spinal cord stimulation (also called dorsal column stimulation) provides low-voltage stimulation inside the spinal cord and may block or decrease the pain signals going to the brain. This technique has been used to treat chronic low back pain, chronic sciatica, and complex regional pain syndrome (reflex sympathetic dystrophy), among other conditions.

Intraspinal drug administration involves the delivery of low doses of analgesic drugs, such as morphine or clonidine, through a catheter inserted directly into the spine. This approach is used often to manage cancer pain and refractory nonmalignant pain.

Rehabilitation Approaches

Physical therapy and occupational therapy may reduce pain and help restore function. Chronic pain sufferers may benefit from a supervised exercise regimen, designed by a physical therapist trained in treating chronic pain, that includes range of motion maneuvers, strengthening techniques, and aerobic conditioning. Heat and cold and other so-called modalities (e.g., vibration or ultrasound) also may help alleviate pain, although they should not be applied to areas without sensation or in patients who are unable to communicate. Sources of heat or cold include heating pads, hot-water baths, ice packs or vapocoolant sprays like ethyl chloride or fluorimethane.

There are also a variety of alternative physical medicine techniques that appear to benefit some patients. The Alexander technique, which focuses on proper body alignment and positioning, is often used to treat chronic pain. Other techniques used include craniosacral manipulation, osteopathic manipulation, and myofascial release, to name just a few.

Stimulatory Approaches

Pain relief also can be achieved through approaches which stimulate nerve pathways to produce analgesia. The invasive approach, spinal cord stimulation, was mentioned before. The best known and most widely prescribed are acupuncture and transcutaneous electrical nerve stimulation (TENS). Patients receiving TENS carry a small, box-shaped device that transmits electrical impulses into the body through the electrodes to interfere with pain signals. A buzzing, tingling or tapping sensation is felt. TENS should not be used on inflamed or infected skin, in the presence of a pacemaker, or if the patient is pregnant.

Psychological Approaches

Distraction is sometimes called cognitive refocusing. Essentially, it is a strategy that directs a person's attention and concentration at other stimuli, thereby shielding them from their pain. Stimuli may be internal (daydreaming) or external (television). They may be self-initiated, such as making phone calls, or passive, as with listening to music or humor. The most effective distraction techniques are those that are unique and changing, those that require input from most or all of the senses—seeing, hearing, tasting, touching and smelling—and those that are interesting to and appropriate for the person practicing them. In some cases, awareness of the pain, as well as fatigue and irritability, increases when the distraction ends.

Relaxation may be used for almost any type of pain, but it is particularly effective for chronic pain by helping to produce a state of relative freedom from anxiety and skeletal muscle tension. Relaxation strategies tend to concentrate on one thing, such as a word, sound, phrase or physical activity, and commonly use music, massage or slow, deep breathing. They also may involve imagery, in which a person focuses mentally on a pleasant or peaceful experience, or superficial body massage, felt to be especially helpful for people with little physical contact or for whom verbal communication is limited or impossible. For maximum relaxation, researchers suggest three 20-minute periods daily, in a quiet environment, assuming a comfortable well-supported position. Practice of a particular technique is suggested to establish a conditioned relaxation response.

Complementary Approaches

Complementary or alternative approaches are often used in combination with traditional analgesic treatments, rather than as substitutes for them. Some therapies that are typically considered alternative are actually considered mainstream by most pain specialists. These include approaches that have been called mind-body (psychologists usually refer to them as cognitive therapies), such as relaxation therapy, distraction techniques, biofeedback, and hypnosis, as well as acupuncture and therapeutic massage. Other complementary therapies include a wide range of practices such as meditation, chiropractic, and nutritional or other remedies that are thought to prompt the body's release of pain-relieving substances. Many of these therapies are readily available, easy to do, inexpensive and low risk. In addition to helping relieve pain, they also may improve sleep, reduce anxiety and increase one's sense of control.

Chapter 48

Ways to Take Pain Medicine

By Mouth

By mouth is often the best way to take pain medicine because it is easy and doesn't require special equipment. Many pain medicines come either in pills or as liquids. In 1997 fentanyl lollipops were made available for breakthrough pain for people with cancer. They have been available in pediatrics for a number of years for use with procedures.

Sustained Release: A number of products are available as sustained release—meaning one pill dissolves over a long period of time—so you don't have to spend your life taking pills. MS Contin is one of the most popular of this type of pain medicine. Recently a new type of sustained release morphine has been introduced that is a capsule filled with tiny pellets. It is the *only* sustained release medicine at this point in time that you can open the capsule and mix the pellets with applesauce. Do not break or crush any other sustained release morphine preparation.

Intramuscular (IM) ("Shots")

Most people, including the nurses who give them, don't like "shots." In many cases people who can't take medicines by mouth, have an IV

"Ways to Take Pain Medicines," an undated fact sheet an undated fact sheet available online at http://www.nursing.uiowa.edu/sites/PedsPain/Routes/Routes.htm (accessed October 2001), © University of Iowa College of Nursing, reprinted with permission.

(intravenous) going and the medicine can be given IV instead of as a "shot." In general, all of us are glad that this is being used less and less.

Intravenous (IV)

One of the nicest things in the last ten years is the use of IV pain medicines. IV provides the quickest help for people in pain, and the pump systems (called PCA) have really made pain control much easier for all involved.

Starting IV Doses

Starting doses of strong pain medicines can also be given IV in what is called a bolus dose that provides pain relief in 1-5 minutes if the medicine used is fentanyl or 15-30 minutes if morphine is used. Try to think of the starting dose as like calling in the fire trucks to put out a fairly large fire. If you only put a garden hose on the fire, then it would take a long time to put out the fire, but if you call the fire department they will bring large hoses and get ahead of the fire most quickly.

After getting the "large fire" put out, a fire department often leaves smaller hoses to sprinkle water on what is left. Continuous drips of strong pain medicines work in a similar way. If they are allowed to drip on the fire of pain then it is less likely the large fire will start again. Pain medicines are usually delivered via a little computer on the IV pole—these devices are called PCA (for patient controlled analgesia).

Transdermal—Skin Patches

Although still relatively new, there is one medicine available as a skin patch. Transdermal Fentanyl has been approved only for cancer pain by the Food and Drug Administration and should not be used for any other type of pain. That's not meant to scare anybody but they are a little difficult to adjust the dosage and are only useful for stable cancer pain. The patches last for 72 hours in most people (48 hours in some). It also takes between 12-16 hours to receive benefit from the patch and 48 hours to maintain a steady level of the drug in your body. (Now, can you see why you really wouldn't want it for the pain from an accident—would you be willing to wait for 12-16 hours for pain relief if you had just broken your leg—I wouldn't!) Nonetheless, the patches seem like a great way to relieve cancer pain because the medicine is "good" and you don't have to mess with taking pills all of the time.

Rectal

If you don't have diarrhea the rectal route is another "low tech"— no joke intended—way to give pain medicine and is used when people can't take medicines by mouth. Children over the age of two and adolescents really don't appreciate medicine given by this route.

Epidural and Intrathecal

Strong analgesics can be given in the space around the spinal cord. It is important to remember that the medicines are placed in the area around the spinal cord, not in the spinal cord itself.

This route of medication administration has been used effectively since the late 1970's, some of you probably have had or know someone who delivered a baby using an epidural for pain relief. Epidurals for long term pain are only tried after other methods have been unsuccessful because the external epidural systems are difficult for some people to maintain and the internal systems are expensive. To place an epidural catheter for long term use a doctor places a small plastic tube in the area next to the spinal column. The tube is connected to a small metal and plastic pump, which automatically delivers a set amount of medication next to the spinal cord. The medication, which is usually morphine, Dilaudid, or fentanyl, after being automatically dosed and delivered next to the spinal cord, crosses the spinal cord and affects central pain receptors giving great pain relief. Some systems may also utilize a member of the "caine" family (similar to what is used to numb your mouth for a filling) to provide long term relief and in some settings combinations of "caines" and strong pain medicines are used. These are outstanding devices for the sufferers of chronic or malignant pain, but may cost up to $7,000 apiece for the pain pumps, and cost nearly $15,000 to surgically implant. When a person suffers chronic pain, the cost may be well worth it.

Chapter 49

Tolerance, Physical Dependence, and Addiction

Together, Pain and Addiction Organizations Recommend New Definitions

Addiction, tolerance, and physical dependence—for decades, the three distinct terms have been confused and used interchangeably by the public, healthcare professionals, scientists, and regulators alike. This confusion has had the tragic consequence of leaving many people with severe pain undertreated because they—or their doctors—fear that opioids will cause addiction.

But in 2001, the American Academy of Pain Medicine (AAPM), the American Pain Society (APS), and the American Society of Addiction Medicine (ASAM) jointly issued a consensus paper called "Definitions Related to the Use of Opioids for the Treatment of Pain." This document clearly defines addiction, tolerance, and physical dependence and discusses how each relates to opioid use in the treatment of pain.

"The importance of the paper is that the three groups—representing both the pain and addiction communities—have come together and agreed upon these recommended definitions. "These are by no means diagnostic criteria. But it's a very important first step," said Albert Ray, MD, President of AAPM.

"Addiction, Physical Dependence, Tolerance. Confused?" in *The Pain Connection*, the newsletter of American Pain Foundation, Spring 2001. © 2001 American Pain Foundation; reprinted with permission.

Addressing Common Concerns

"The three organizations formed a liaison committee in response to the perception that there's an overlap in the pain population—some people with pain have addictive disorders. And there was uncertainty about treatment and diagnosis in these cases," said Edward Covington, MD, Director of the Chronic Pain Rehabilitation Program at the Cleveland Clinic and past president of AAPM, who was one of the paper's authors. "Also, we needed agreement about what is and what is not an addictive disorder."

"The addiction community was concerned because of inaccurate diagnosis. The pain community was concerned about over-diagnosis of addiction when it didn't exist, and how this misdiagnosis interfered with treatment with opioids," Dr. Covington pointed out.

But, how do these definitions of addiction, physical dependence, and tolerance differ from others?

"The definitions of addiction used by the American Psychiatric Association and the World Health Organization (WHO) rely heavily on the concepts of tolerance and withdrawal as indicators of addiction," Dr. Covington said. "We believe this is erroneous. Also, to make matters more confusing, the WHO got away from using the word 'addiction' and they use 'dependence' instead—a term which has an entirely different meaning to us."

Addiction, Physical Dependence, and Tolerance Defined

Addiction is a primary, chronic, neurobiologic disease, with genetic, psychosocial, and environmental factors influencing its development and manifestations. It is characterized by behaviors that include one or more of the following: impaired control over drug use, compulsive use, continued use despite harm, and craving.

Physical Dependence is a state of adaptation that is manifested by a drug class specific withdrawal syndrome that can be produced by abrupt cessation, rapid dose reduction, decreasing blood level of the drug, and/or administration of an antagonist.

Tolerance is a state of adaptation in which exposure to a drug induces changes that result in a diminution of one or more of the drug's effects over time.

362

Addiction—What It Is

According to the new definition, "Addiction is a primary, chronic, neurobiologic disease, with genetic, psychosocial, and environmental factors...."

"Addiction," Dr. Covington explained, "can be identified by the three "C's"—craving or compulsive use, loss of control, and use despite adverse consequences, such as divorce, liver disease, or waking up in strange places."

Other behaviors that signal addiction include "drug seeking," taking multiple doses of medications and an inability to take them on schedule, "doctor shopping," and frequent reports of lost or stolen prescriptions. Isolation from friends and family members, taking analgesic medications for sedation or increased energy, or to get "high" are other behaviors that indicate addictive disorder.

Both pain and addiction specialists agree that, in most cases, patients taking opioids do develop physical dependence. Less often they develop tolerance. But they rarely develop an addictive disorder. Unlike tolerance and physical dependence, addiction is not a predictable effect of a drug, but an adverse reaction in biologically and psychosocially vulnerable individuals.

Addiction—What It's Not

Pseudoaddiction

Often, when patients are undertreated for pain, they will behave "like addicts" to get the relief they need. They will focus on getting medication, appear to be engaging in "drug-seeking" behaviors, "clock watch," and even lie to get drugs. But unlike a person with true addictive disorder, once their pain is properly managed, these behaviors stop immediately.

Dr. Ray believes it's important for doctors to recognize the difference between true addiction and pseudoaddiction. "We don't want to frighten practitioners out of giving appropriate opioid treatment when it's indicated—nor do we want to misdiagnosis addiction when it's staring us in the face. We want to present something to the medical world on what addiction really is so that it's not confused with pseudoaddiction—which is mostly what we see," said Dr. Ray. "These distinctions are particularly important for family practitioners who deal with these issues everyday."

Physical Dependence and Tolerance

Physical dependence and tolerance are also often confused with addiction. But, according to the consensus paper, both of these are normal responses to regular use of some prescribed medications (including opioids), and are not evidence of an addictive disorder.

Physical dependence refers to the fact that when some drugs are stopped or the blood level of the drug is decreased, withdrawal symptoms emerge. Withdrawal symptoms can occur from a number of drugs (e.g. beta blockers and antidepressants as well as opioids). The paper cautions that the term detoxification should not be used when a medication is being stopped or tapered off.

Tolerance develops when the effects of a drug diminish with exposure, or when greater doses are needed to produce the same effect. "The body is designed to develop tolerance to almost anything it's exposed to. It's a compensatory response," said Dr. Covington. "Patients develop tolerance to all kinds of drugs that are in no way habit forming."

"In terms of opioids, tolerance doesn't develop at the same rate for all of the effects of the drug. For example, a patient will develop tolerance to sleepiness and respiratory depression [trouble breathing] very quickly, but not to constipation or the analgesic effects. Many people can take high doses [of opioids] with no mental impairment and retain good analgesia. But this is not true of everyone. It takes about a six-month trial with the drug to determine the assets and liabilities for the patient."

Need for Universal Agreement Terms

"Our next step is to get buy-in on the definitions from various organizations with influence in our arena, such as the American Psychiatric Association and the WHO, as well as federal regulatory agencies and medical boards," Dr. Covington said. "Once we get agreement on definitions, we hope to develop some sensible, evidence-based policy recommendations for patients who have co-morbid pain and addictive disorders. It will help us manage patients with 'double trouble.'"

The ultimate goal of the three organizations, according to the consensus statement, is "...to promote better care of patients with pain and other conditions where the use of dependence-producing drugs is appropriate, and to encourage appropriate regulatory policies and enforcement strategies."

Chapter 50

Risks of Prescription Drug Abuse

Pain and Opiophobia

It is estimated that more than 50 million Americans suffer from chronic pain. When treating pain, health care providers have long wrestled with a dilemma: How to adequately relieve a patient's suffering while avoiding the potential for that patient to become addicted to pain medication?

Many health care providers underprescribe painkillers because they overestimate the potential for patients to become addicted to medications such as morphine and codeine. Although these drugs carry a heightened risk of addiction, research has shown that providers' concerns that patients will become addicted to pain medication are largely unfounded. This fear of prescribing opioid pain medications is known as "opiophobia."

Most patients who are prescribed opioids for pain, even those undergoing long-term therapy, do not become addicted to the drugs. The few patients who do develop rapid and marked tolerance for and addiction to opioids usually have a history of psychological problems or prior substance abuse. In fact, studies have shown that abuse potential of

This chapter includes text excerpted from "Pain and Opiophobia," *Research Report Series*, National Institute on Drug Abuse (NIDA), July 2001; "Pain Medications and Other Prescription Drugs," Document No. 13553, NIDA, September 2001; "NIDA Scientific Panel Reports on Prescription Drug Misuse and Abuse," by Patrick Zickler, *NIDA Notes*, vol,. 13, no. 3, 2001; and "Prescription Drugs: Abuse and Addiction," *Research Report Series*, NIDA, June 2001.

opioid medications is generally low in healthy, nondrug-abusing volunteers. One study found that only 4 out of about 12,000 patients who were given opioids for acute pain became addicted. In a study of 38 chronic pain patients, most of whom received opioids for 4 to 7 years, only 2 patients became addicted, and both had a history of drug abuse.

Pain Medications and Other Prescription Drugs

Addiction rarely occurs among people who use a pain reliever, central nervous system (CNS) depressant, or stimulant as prescribed; however, inappropriate use of prescription drugs can lead to addiction in some cases. Patients, healthcare professionals, and pharmacists all have roles in preventing misuse and addiction. For example, if a doctor prescribes a pain medication, CNS depressant, or stimulant, the patient should follow the directions for use carefully, and also learn what effects the drug could have and potential interactions with other drugs by reading all information provided by the pharmacist. Physicians and other health care providers should screen for any type of substance abuse during routine history-taking with questions about what prescriptions and over-the-counter medicines the patient is taking and why.

Opioids

Opioids are commonly prescribed because of their effective analgesic, or pain relieving, properties. Many studies have shown that properly managed medical use of opioid analgesic drugs is safe and rarely causes clinical addiction, which is defined as compulsive, often uncontrollable use. Taken exactly as prescribed, opioids can be used to manage pain effectively.

Among the drugs that fall within this class—sometimes referred to as narcotics—are morphine, codeine, and related drugs. Morphine is often used before or after surgery to alleviate severe pain. Codeine is used for milder pain. Other examples of opioids that can be prescribed to alleviate pain include oxycodone (OxyContin—an oral, controlled release form of the drug); propoxyphene (Darvon); hydrocodone (Vicodin); hydromorphone (Dilaudid); and meperidine (Demerol), which is used less often because of its side effects. In addition to their effective pain relieving properties, some of these drugs can be used to relieve severe diarrhea (Lomotil, for example, which is diphenoxylate) or severe coughs (codeine).

Opioids act by attaching to specific proteins called opioid receptors, which are found in the brain, spinal cord, and gastrointestinal tract. When these drugs attach to certain opioid receptors in the brain and spinal cord they can effectively block the transmission of pain messages to the brain.

In addition to relieving pain, opioid drugs can affect regions of the brain that mediate what we perceive as pleasure, resulting in the initial euphoria that many opioids produce. They can also produce drowsiness, cause constipation, and, depending upon the amount of drug taken, depress breathing. Taking a large single dose could cause severe respiratory depression or be fatal.

Opioids may interact with other drugs and are only safe to use with other drugs under a physician's supervision. Typically, they should not be used with substances such as alcohol, antihistamines, barbiturates, or benzodiazepines. These drugs slow down breathing, and their combined effects could risk life-threatening respiratory depression.

Chronic use of opioids can result in tolerance to the drugs so that higher doses must be taken to obtain the same initial effects. Long-term use also can lead to physical dependence—the body adapts to the presence of the drug and withdrawal symptoms occur if use is reduced abruptly. Symptoms of withdrawal can include restlessness, muscle and bone pain, insomnia, diarrhea, vomiting, cold flashes with goose bumps ("cold turkey"), and involuntary leg movements.

Reports on Prescription Drug Misuse and Abuse

The National Institute on Drug Addiction (NIDA) launched a new initiative on prescription drug abuse, misuse, and addiction at a press conference in Washington, D.C., in April 2001. NIDA developed the initiative in response to reports of increased abuse of prescription pain relievers and concern over abuse of other prescription drugs. A scientific program following the press conference provided an overview of current research into issues associated with prescription opioid drugs used in pain relief, central nervous system depressants prescribed for anxiety and sleep disorders, and stimulants used to treat attention-deficit/hyperactivity disorder (ADHD) and obesity. Dr. Alice Young, a NIDA-supported researcher at Wayne State University in Detroit, presented a discussion of the neurobiology of addiction. In subsequent presentations, researchers focused on investigations into specific aspects of prescription drug abuse.

Dr. Howard Chilcoat of the Johns Hopkins University School of Public Health and Hygiene in Baltimore discussed research into the epidemiology of prescription drug abuse. Overall, he said, the number of people who abuse prescription drugs each year roughly equals the number who abuse cocaine—about 2 to 4 percent of the population. Whites are more likely than other racial or ethnic groups to abuse prescription drugs, and many people who abuse these drugs also have psychiatric disorders. Persons age 18 to 25 are more likely than persons in other age groups to begin abusing prescription drugs. Between the ages of 12 and 17, girls are more likely than boys to begin prescription drug abuse and are more likely to abuse stimulants and sedatives than other prescription drugs.

Dr. Kenneth Schmader of Duke University in Durham, North Carolina, said that the elderly (persons age 65 or older) represent about 13 percent of the U.S. population but consume one-third of all prescription drugs. These patients are generally less healthy than younger persons and often suffer from multiple diseases for which they take multiple drugs, Dr. Schmader said, and are therefore more vulnerable than are younger patients to unintentionally misusing and becoming habituated to prescription medications. In one study of more than 1,500 elderly patients, 50 patients, roughly 3 percent, were abusing prescription drugs. In a study of consecutive admissions to a treatment program, 70 of 100 elderly patients admitted for prescription drug abuse were women. Eighty were dependent (that is, they experienced withdrawal symptoms if they tried to stop taking the drugs) on sedatives, 49 on opioids, and 3 on stimulants. Thirty-six were dependent on 2 drugs and 8 were dependent on 3.

Dr. Richard Brown of the University of Wisconsin Medical School in Madison said that physicians' misunderstanding of the risks associated with prescription drugs can lead to inadequate treatment of some illnesses. Dr. Brown based his statement on research in which he and his colleagues asked physicians how they would treat a set of hypothetical patients who suffered anxiety disorders, pain associated with cancer, or back pain. The researchers gave the clinicians detailed profiles of the hypothetical patients that included a treatment history and characteristics, such as use of alcohol and history of substance abuse, related to possible misuse of prescription medication. The researchers compared the physicians' treatment plans with a plan developed by a panel of experts. Compared to the experts, the 2,000 physicians who participated in the study were more reluctant to provide opioids and less cautious about prescribing sedatives. For example, 5 percent of the respondents would not prescribe opioids for severe cancer pain and nearly 80 percent would avoid opioids for severe, chronic back pain that had not responded to other treatments. About 25 percent of the physicians would prescribe benzodiazepines (sedatives such as Valium or Xanax) for a hypothetical patient with an adjustment disorder (anxiety or sadness associated with a particular situation), even though they showed several signs and symptoms of a current alcohol use disorder.

Dr. Steven Passik of Community Cancer Care, Inc., in Indianapolis, Indiana, discussed a study designed to evaluate the risks of misuse or abuse of drugs prescribed for management of chronic pain and to compare the risks with the drugs' benefits. The research involved 264 patients being treated with opioids for chronic pain not associated with cancer. On average, patients reported that the drugs relieved nearly 60 percent of their pain, and more than 90 percent said the pain relief made a significant improvement in their quality of life. Nearly 80 percent reported improvement in overall aspects of daily life such as mood, physical functioning, relationships, and sleep patterns. More than 60 percent of patients reported some adverse side effects from their medication, but only 1.2 percent described the side effects as intolerable. Overall, roughly 6 percent of patients (or their physicians) reported abuse or misuse of prescribed drugs. Drug abuse issues in pain management are complex, Dr. Passik said, but his study results suggest that the risk of opioid abuse is low compared with the benefits of the drugs in chronic pain management.

Trends in Prescription Drug Abuse

Several indicators suggest that prescription drug abuse is on the rise in the United States. According to the 1999 National Household Survey on Drug Abuse, in 1998, an estimated 1.6 million Americans used prescription pain relievers nonmedically for the first time. This represents a significant increase since the 1980s, when there were generally fewer than 500,000 first-time users per year. From 1990 to 1998, the number of new users of pain relievers increased by 181 percent; the number of individuals who initiated tranquilizer use increased by 132 percent; the number of new sedative users increased by 90 percent; and the number of people initiating stimulant use increased by 165 percent. In 1999, an estimated 4 million people—almost 2 percent of the population aged 12 and older—were currently (use in past month) using certain prescription drugs nonmedically: pain relievers (2.6 million users), sedatives and tranquilizers (1.3 million users), and stimulants (0.9 million users).

Although prescription drug abuse affects many Americans, some trends of concern can be seen among older adults, adolescents, and women. In addition, health care professionals—including physicians, nurses, pharmacists, dentists, anesthesiologists, and veterinarians—

may be at increased risk of prescription drug abuse because of ease of access, as well as their ability to self-prescribe drugs. In spite of this increased risk, recent surveys and research in the early 1990s indicate that health care providers probably suffer from substance abuse, including alcohol and drugs, at a rate similar to rates in society as a whole, in the range of 8 to 12 percent.

Older Adults

The misuse of prescription drugs may be the most common form of drug abuse among the elderly. Elderly persons use prescription medications approximately three times as frequently as the general population and have been found to have the poorest rates of compliance with directions for taking a medication. In addition, data from the Veterans Affairs Hospital System suggest that elderly patients may be prescribed inappropriately high doses of medications such as benzodiazepines and may be prescribed these medications for longer periods than are younger adults. In general, older people should be prescribed lower doses of medications, because the body's ability to metabolize many medications decreases with age.

An association between age-related morbidity and abuse of prescription medications likely exists. For example, elderly persons who take benzodiazepines are at increased risk for falls that cause hip and thigh fractures, as well as for vehicle accidents. Cognitive impairment also is associated with benzodiazepine use, although memory impairment may be reversible when the drug is discontinued. Finally, use of benzodiazepines for longer than 4 months is not recommended for elderly patients because of the possibility of physical dependence.

Adolescents and Young Adults

Data from the National Household Survey on Drug Abuse indicate that the most dramatic increase in new users of prescription drugs for nonmedical purposes occurs in 12- to 17-year-olds and 18- to 25-year-olds. In addition, 12- to 14-year-olds reported psychotherapeutics (for example, painkillers or stimulants) as one of two primary drugs used. The 1999 Monitoring the Future survey showed that for barbiturates, tranquilizers, and narcotics other than heroin, the general, long-term declines in use among young adults in the 1980s leveled off in the early 1990s, with modest increases again in the mid- to late 1990s. For example, the use of methylphenidate (Ritalin) among high school seniors increased from an annual prevalence (use of the drug within the preceding year) of 0.1 percent in 1992 to an annual prevalence of 2.8 percent in 1997 before reaching a plateau.

It also appears that college students' nonmedical use of pain relievers such as oxycodone with aspirin (Percodan) and hydrocodone (Vicodin) is on the rise. The 1999 Drug Abuse Warning Network, which collects data on drug-related episodes in hospital emergency departments, reported that mentions of hydrocodone as a cause for visiting an emergency room increased by 37 percent among all age groups from 1997 to 1999. Mentions of the benzodiazepine clonazepam (Klonopin) increased by 102 percent since 1992.

Gender Differences

Studies suggest that women are more likely than men to be prescribed an abusable prescription drug, particularly narcotics and anti-anxiety drugs—in some cases 48 percent more likely.

Overall, men and women have roughly similar rates of nonmedical use of prescription drugs. An exception is found among 12- to 17-year-olds: In this age group, young women are more likely than young men to use psychotherapeutic drugs nonmedically.

In addition, research has shown that women and men who use prescription opioids are equally likely to become addicted. However, among women and men who use either a sedative, anti-anxiety drug, or hypnotic, women are almost two times more likely to become addicted.

Chapter 51

Opioids for People with Severe Pain

Note: The terms "opiate" and "opioid" are similar, but not quite the same. Opiates are narcotic drugs derived from opium; "opioids" include both these natural opiates and synthetic narcotics that function in the same manner.

How Opiates Work

Opiates are powerful drugs derived from the poppy plant that have been used for centuries to relieve pain. They include opium, heroin, morphine, and codeine. Even centuries after their discovery, opiates are still the most effective pain relievers available to physicians for treating pain. Although heroin has no medicinal use, other opiates, such as morphine and codeine, are used in the treatment of pain related to illnesses (for example, cancer) and medical and dental procedures. When used as directed by a physician, opiates are safe and generally do not produce addiction. But opiates also possess very

This chapter contains text excerpted from "Opiates" in *Mind Over Matter: Teachers Guide*, National Institute on Drug Abuse, NIH Pub. No. 98-3592, 1998 (copies of the complete guide can be obtained by calling 1-800-729-6686) and "Balancing News Stories about Opioids: A Statement on the Value of Opioids for People with Severe Pain," © 2001 American Pain Foundation; reprinted with permission. For more information from the American Pain Foundation visit http://www.painfoundation.org.

strong reinforcing properties and can quickly trigger addiction when used improperly.

Mechanism of Action

Opiates elicit their powerful effects by activating opiate receptors that are widely distributed throughout the brain and body. Once an opiate reaches the brain, it quickly activates the opiate receptors that are found in many brain regions and produces an effect that correlates with the area of the brain involved. Two important effects produced by opiates, such as morphine, are pleasure (or reward) and pain relief. The brain itself also produces substances known as endorphins that activate the opiate receptors. Research indicates that endorphins are involved in many things, including respiration, nausea, vomiting, pain modulation, and hormonal regulation.

When opiates are prescribed by a physician for the treatment of pain and are taken in the prescribed dosage, they are safe and there is little chance of addiction. However, when opiates are abused and taken in excessive doses, addiction can result. Findings from animal research indicate that, like cocaine and other abused drugs, opiates can also activate the brain's reward system. When a person injects, sniffs, or orally ingests heroin (or morphine), the drug travels quickly to the brain through the bloodstream. Once in the brain, the heroin is rapidly converted to morphine, which then activates opiate receptors located throughout the brain, including within the reward system. (Note: Because of its chemical structure, heroin penetrates the brain more quickly than other opiates, which is probably why many addicts prefer heroin.) Within the reward system, the morphine activates opiate receptors. Research suggests that stimulation of opiate receptors by morphine results in feelings of reward and activates the pleasure circuit by causing greater amounts of dopamine to be released within the nucleus accumbens. This causes an intense euphoria, or rush, that lasts only briefly and is followed by a few hours of a relaxed, contented state. This excessive release of dopamine and stimulation of the reward system can lead to addiction.

Opiates also act directly on the respiratory center in the brainstem, where they cause a slowdown in activity. This results in a decrease in breathing rate. Excessive amounts of an opiate, like heroin, can cause the respiratory centers to shut down breathing altogether. When someone overdoses on heroin, it is the action of heroin in the brainstem respiratory centers that can cause the person to stop breathing and die.

The brain itself produces endorphins that have an important role in the relief or modulation of pain. Sometimes, though, particularly when pain is severe, the brain does not produce enough endorphins to provide pain relief. Fortunately, opiates, such as morphine are very powerful pain relieving medications. When used properly under the care of a physician, opiates can relieve severe pain without causing addiction.

Relieving Pain

Feelings of pain are produced when specialized nerves are activated by trauma to some part of the body, either through injury or illness. These specialized nerves, which are located throughout the body, carry the pain message to the spinal cord. After reaching the spinal cord, the message is relayed to other neurons, some of which carry it to the brain. Opiates help to relieve pain by acting in both the spinal cord and brain. At the level of the spinal cord, opiates interfere with the transmission of the pain messages between neurons and therefore prevent them from reaching the brain. This blockade of pain messages protects a person from experiencing too much pain. This is known as analgesia.

Opiates also act in the brain to help relieve pain, but the way in which they accomplish this is different than in the spinal cord.

There are several areas in the brain that are involved in interpreting pain messages and in subjective responses to pain. These brain regions are what allow a person to know he or she is experiencing pain and that it is unpleasant. Opiates also act in these brain regions, but they don't block the pain messages themselves. Rather, they change the subjective experience of the pain. This is why a person receiving morphine for pain may say that they still feel the pain but that it doesn't bother them anymore.

Endorphins and Research

Although endorphins are not always adequate to relieve pain, they are very important for survival. If an animal or person is injured and needs to escape a harmful situation, it would be difficult to do so while experiencing severe pain. However, endorphins that are released immediately following an injury can provide enough pain relief to allow escape from a harmful situation. Later, when it is safe, the endorphin levels decrease and intense pain may be felt. This also is important for survival. If the endorphins continued to blunt the pain, it would be easy to ignore an injury and then not seek medical care.

There are several types of opiate receptors, including the delta, mu, and kappa receptors. Each of these three receptors is involved in controlling different brain functions. For example, opiates and endorphins are able to block pain signals by binding to the mu receptor site. The powerful new technology of cloning has enabled scientists to copy the genes that make each of these receptors. This in turn is allowing researchers to conduct laboratory studies to better understand how opiates act in the brain and, more specifically, how opiates interact with each opiate receptor to produce their effects. This information may eventually lead to more effective treatments for pain and opiate addiction.

A Statement on the Value of Opioids for People with Severe Pain

From the American Pain Foundation

The diversion and abuse of opioids—strong medications used to treat people suffering with severe pain—is now making front-page news. While these often-sensationalized stories have focused primarily on the illegal and dangerous use of these medications by drug abusers, they have often failed to balance the problem of abuse with the real news about these drugs—that they provide valuable relief for people suffering with serious pain. The danger of these stories is that they perpetuate long-standing myths and misconceptions about pain management and have the potential to discourage people with pain from receiving treatment that works.

According to Dr. James Campbell, Professor of Neurosurgery at Johns Hopkins Medical Center, past president of the American Pain Society, and Chairman of the American Pain Foundation, "Taking legal, FDA-approved opioid medications as prescribed, under the direction of a physician for pain relief, is safe and effective, and only in rare cases, leads to addiction. When properly used, these medications rarely give a "high" —they give relief. And, most importantly, they allow many people to resume their normal lives."

The management of pain is finally starting to achieve the status it deserves in healthcare. Healthcare professionals, policy makers, the public, and the media are becoming more aware of the undertreatment of pain and are beginning to take steps to address the problem. On January 1, 2001, for example, the new pain standards of the Joint Commission on Accreditation of Healthcare Organizations (JCAHO), the largest accrediting body in the United States, now require all of its 19,000 hospitals, nursing homes, and other healthcare facilities to assess and treat pain, and inform patients about their right to effective pain care. If they don't comply, they can lose their accreditation.

In spite of these advances, over 50 million Americans still live with malignant or non-malignant chronic pain. And although most pain can be managed, it often goes untreated, improperly treated, or undertreated. For example, studies show that while cancer pain can almost always be relieved, more than 40% of cancer patients are undertreated for pain. Why? One reason is a false fear that opioid medications taken for pain are dangerous or addictive.

Doctors and pharmacists need to be diligent in taking security measures to keep opioid medications out of illegal and improper hands. Regulators and law enforcement officers should be tough in combating the illegal diversion of opioids into street traffic, but they should do it in a balanced way that doesn't discourage the safe and legal use of opioid medications for pain care. And the news media should always balance news about opioids with information about their value to people with severe chronic pain.

Chapter 52

Patient Controlled Analgesia (PCA)

Every attempt has been made to insure the accuracy of this material, however, medical science is constantly changing—if the information in this chapter differs from what you have been told by a nurse, pharmacist or physician, consult the person who told you differently or the manufacturer.

What is PCA?

Patient Controlled Analgesia is a pump which allows you or your family member to give yourself pain medication. A PCA pump will be set up for you to give a small amount of pain medication using a hand-held button and/or there can be a continuous infusion of medication. When you push the button a small amount of the medication goes into your intravenous line (IV).

Who can use a PCA pump?

Most patients can use a PCA pump. PCA pumps have been used for children as young as three years old with the parents pushing the button up to the elderly with a family member assisting with pushing the button. Many patients can use them without any help from others.

"Patient Controlled Analgesia (PCA)," (Patient and Family Version), by Julie Hensley RN, an undated fact sheet available online at http://www.nursing.uiowa.edu/sites/PedsPain/Routes/PCAnonte.htm (accessed October 2001), © University of Iowa College of Nursing, reprinted with permission.

When should I use the PCA and how long until works?

Try to anticipate when you need the pain medication rather than trying to play catch up with the pain increasing. A good time to use your PCA pump is before therapies or procedures—like walking down the hall or sitting in a chair the first few times after surgery. Allow at least 15 to 20 minutes before the activity. If you have major surgery, a severe injury or cancer pain you may not be able to totally eliminate your pain, but you will be much better able to control the pain and it will allow you to do more of the things you want to do. If you feel the pain medication is not helping enough, please notify your nurse so that she can call your doctor and request a change in your medication. Your nurse may explain to you how long before you will begin to feel some relief. Usually it takes approximately 10 to 45 minutes before the onset of relief after receiving the medication through the IV.

What are the benefits of using a PCA?

1. You don't have to wait for a nurse to go get your medication, and with most systems you get a small amount of medicine all of the time and it is available at your convenience.

2. You can get ahead and stay ahead of your pain, which allows you to be more alert, heal faster, breathe deeper, move more and do the things you want to do.

What are some common fears of pain medications?

*   *Fear of overdosing when giving the pain medicine to myself.* The PCA pumps delivers only small dose of medicine that can be given at pre-set intervals or a low continuous rate. The pre-set dose of medication is set by your doctor or advanced practice nurse. You will be closely monitored for your response to the pain medication by your nurse.

*   *Fear of becoming addicted to pain medicine.* Studies have shown that when pain medication is taken for real pain there is very little chance of becoming addicted unless you have had some problems with addiction in the past.

Some Advice to Patients

Be honest with your nurse and doctor about your pain.

Learn to rate your pain using a pain scale from 0-10 to let your nurse know how this pain feels to you. For pediatric patients, some special scales have been made to help rate their pain (faces from sad with tears to happy and smiling).

Good news, this is not a time to be a tough guy. If you need your pain medication and take it to control your pain you will do better and heal faster. Pain is not good—keep it under control!

Reference

Clinical Reference System. (1998), North Iowa Mercy Health Center.

AHCPR, *Acute Pain Management: Operative or Medical Procedures and Trauma; Clinical Practice Guideline*, DHHS. Pub. No. 92-0032, pp. 5, 15, 20, 21, 31-32, 51, 59, 61, 64, 71, 75, 80, 85, 97, 104-105.

Dickson, Carol J., *Pharmacy & Therapeutics*, May '93, p. 517.

Facts and Comparisons, St Louis, p.242-243.

Iowa Health Book: Pediatrics, Pediatric Use of Patient Controlled Analgesia Sept. '93 Virtual Children's Hospital UIHC.

Chapter 53

OxyContin

Questions and Answers about OxyContin

What kind of medicine is OxyContin?

OxyContin contains oxycodone, a very strong narcotic pain reliever similar to morphine. OxyContin is designed so that the oxycodone is slowly released over time, allowing it to be used twice daily. You should never break, chew, or crush the OxyContin tablet since this causes a large amount of oxycodone to be released from the tablet all at once, potentially resulting in a dangerous or fatal drug overdose.

What kind of pain is appropriate to treat with OxyContin?

OxyContin is intended to help relieve pain that is moderate to severe in intensity, when that pain is present all the time, and expected to continue for a long time. This level of pain severity may be caused by a variety of different medical conditions.

How do I know if I have the right kind of pain to use OxyContin?

Only a physician can determine if OxyContin is a good choice to manage a your pain. If you have pain every day that lasts for a large

"OxyContin Questions and Answers," Food and Drug Administration (FDA), Center for Drug Evaluation and Research, updated August 2, 2001.

part of the day, and the pain is moderate or severe in intensity, depending upon other factors in your medical history, OxyContin may be a good choice for you. Speak with your physician.

If you feel you only need to take a pain reliever occasionally and this adequately treats your pain, OxyContin is **not** the right drug for you. If you only need a pain reliever for a few days, for example following a dental or surgical procedure, OxyContin is not the right drug for you.

Are there any activities that I should not perform while using OxyContin for pain relief?

OxyContin may interfere with your ability to do certain things that require your full attention. You should not drive a car, operate heavy machinery, or do other possibly dangerous activities while taking OxyContin.

What should I do if I still have pain after I take the OxyContin?

Because OxyContin is a very strong medication, you should not adjust the dose without first speaking with your physician.

Can I take other medicines while I am using OxyContin for pain relief?

Combining OxyContin with some other types of medication such as sleeping pills, tranquilizers, and other pain medications may be dangerous due to the risk of interactions of these medications that can result in injury or death. You should speak with your physician before taking any other medicines with OxyContin. You should also tell your physician about all prescription drugs, over-the-counter drugs, and dietary supplements/herbal remedies that you are taking before starting OxyContin.

Can I drink an alcoholic beverage while I am using OxyContin for pain relief?

You should not drink any beverage that contains alcohol while you are taking OxyContin. This includes beer, wine, and all distilled liquors. OxyContin and alcoholic beverages may have dangerous interactions that can result in serious injury or death.

Will I become addicted to OxyContin if I take it every day?

OxyContin is only intended for moderate to severe pain that is present on a daily basis and that requires a very strong pain reliever. Patients with this type of severe pain condition require daily pain treatment. Taking OxyContin daily can result in physical dependence, a condition in which the body shows signs of narcotic withdrawal if the OxyContin is stopped suddenly. This is not the same thing as addiction, which represents a situation in which people obtain and take narcotics because of a psychological need, and not just to treat a legitimate painful condition. Physical dependence can be treated under the advice of a physician by slowly decreasing the OxyContin dose when it is no longer needed for the treatment of pain. Concerns of addiction should not prevent patients with appropriate pain conditions from using OxyContin or other narcotics for pain relief.

What should I do when I no longer need the OxyContin for pain relief?

When you no longer need OxyContin, the dose should be gradually reduced so that you do not feel sick with withdrawal symptoms. You should ask your physician for a plan on how to gradually decrease the dose and when to stop the OxyContin.

Haven't there been press reports about the misuse of OxyContin?

OxyContin is a safe and effective pain medication when properly prescribed and used as directed. OxyContin has also been used as a drug of abuse. You should protect your prescription and your medication from theft and never give OxyContin to anyone else. You should destroy any left over OxyContin tablets that you may have once your physician instructs you to stop taking the medication.

Can I take OxyContin if I am pregnant, planning to become pregnant, or planning to nurse my baby?

Your should speak to your physician about the effects of drugs like OxyContin on an unborn or newborn child.

Are there any other special precautions I should take with my OxyContin?

Because there is a large dose of medication in each OxyContin tablet, you must be very careful to keep OxyContin stored in a secure location, out of the reach of children. When you no longer need OxyContin for pain relief, you should flush the unused tablets down the toilet.

Chapter 54

Actiq for Breakthrough Cancer Pain

FDA approved for marketing Actiq, a new product developed specifically for cancer patients with severe pain that breaks through their regular narcotic therapy. Actiq is a dosage form of fentanyl citrate, an opioid narcotic more powerful than morphine. The medicine is in the form of a flavored sugar lozenge that dissolves in the mouth while held by an attached handle.

While Actiq is an effective treatment for breakthrough cancer pain, it is not without risk. Because Actiq may be fatal to children (as well as to adults not already taking opioid narcotics), FDA approved Actiq under special regulations that restrict distribution as defined in a comprehensive risk management plan.

Many patients with cancer experience persistent pain which is treated with oral narcotics. These patients, however, often also experience breakthrough pain. Breakthrough cancer pain is acute, with sudden onset, and can occur spontaneously or as a result of activity.

Actiq is designed to be dissolved slowly in the mouth until the medicine is consumed. The unit is consumed in approximately 15 minutes, with pain relief beginning in some cases while Actiq is still

From "FDA Approves Actiq for Marketing: Drug Offers Cancer Patients Relief from Breakthrough Cancer Pain," *Talk Paper*, U.S. Food and Drug Administration (FDA), November 5, 1998. FDA *Talk Papers* are prepared by the Press Office to guide FDA personnel in responding with consistency and accuracy to questions from the public on subjects of current interest. *Talk Papers* are subject to change as more information becomes available.

being consumed. Patients may obtain further relief for up to several hours after taking Actiq.

This approval follows the September 17, 1997 recommendation of the Drug Abuse Drugs Advisory Committee to ensure that a comprehensive risk management plan be in place when this product was approved. These measures are now in place.

Because of the uniqueness of the dosage form and because fentanyl is a potent schedule II narcotic, FDA advisory committee members and the Agency were extremely concerned that this product be packaged and marketed to minimize the opportunity for diversion, abuse, or access by children.

During clinical trials, the most common reported side effects were sleepiness, dizziness, nausea, and constipation. Anesta Corporation of Salt Lake city, Utah will market Actiq with partner Abbott Laboratories.

Chapter 55

Vioxx for Osteoarthritis and Menstrual Pain

The Food and Drug Administration (FDA) has approved Vioxx (rofecoxib), a new drug for treatment of osteoarthritis, menstrual pain and for the management of acute pain in adults. Vioxx is a non-steroidal anti-inflammatory drug or NSAID, and is the second approved version in a class of drugs commonly referred to as a "Cox-2 inhibitor". (Celebrex, the first, was approved in December 1998.)

NSAID drugs temporarily relieve pain by blocking the body's production of prostaglandins, chemicals which are believed to be associated with the pain and inflammation of injuries and immune reactions.

An enzyme called cyclo-oxygenase is needed for the production of prostaglandins. People have two such enzymes, called cyclo-oxygenase-1 (Cox 1) and cyclo-oxygenase-2 (Cox-2). Most NSAIDS inhibit both these enzymes, but Vioxx and other selective Cox-2 inhibitors do not inhibit cyclo-oxygenase-1. Based on what is known about the role of Cox-1 and Cox-2, it is hoped that NSAIDS that selectively inhibit Cox-2 will have a lower incidence of some side effects (particularly certain adverse effects on the gastrointestinal system such as ulcers and bleeding), while still providing effective treatment for conditions such as pain and osteoarthritis.

From "FDA Approves Vioxx for Osteoarthritis, Pain and Menstrual Pain," *Talk Paper*, U.S. Food and Drug Administration (FDA), May 21, 1999. FDA *Talk Papers* are prepared by the Press Office to guide FDA personnel in responding with consistency and accuracy to questions from the public on subjects of current interest. *Talk Papers* are subject to change as more information becomes available.

In clinical trials of about 3600 people, Vioxx was found to be an effective treatment for the signs and symptoms of osteoarthritis—the most common form of arthritis—which is also known as a degenerative joint disease and tends to affect older people. Vioxx was also found effective for management of acute pain in adults, in studies conducted in people with post-operative pain following dental extractions or post-operative pain following orthopedic surgery; and for the management of pain related to the menstrual cycle.

Vioxx was compared to ibuprofen (a commonly used NSAID) and to placebo in two clinical trials by using endoscopes (devices to examine the upper gastrointestinal tract) to determine the incidence of stomach and upper intestinal ulcerations following use of these products. Treatment with 25 to 50 mg of Vioxx daily was associated with a significantly lower percentage of patients with endoscopic gastroduodenal ulcers than treatment with ibuprofen 2400 mg daily.

However, NSAID products can cause a range of gastrointestinal problems; and patients with asymptomatic ulcers found with endoscopy often recover without special treatment and without experiencing any serious symptoms or complications. A few cases of serious gastrointestinal bleeding and one case of obstruction occurred among patients taking Vioxx in clinical studies. Additional studies in a larger population would be needed to see whether Vioxx actually causes fewer serious gastrointestinal complications than older NSAID products. Until such studies are done, the drug labeling for Vioxx will include a warning for doctors and their patients about the risks associated with all NSAIDS, including risks of GI ulceration, bleeding and perforation. Patients are advised to promptly report signs and symptoms of gastrointestinal ulceration or bleeding, skin rash, unexplained weight gain, or swelling to their physicians.

In addition, Vioxx does not affect the platelet aggregation (clumping), an important part of the blood clotting process. Many other NSAID products can interfere with this platelet function, which may increase the risk of bleeding complications in some patients. However, like other NSAIDS, Vioxx appears to have some potential for causing adverse effects on the kidney, particularly at higher doses.

Chapter 56

New Arthritis Drugs

Arthritis treatments aim to relieve pain, reduce inflammation, and slow or stop joint damage to maintain or restore the patient's functional ability and quality of life. Arthritis therapies generally used today address the medical needs of many patients. However, these therapies are occasionally associated with harmful side effects ranging from mild to severe. Medical research continues to search for effective, fast-acting treatments with fewer side effects.

New arthritis drugs designed to meet these treatment needs are presently available or awaiting approval by the U.S. Food and Drug Administration (FDA). The foundation for these new drugs was laid in basic biomedical research supported by the National Institutes of Health.

Drug Category: Biological Response Modifiers for Rheumatoid Arthritis

Description: One class of drugs in this category reduces inflammation in the joints by blocking the action of a substance called tumor necrosis factor (TNF). TNF is a protein of the body's immune system that triggers inflammation during normal immune responses; however, when overproduced, TNF can lead to excessive inflammation such as that experienced by patients with rheumatoid arthritis.

"New Arthritis Drugs for Rheumatoid Arthritis and Osteoarthitis," National Institute of Arthritis and Musculoskeletal and Skin Diseases (NIAMS), March 2000, updated August 2001.

Medication (drug name): Enbrel® (etanercept)

How taken: twice-weekly subcutaneous (under the skin) injections by the patient or health care provider

Most common side effects: mild to moderate injection-site reactions (itching, pain, swelling)

Drug status: approved by the FDA; not recommended for patients with active infections; caution should be used in patients with a history of infections or those who develop new infections while taking Enbrel®; not recommended for pregnant women.

For more information:

Immunex Corporation
51 University Street
Seattle, WA 98101
Phone: (800) 436–2735
website: http://www.enbrelinfo.com/

Medication (drug name): Remicade® (infliximab)

How taken: intravenous (in the vein) injections by the health care provider once every 8 weeks

Most common side effects: mild infusion reactions

Drug status: approved by the FDA for use in combination with methotrexate; not recommended for pregnant women

For more information:

Centocor
200 Great Valley Parkway
Malvern, PA 19355
Phone: (800) 457–6399
website: http://www.centocor.com/

Drug Category: Disease-Modifying Antirheumatic Drugs (DMARDs) for Rheumatoid Arthritis

Description: These are the mainstay arthritis drugs that are known to relieve painful, swollen joints and to slow joint damage.

Medication (drug name): Arava® (leflunomide)

How taken: orally, once daily

Most common side effects: diarrhea, hair loss, rash

Drug status: approved by the FDA; not recommended for pregnant women

For more information:

Aventis
P.O. Box 9627
Kansas City, MO 64134–0627
Phone: (816) 966–4000
website: http://www.aventis.com/

Drug Category: Nonsteroidal Anti-Inflammatory Drugs (NSAIDs), Specifically Cyclo-Oxygenase-2 (COX-2) Inhibitors, for Rheumatoid Arthritis and Osteoarthritis

Description: COX-2 inhibitors, like traditional NSAIDs, block COX-2, an enzyme in the body known to stimulate an inflammatory response. Unlike traditional NSAIDs, however, they do not block the action of COX-1, an enzyme known to protect the stomach lining. Therefore, drugs in this category reduce joint pain and inflammation with reduced risk of gastrointestinal ulceration and bleeding.

Medication (drug name): Celebrex® (celecoxib) for rheumatoid arthritis and osteoarthritis

How taken: orally once or twice daily, dosage determined by the physician

Most common side effects: abdominal pain, nausea, indigestion, diarrhea

Drug status: approved by the FDA

For more information:

G.D. Searle & Company
5200 Old Orchard Road
Skokie, IL 60077
website: http://www.searle.com/

Medication (drug name): Vioxx® (rofecoxib) for rheumatoid arthritis and osteoarthritis, as well as acute pain associated with primary dysmenorrhea (painful menstruation) and post-surgical pain

How taken: orally, once daily

Most common side effects: abdominal pain, diarrhea, indigestion, insomnia, edema

Drug status: approved by the FDA

For more information:

Merck & Co., Inc.
One Merck Drive
Whitehouse Station, NJ 08889–0100
website: http://www.merck.com/product/usa/

Drug Category: Other Products

Description: Hyaluronic acid viscosupplementation products for osteoarthritis. These products mimic a naturally occurring substance in the body called hyaluronic acid by providing lubrication to the knee joint, thus permitting flexible joint movement without pain.

Medication (drug name): Hyalgan® (hyaluronan)

How taken: a series of five injections per knee by a health care provider over 4 weeks

Most common side effects: some pain and swelling at the injection site

Drug status: approved by the FDA

For more information:

Sanofi~Synthelabo, Inc.
90 Park Avenue
New York, NY 10016
Phone: (800) 446–6267
website: http://www.hyalgan.com/

Medication (drug name): Synvisc® (hylan G-F20)

How taken: a series of three injections per knee by a health care provider over a 15-day period

Most common side effects: some pain and swelling at the injection site

Drug status: approved by the FDA

For more information:

Biomatrix, Inc.
65 Railroad Avenue
Ridgefield, NJ 07657
Phone: (800) 666–7248

Description: Blood filtering device for severe rheumatoid arthritis. This device is designed to remove harmful antibodies from the patient's immune system, thus lowering disease activity associated with severe rheumatoid arthritis.

Device (device name): Prosorba Column® (apheresis)

How used: The device consists of a catheter, tubing, and a column. The catheter and tubing are used to filter the patient's blood through the column (which is coated with protein A, a substance that attracts harmful antibodies), then reinfuse it into the patient's body. The procedure takes 2 hours and is performed weekly at a health care facility for 12 weeks.

Most common side effects: flu-like symptoms (chills, fever, nausea, and joint/muscle pain)

Drug status: approved by the FDA

For more information:

Frenesius HemoCare, Inc.
6675 185th Avenue NE, Suite 100
Redmond, WA 98052
Phone: (800) 909–3872 or 425-497-1197
website: http://www.freseniushc.com/

Additional Resources

To find out more about these drugs and devices, including dosage, full range of side effects, and study results, check the following resources:

National Library of Medicine's (NLM's) Internet Grateful Med is a computer system that allows users to search through 15 of the NLM's databases for bibliographic references and abstracts on medical and scientific information pertaining to rheumatic diseases, including treatments.

website: http://www.nlm.nih.gov/

U.S. Food and Drug Administration (FDA), Center for Evaluation and Research, provides information on drugs that have been approved, as well as those undergoing the approval process.

website: http://www.fda.gov/cder/

The Arthritis Foundation offers "The Drug Guide," a reprint from *Arthritis Today*.

website: http://www.arthritis.org/

Local public university libraries have journals on rheumatic diseases and pharmaceutical (drug) therapies, as well as reference books such as the *Physician's Desk Reference*, an annually updated guide that describes the use, effects, dosages, and administration of FDA-approved drugs, as well as warnings, side effects, and precautions. Many libraries also provide computers with public access to the internet.

Note: Brand names included in this document are provided as examples only, and their inclusion does not mean that these products are endorsed by the National Institutes of Health or any other Government agency. Also, if a particular brand name is not mentioned, this does not mean or imply that the product is unsatisfactory.

Chapter 57

Non-Drug Adjuncts to Pain Medication

There are a number of non drug measures that can be very useful in relieving pain. This chapter will tell you about a few of them and their uses.

In general, if pain is a major problem in your life these interventions will work best if used in combination with pain medicine. Before using any of these non drug measures it would be a great idea to check with the health professionals taking care of you—there may be some things that make an intervention wrong for you.

Ice

Ice is a perfect example of why it's a good idea to check with your healthcare provider. As you know, ice can be great for aches and sprains associated with acute injury and it is also great for some kinds of pain you may be having.

However you have to be *very careful* in using ice if you have had neuropathy from chemotherapy or if you are diabetic. Neuropathy makes your hands and feet tingle and burn. If you have neuropathy and then accidentally sprain an ankle, you will have difficulty in telling just how cold an ice pack is and will have to check more frequently than you would under ordinary circumstances. *You could frostbite your*

"Non Drug Measures," an undated fact sheet an undated fact sheet available online at http://www.nursing.uiowa.edu/sites/PedsPain/Nonpharm/general.htm (accessed October 2001), © University of Iowa College of Nursing, reprinted with permission.

*foot and not know it because your temperature feelers have been al-
tered.*

Warm Baths

Sometimes a bath can help decrease the muscle tension that you
get from holding your body in one place for a long time because of pain.
If you need some help getting in and out of the tub, don't be afraid to
ask for it.

A relaxing bath for a painful body can be wonderful but again, *if
you've had trouble with neuropathies — be very careful about the temperature of that bath.*

Religion

Religion may play an important part in your life. Some patients
find that prayer helps them cope with pain. Others read their Bibles
and look to religion for guidance at this difficult period in their lives.
For whatever reasons, for some people religion helps them deal with
illness and pain.

It is also important to state that the organized religions of the world
have specifically stated formally that pain should be relieved whenever possible.

Pets

Pets can also be a source of great comfort in the time of illness.
Their vigilance when you are ill has probably already been a comfort
to you. Even if you don't have a pet right now, maybe one you can remember from the past — it can keep your mind occupied and perhaps
keep pain out of your thoughts for at least a little while. A discussion
with your family of famous pets in your lives also passes the time
pleasantly.

Music

I have always loved music and easily escape into it either for pure
pleasure or when I'm troubled and need to clear my head. Most of the
time I use music that I like and it often reminds me of a pleasant time
or place. Several years ago a patient who had been badly burned re-
quested loud country western music be used when he had to go to hydro-
therapy to have dead tissue removed. I said "Oh, you like country?"

He replied, "No, actually I hate it but if it is played loudly I keep my mind on how much I hate it and don't think of anything else."

Massage

Massaging aching body parts can make them feel better. If you have been in bed a lot or if you hold your body in such a way to prevent pain many of your muscles probably ache. Massage might help you but again you should probably ask those in charge of your care if it's okay.

Massage therapists are professionals and have a professional organization whose initials are CMTA. If you need a massage therapist, the yellow pages in the phone book are a good source under the topic "massage" or "therapeutic massage." Also the person usually identifies that they are a member of CMTA.

Massage therapists are professional—your privacy is completely respected. When I've been working too hard on projects like this one, or the stress of working with patients gets me down, this is where I go and for an hour or so I let the cares of the world leave me, listen to wonderful music, have massage with wonderful oils and leave a whole new person.

Acupuncture and Acupressure

I imagine you know what acupuncture is but you may not know that many of the same points can be massaged or stimulated with heat or cold for pain relief. Some of you reading this may not believe a tiny needle in the body can stop pain. That's okay—but for some people it is a powerful pain relief intervention. Many individuals who practice holistic nursing and medicine know acupuncture or acupressure.

Reading

Reading a good book or even having someone read it to you can be a wonderful escape from a world full of pain. Remember if you can't read, it can be a joy for someone else to read to you—and if you are at that point in your life it may make the person who is reading to you feel good because of sharing a good book and because of being able to help.

Scrapbooks

Scrapbooks are one of the best things I know to take your mind off of mild to moderate pain. They remind us of better times, of great fun, and things we've done. Dig them out of wherever you put them—or for that matter maybe you could put a few of those pictures that are laying around in boxes into a scrapbook. It doesn't take a lot of energy and the photos serve as a point of conversation and good memories.

Chapter 58

Acupuncture

Acupuncture is one of the oldest, most commonly used medical procedures in the world. Originating in China more than 2,000 years ago, acupuncture became widely known in the United States in 1971 when New York Times reporter James Reston wrote about how doctors in Beijing, China, used needles to ease his abdominal pain after surgery. Research shows that acupuncture is beneficial in treating a variety of health conditions.

In the past two decades, acupuncture has grown in popularity in the United States. In 1993, the U.S. Food and Drug Administration (FDA) estimated that Americans made 9 to 12 million visits per year to acupuncture practitioners and spent as much as $500 million on acupuncture treatments.[1] In 1995, an estimated 10,000 nationally certified acupuncturists were practicing in the United States. An estimated one-third of certified acupuncturists in the United States are medical doctors.[2]

The National Institutes of Health (NIH) has funded a variety of research projects on acupuncture that have been awarded by its National Center for Complementary and Alternative Medicine (NCCAM), National Institute on Alcohol Abuse and Alcoholism, National Institute

From "Acupuncture Information and Resources," National Center for Complementary and Alternative Medicine (NCCAM), NIH Pub. No. D003, April 1999, web version updated March 2001, contact information updated February 2002. Inclusion of a treatment or resource does not imply endorsement by the National Center for Complementary and Alternative Medicine, National Institutes of Health, or U.S. Public Health Service.

of Dental Research, National Institute of Neurological Disorders and Stroke, and National Institute on Drug Abuse.

This chapter provides general information about acupuncture, summaries of NIH research findings on acupuncture, information for the health consumer, a list of additional information resources, and a glossary of terms used in this text. It also lists books, journals, organizations, and Internet resources to help you learn more about acupuncture and traditional Chinese medicine.

Acupuncture Theories

Traditional Chinese medicine theorizes that the more than 2,000 acupuncture points on the human body connect with 12 main and 8 secondary pathways, called meridians. Chinese medicine practitioners believe these meridians conduct energy, or qi, between the surface of the body and internal organs.

Qi regulates spiritual, emotional, mental, and physical balance. Qi is influenced by the opposing forces of yin and yang. According to traditional Chinese medicine, when yin and yang are balanced, they work together with the natural flow of qi to help the body achieve and maintain health. Acupuncture is believed to balance yin and yang, keep the normal flow of energy unblocked, and restore health to the body and mind.

Traditional Chinese medicine practices (including acupuncture, herbs, diet, massage, and meditative physical exercises) all are intended to improve the flow of qi.[3]

Western scientists have found meridians hard to identify because meridians do not directly correspond to nerve or blood circulation pathways. Some researchers believe that meridians are located throughout the body's connective tissue;[4] others do not believe that qi exists at all.[5,6] Such differences of opinion have made acupuncture a source of scientific controversy.

Preclinical Studies

Preclinical studies have documented acupuncture's effects, but they have not been able to fully explain how acupuncture works within the framework of the Western system of medicine.[7,8,9,10,11,12]

Mechanisms of Action

Several processes have been proposed to explain acupuncture's effects, primarily those on pain. Acupuncture points are believed to stimulate the central nervous system (the brain and spinal cord) to release chemicals into the muscles, spinal cord, and brain. These chemicals either change the experience of pain or release other chemicals, such as hormones, that influence the body's self-regulating systems. The biochemical changes may stimulate the body's natural healing abilities and promote physical and emotional well-being.[13] There are three main mechanisms:

1. **Conduction of electromagnetic signals.** Western scientists have found evidence that acupuncture points are strategic conductors of electromagnetic signals. Stimulating points along these pathways through acupuncture enables electromagnetic signals to be relayed at a greater rate than under normal conditions. These signals may start the flow of pain-killing biochemicals, such as endorphins, and of immune system cells to specific sites in the body that are injured or vulnerable to disease.[14,15]

2. **Activation of opioid systems.** Research has found that several types of opioids may be released into the central nervous system during acupuncture treatment, thereby reducing pain.[16]

3. **Changes in brain chemistry, sensation, and involuntary body functions.** Studies have shown that acupuncture may alter brain chemistry by changing the release of neurotransmitters and neurohormones in a good way. Acupuncture also has been documented to affect the parts of the central nervous system related to sensation and involuntary body functions, such as immune reactions and processes whereby a person's blood pressure, blood flow, and body temperature are regulated.[3,17,18]

Clinical Studies

According to an NIH consensus panel of scientists, researchers, and practitioners who convened in November 1997, clinical studies have shown that acupuncture is an effective treatment for nausea caused by surgical anesthesia and cancer chemotherapy as well as for dental pain experienced after surgery. The panel also found that acupuncture is useful by itself or combined with conventional therapies to treat addiction, headaches, menstrual cramps, tennis elbow, fibromyalgia, myofascial pain, osteoarthritis, lower back pain, carpal tunnel syndrome, and asthma; and to assist in stroke rehabilitation.[19]

Increasingly, acupuncture is complementing conventional therapies. For example, doctors may combine acupuncture and drugs to control surgery-related pain in their patients.[20] By providing both acupuncture and certain conventional anesthetic drugs, doctors have found it possible to achieve a state of complete pain relief for some patients.[16] They also have found that using acupuncture lowers the need for conventional pain-killing drugs and thus reduces the risk of side effects for patients who take the drugs.[21,22]

Outside the United States, the World Health Organization (WHO), the health branch of the United Nations, lists more than 40 conditions for which acupuncture may be used.[23]

Currently, one of the main reasons Americans seek acupuncture treatment is to relieve chronic pain, especially from conditions such as arthritis or lower back disorders.[24,25] Some clinical studies show that acupuncture is effective in relieving both chronic (long-lasting) and acute or sudden pain, but other research indicates that it provides no relief from chronic pain.[27] Additional research is needed to provide definitive answers.

FDA's Role

The FDA approved acupuncture needles for use by licensed practitioners in 1996. The FDA requires manufacturers of acupuncture needles to label them for single use only.[28] Relatively few complications from the use of acupuncture have been reported to the FDA when one considers the millions of people treated each year and the number of acupuncture needles used. Still, complications have resulted from inadequate sterilization of needles and from improper delivery of treatments. When not delivered properly, acupuncture can cause serious adverse effects, including infections and puncturing of organs.[1]

NCCAM-Sponsored Clinical Research

Originally founded in 1992 as the Office of Alternative Medicine (OAM), the NCCAM facilitates the research and evaluation of unconventional medical practices and disseminates this information to the public. The NCCAM, established in 1998, supports nine Centers, where researchers conduct studies on complementary and alternative medicine for specific health conditions and diseases. Scientists at several Centers are investigating acupuncture therapy.

Researchers at the NCCAM Center at the University of Maryland in Baltimore conducted a randomized controlled clinical trial and found that patients treated with acupuncture after dental surgery had less intense pain than patients who received a placebo.[20] Other scientists at the Center found that older people with osteoarthritis experienced significantly more pain relief after using conventional drugs and acupuncture together than those using conventional therapy alone.[29]

Researchers at the Minneapolis Medical Research Foundation in Minnesota are studying the use of acupuncture to treat alcoholism and addiction to benzodiazepines, nicotine, and cocaine. Scientists at the Kessler Institute for Rehabilitation in New Jersey studied acupuncture to treat a stroke-related swallowing disorder and the pain associated with spinal cord injuries.

The OAM, now the NCCAM, also funded several individual researchers in 1993 and 1994 to conduct preliminary studies on acupuncture. In one small randomized controlled clinical trial, more than half of the 11 women with a major depressive episode who were treated with acupuncture improved significantly.[30]

In another controlled clinical trial, nearly half of the seven children with attention deficit hyperactivity disorder who underwent acupuncture treatment showed some improvement in their symptoms. Researchers concluded that acupuncture was a useful alternative to standard medication for some children with this condition.[31]

In a third small controlled study, eight pregnant women were given a type of acupuncture treatment, called moxibustion, to reduce the rate of breech births, in which the fetus is positioned for birth feet-first instead of the normal position of head-first. Researchers found the treatment to be safe, but they were uncertain whether it was effective.[32] Then, researchers reporting in the November 11, 1998, issue of the *Journal of the American Medical Association* conducted a larger randomized controlled clinical trial using moxibustion. They found that moxibustion applied to 130 pregnant women presenting breech significantly increased the number of normal head-first births.[33]

Acupuncture and You

The use of acupuncture, like many other complementary and alternative treatments, has produced a good deal of anecdotal evidence. Much of this evidence comes from people who report their own successful use of the treatment. If a treatment appears to be safe and patients report recovery from their illness or condition after using it, others may decide to use the treatment. However, scientific research may not substantiate the anecdotal reports.

Lifestyle, age, physiology, and other factors combine to make every person different. A treatment that works for one person may not work for another who has the very same condition. You, as a health care consumer (especially if you have a preexisting medical condition); should discuss acupuncture with your doctor. Do not rely on a diagnosis of disease by an acupuncturist who does not have substantial conventional medical training. If you have received a diagnosis from a doctor and have had little or no success using conventional medicine, you may wish to ask your doctor whether acupuncture might help.

Finding a Licensed Acupuncture Practitioner

Doctors are a good resource for referrals to acupuncturists. Increasingly, doctors are familiar with acupuncture and may know of a certified practitioner. In addition, more medical doctors, including neurologists, anesthesiologists, and specialists in physical medicine, are becoming trained in acupuncture, traditional Chinese medicine, and other alternative and complementary therapies. Friends and family members may be a source of referrals as well. In addition, national referral organizations provide the names of practitioners, although these organizations may be advocacy groups for the practitioners to whom they refer. See "Acupuncture Resources" below for a list of these organizations.

Check a Practitioner's Credentials

A practitioner who is licensed and credentialed may provide better care than one who is not. About 30 states have established training standards for certification to practice acupuncture, but not all states require acupuncturists to obtain a license to practice. Although proper credentials do not ensure competency, they do indicate that the practitioner has met certain standards to treat patients with acupuncture.

The American Academy of Medical Acupuncture can give you a referral list of doctors who practice acupuncture. The National Acupuncture and Oriental Medicine Alliance lists thousands of acupuncturists on its website and provides the list to callers to their information and referral line. The Alliance requires documentation of state license or national board certification from its listed acupuncturists. The American Association of Oriental Medicine can tell you the state licensing status of acupuncture practitioners across the United States as well. To contact these and other organizations, see "Acupuncture Resources" below.

Check Treatment Cost and Insurance Coverage

Reflecting public demand, an estimated 70 to 80 percent of the nation's insurers covered some acupuncture treatments in 1996. An acupuncturist may provide information about the number of treatments needed and how much each will cost. Generally, treatment may take place over a few days or several weeks. The cost per treatment typically ranges between $30 and $100, but it may be appreciably more. Physician acupuncturists may charge more than nonphysician practitioners.[13]

Check Treatment Procedures

To find out about the treatment procedures that will be used and their likelihood of success. You also should make certain that the practitioner uses a new set of disposable needles in a sealed package every time. The FDA requires the use of sterile, nontoxic needles that bear a labeling statement restricting their use to qualified practitioners. The practitioner also should swab the puncture site with alcohol or another disinfectant before inserting the needle.

Some practitioners may use electroacupuncture; others may use moxibustion. These approaches are part of traditional Chinese medicine, and Western researchers are beginning to study whether they enhance acupuncture's effects.

During your first office visit, the practitioner may ask you at length about your health condition, lifestyle, and behavior. The practitioner will want to obtain a complete picture of your treatment needs and behaviors that may contribute to the condition. This holistic approach is typical of traditional Chinese medicine and many other alternative and complementary therapies.

Let the acupuncturist, or any doctor for that matter, know about all treatments or medications you are taking and whether you have a pacemaker, are pregnant, or have breast or other implants. Acupuncture may be risky to your health if you fail to tell the practitioner about any of these matters.

The Sensation of Acupuncture

Acupuncture needles are metallic, solid, and hair-thin, unlike the thicker, hollow hypodermic needles used in Western medicine to administer treatments or take blood samples. People experience acupuncture differently, but most feel minimal pain as the needles are inserted. Some people are energized by treatment, while others feel relaxed.[34] Some patients may fear acupuncture because they are afraid of needles. Improper needle placement, movement of the patient, or a defect in the needle can cause soreness and pain during treatment.[35] This is why it is so important to seek treatment from a qualified acupuncture practitioner.

As important research advances continue to be made on acupuncture worldwide, practitioners and doctors increasingly will work together to give you the best care available.

For More Information

For more information about acupuncture research sponsored by different parts of NIH, contact the respective Information Office or Clearinghouse. Call the NIH operator for assistance at (301) 496-4000.

For more information about research on acupuncture, contact the NIH National Library of Medicine (NLM), which has published a bibliography of more than 2,000 citations to studies conducted on acupuncture. The bibliography is available on the Internet at http://www.nlm.nih.gov/pubs/cbm/acupuncture.html or by writing the NLM, 8600 Rockville Pike, Bethesda, MD 20894. The NLM also has a toll-free telephone number: (888) 346-3656.

For a database of research on complementary and alternative medicine, including acupuncture, access CAM on PubMed at www.nlm.nih.gov/nccam/camonpubmed.html.

Glossary of Terms

Acupuncture: An ancient Chinese health practice that involves puncturing the skin with hair-thin needles at particular locations, called acupuncture points, on the patient's body. Acupuncture is believed to help reduce pain or change a body function. Sometimes the needles are twirled, given a slight electric charge (see electroacupuncture), or warmed (see moxibustion).

Attention deficit hyperactivity disorder: A syndrome primarily found in children and teenagers that is characterized by excessive physical movement, impulsiveness, and lack of attention.

Clinical studies: (Also clinical trials, clinical outcomes studies, controlled trials, case series, comparative trials, or practice audit evidence.) Tests of a treatment's effects in humans. Treatments undergo clinical studies only after they have shown promise in laboratory studies of animals. Clinical studies help researchers find out whether a promising treatment is safe and effective for people. They also tell scientists which treatments are more effective than others.

Electroacupuncture: A variation of traditional acupuncture treatment in which acupuncture or needle points are stimulated electronically.

Electromagnetic signals: The minute electrical impulses that transmit information through and between nerve cells. For example, electromagnetic signals convey information about pain and other sensations within the body's nervous system.

Fibromyalgia: A complex chronic condition having multiple symptoms, including muscle pain, weakness, and stiffness; fatigue; metabolic disorders; allergies; and headaches.

Holistic: Describes therapies based on facts about the "whole person," including spiritual and mental aspects, not only the specific part of the body being treated. Holistic practitioners may advise changes in diet, physical activity, and other lifestyle factors to help treat a patient's condition.

Meridians: A traditional Chinese medicine term for the 14 pathways throughout the body for the flow of qi, or vital energy, accessed through acupuncture points.

Moxibustion: The use of dried herbs in acupuncture. The herbs are placed on top of acupuncture needles and burned. This method is believed to be more effective at treating some health conditions than using acupuncture needles alone.

Neurohormones: Chemical substances made by tissue in the body's nervous system that can change the structure or function or direct the activity of an organ or organs.

Neurological: A term referring to the body's nervous system, which starts, oversees, and controls all body functions.

Neurotransmitters: Biochemical substances that stimulate or inhibit nerve impulses in the brain that relay information about external stimuli and sensations, such as pain.

Opioids: Synthetic or naturally occurring chemicals in the brain that may reduce pain and induce sleep.

Placebo: An inactive substance given to a participant in a research study as part of a test of the effects of another substance or treatment. Scientists often compare the effects of active and inactive substances to learn more about how the active substance affects participants.

Preclinical studies: Tests performed after a treatment has been shown in laboratory studies to have a desirable effect. Preclinical studies provide information about a treatment's harmful side effects and safety at different doses in animals.

Qi: (Pronounced "chee.") The Chinese term for vital energy or life force.

Randomized controlled clinical trials: A type of clinical study that is designed to provide information about whether a treatment is safe and effective in humans. These trials generally use two groups of people; one group receives the treatment and the other does not. The participants being studied do not know which group receives the actual treatment.

Traditional Chinese medicine: An ancient system of medicine and health care that is based on the concept of balanced qi, or vital energy, that flows throughout the body. Components of traditional Chinese medicine include herbal and nutritional therapy, restorative physical exercises, meditation, acupuncture, acupressure, and remedial massage.

Yang: The Chinese concept of positive energy and forces in the universe and human body. Acupuncture is believed to remove yang imbalances and bring the body into balance.

Yin: The Chinese concept of negative energy and forces in the universe and human body. Acupuncture is believed to remove yin imbalances and bring the body into balance.

References

1. Lytle, C.D. *An Overview of Acupuncture*. 1993. Washington, DC: United States Department of Health and Human Services, Health Sciences Branch, Division of Life Sciences, Office of Science and Technology, Center for Devices and Radiological Health, Food and Drug Administration.

2. Culliton, P.D. "Current Utilization of Acupuncture by United States Patients." *National Institutes of Health Consensus*

Development Conference on Acupuncture, Program & Abstracts (Bethesda, MD, November 3-5, 1997). Sponsors: Office of Alternative Medicine and Office of Medical Applications Research. Bethesda, MD: National Institutes of Health, 1997.

3. Beinfield, H. and Korngold, E.L. *Between Heaven and Earth: A Guide to Chinese Medicine.* New York, NY: Ballantine Books, 1991.

4. Brown, D. "Three Generations of Alternative Medicine: Behavioral Medicine, Integrated Medicine, and Energy Medicine." *Boston University School of Medicine Alumni Report.* Fall 1996.

5. Senior, K. "Acupuncture: Can It Take the Pain Away? " *Molecular Medicine Today.* 1996. 2(4):150-3.

6. Raso, J. *Alternative Health Care: A Comprehensive Guide.* Buffalo, NY: Prometheus Books, 1994.

7. Eskinazi, D.P. "National Institutes of Health Technology Assessment Workshop on Alternative Medicine: Acupuncture." *Journal of Alternative and Complementary Medicine.* 1996. 2(1):1-253.

8. Tang, N.M., Dong, H.W., Wang, X.M., Tsui, Z.C., and Han, J.S. "Cholecystokinin Antisense RNA Increases the Analgesic Effect Induced by Electroacupuncture or Low Dose Morphine: Conversion of Low Responder Rats into High Responders." *Pain.* 1997. 71(1):71-80.

9. Cheng, X.D., Wu, G.C., He, Q.Z., and Cao, X.D. "Effect of Electroacupuncture on the Activities of Tyrosine Protein Kinase in Subcellular Fractions of Activated T Lymphocytes from the Traumatized Rats." *Acupuncture and Electro-Therapeutics Research.* 1998. 23(3-4):161-170.

10. Chen, L.B. and Li, S.X. "The Effects of Electrical Acupuncture of Neiguan on the PO2 of the Border Zone Between Ischemic and Non-Ischemic Myocardium in Dogs." *Journal of Traditional Chinese Medicine.* 1983. 3(2):83-8.

11. Lee, H.S. and Kim, J.Y. "Effects of Acupuncture on Blood Pressure and Plasma Renin Activity in Two-Kidney One Clip Goldblatt Hypertensive Rats." *American Journal of Chinese Medicine.* 1994. 22(3-4):215-9.

12. Okada, K., Oshima, M., and Kawakita, K. "Examination of the Afferent Fiber Responsible for the Suppression of Jaw-Opening Reflex in Heat, Cold and Manual Acupuncture Stimulation in Anesthetized Rats." *Brain Research*. 1996. 740(1-2):201-7.

13. National Institutes of Health. *Frequently Asked Questions About Acupuncture*. Bethesda, MD: National Institutes of Health, 1997.

14. Dale, R.A. "Demythologizing Acupuncture. Part 1. The Scientific Mechanisms and the Clinical Uses." *Alternative & Complementary Therapies Journal*. April 1997. 3(2):125-31.

15. Takeshige, C. "Mechanism of Acupuncture Analgesia Based on Animal Experiments." *Scientific Bases of Acupuncture*. Berlin, Germany: Springer-Verlag, 1989.

16. Han, J. S. "Acupuncture Activates Endogenous Systems of Analgesia." *National Institutes of Health Consensus Conference on Acupuncture, Program & Abstracts* (Bethesda, MD, November 3-5, 1997). Sponsors: Office of Alternative Medicine and Office of Medical Applications of Research. Bethesda, MD: National Institutes of Health, 1997.

17. Wu, B., Zhou, R.X., and Zhou, M.S. "Effect of Acupuncture on Interleukin-2 Level and NK Cell Immunoactivity of Peripheral Blood of Malignant Tumor Patients." *Chung Kuo Chung Hsi I Chieh Ho Tsa Chich*. 1994. 14(9):537-9.

18. Wu, B. "Effect of Acupuncture on the Regulation of Cell-Mediated Immunity in Patients With Malignant Tumors." *Chen Tzu Yen Chiu*. 1995. 20(3):67-71.

19. National Institutes of Health Consensus Panel. Acupuncture. *National Institutes of Health Consensus Development Statement* (Bethesda, MD, November 3-5, 1997). Sponsors: Office of Alternative Medicine and Office of Medical Applications of Research. Bethesda, MD: National Institutes of Health, 1997.

20. Lao, L., Bergman, S., Langenberg, P., Wong, R., and Berman, B. "Efficacy of Chinese Acupuncture on Postoperative Oral Surgery Pain." *Oral Surgery, Oral Medicine, Oral Pathology*. 1995. 79(4):423-8.

21. Lewith, G.T. and Vincent, C. "On the Evaluation of the Clinical Effects of Acupuncture: A Problem Reassessed and a Framework for Future Research." *Journal of Alternative and Complementary Medicine.* 1996. 2(1):79-90.

22. Tsibuliak, V.N., Alisov, A.P., and Shatrova, V.P. "Acupuncture Analgesia and Analgesic Transcutaneous Electroneurostimulation in the Early Postoperative Period." *Anesthesiology and Reanimatology.* 1995. 2:93-8.

23. World Health Organization. *Viewpoint on Acupuncture.* Geneva, Switzerland: World Health Organization, 1979.

24. Bullock, M.L., Pheley, A.M., Kiresuk, T.J., Lenz, S.K., and Culliton, P.D. "Characteristics and Complaints of Patients Seeking Therapy at a Hospital-Based Alternative Medicine Clinic." *Journal of Alternative and Complementary Medicine.* 1997. 3(1):31-7.

25. Diehl, D.L., Kaplan, G., Coulter, I., Glik, D., and Hurwitz, E.L. "Use of Acupuncture by American Physicians." *Journal of Alternative and Complementary Medicine.* 1997. 3(2):119-26.

26. Levine, J.D., Gormley, J., and Fields, H.L. "Observations on the Analgesic Effects of Needle Puncture (Acupuncture)." *Pain.* 1976. 2(2):149-59.

27. Ter Reit, G., Kleijnen, J., and Knipschild, P. "Acupuncture and Chronic Pain: A Criteria-Based Meta-Analysis." *Clinical Epidemiology.* 1990. 43:1191-9.

28. U.S. Food and Drug Administration. "Acupuncture Needles No Longer Investigational." *FDA Consumer Magazine.* June 1996. 30(5).

29. Berman, B., Lao, L., Bergman, S., Langenberg, P., Wong, R., Loangenberg, P., and Hochberg, M. "Efficacy of Traditional Chinese Acupuncture in the Treatment of Osteoarthritis: A Pilot Study." *Osteoarthritis and Cartilage.* 1995. (3):139-42.

30. Allen, John J.B. "An Acupuncture Treatment Study for Unipolar Depression." *Psychological Science.* 1998. 9:397-401.

31. Sonenklar, N. *Acupuncture and Attention Deficit Hyperactivity Disorder.* National Institutes of Health, Office of Alternative Medicine Research Grant #R21 RR09463. 1993.

32. Milligan, R. *Breech Version by Acumoxa*. National Institutes of Health, Office of Alternative Medicine Research Grant #R21 RR09527. 1993.

33. Cardini, F. and Weixin, H. "Moxibustion for Correction of Breech Presentation: A Randomized Controlled Trial." *Journal of the American Medical Association*. 1998. 280:1580-4.

34. American Academy of Medical Acupuncture. *Doctor, What's This Acupuncture All About? A Brief Explanation for Patients*. Los Angeles, CA: American Academy of Medical Acupuncture, 1996.

35. Lao, L. "Safety Issues in Acupuncture." *Journal of Alternative and Complementary Medicine*. 1996. 2(1):27-9.

Acupuncture Information Resources

The NIH does not endorse any of the resources listed below. You, as a health care consumer, are encouraged to explore these resources fully to determine their relevancy, position on treatment, relative cost, and background of authors or staff. You may wish to discuss this information with your doctor, who can assist you in critically evaluating all resources for their relevance to your diagnoses and circumstances.

Introduction

The Information resources below are listed by title in the following categories:

- National Institutes of Health
- Publications
- Organizations (including Training and Credentialing Organizations)
- Online Resources

National Institutes of Health

Combined Health Information Database (CHID)
7830 Old Georgetown Road, Suite 204
Bethesda, MD 20814
Website: http://chid.nih.gov
E-mail: chid@aerie.com

CHID Online is a searchable and user-friendly database produced by more than a dozen health-related agencies of the Federal Government. This database provides titles, abstracts, and availability information for health information and health education resources, including acupuncture and Chinese medicine.

National Center for Complementary and Alternative Medicine (NCCAM) Clearinghouse
P.O. Box 7923
Gaithersburg, MD 20898
Phone: (888) 644-6226
TTY: (866) 464-3615 (Toll-Free)
Fax: (866) 464-3616 (Toll-Free)
Website: http://nccam.nih.gov
E-mail: info@nccam.nih.gov

The NCCAM Clearinghouse, the information arm of NIH's NCCAM, provides information about complementary and alternative medicine (CAM), including acupuncture, and the activities of the NCCAM. The NCCAM website has acupuncture information and provides links to the websites of several CAM research centers (sponsored by the NCCAM), some of which are conducting acupuncture research.

NIH Consensus Program Information Center
P.O. Box 2577
Kensington, MD 20891
Phone: (888) 644-2667
Fax: (301) 593-9485
E-mail: consensus_statement@nih.gov

The NIH organized a conference that produced a consensus statement about acupuncture (November 3-5, 1997).

U.S. National Library of Medicine (NLM)
MEDLINE
8600 Rockville Pike
Bethesda, MD 20894
Phone: (888) 346-3656
Fax: (301) 402-1384
Website: http://www.nlm.nih.gov/databases/freemedl.html
E-mail: custserv@nlm.nih.gov

The world's largest biomedical library containing more than nine million scientific and biomedical articles.

MEDLINEplus
Website: http://www.nlm.nih.gov/medlineplus

An online consumer health information tool.

Publications

Books

A Manual of Acupuncture, by Peter Deadman and Mazin Al-Khafaji (East Sussex, England: *Journal of Chinese Medicine Publications*, 1998). A detailed guidebook to descriptions of the theories and actual specific methods of acupuncture. It provides information on the channels, collaterals, point categories, point selection methods, point location, and needling.

Basics of Acupuncture, by Gabriel Stux (Editor) and Bruce Pomerantz (Berlin, Germany: Springer Verlag, 1995). The most recent of several widely used texts by acupuncture researchers.

Between Heaven and Earth: A Guide to Chinese Medicine, by Harriet Beinfield and Efrem Korngold (New York, NY: Ballantine Books, 1991). An overview of Chinese medicine, with case histories of treatments and illustrated explanations of philosophy, components, and treatments.

Principles and Practice of Contemporary Acupuncture, by Sung J. Liao, Matthew Lee, and Lorenz K.Y. Ng (New York, NY: Marcel Dekker, 1994). Contains translations of ancient Chinese medical classics previously unavailable in English. Compares and contrasts traditional Chinese and Western scientific medicine.

The Chinese Way to Healing: Many Paths to Wholeness, by Misha Ruth Cohen (New York, NY: The Berkeley Publishing Group, 1996). A guidebook to Chinese medicine in the United States, with information about diet, herbs, acupuncture, and finding qualified practitioners.

The Web That Has No Weaver, by Ted Kaptchuk (New York, NY: Congdon and Weed, 1992). An introduction to traditional Chinese medicine, with comparisons of Eastern and Western medical treatments.

The Yellow Emperor's Classic of Internal Medicine, by Maoshing Ni (Boston, MA: Shambala Press, 1995). A contemporary translation of the classic traditional Chinese medicine text that dates from 2000 B.C.

Periodicals

These periodicals contain information about acupuncture research studies, techniques, effects, and use. Look for "peer reviewed" journals, which publish studies reviewed by researchers in the field to ensure suitability for publication.

Acupuncture and Electro-Therapeutics Research
Cognizant Communication Corporation
3 Hartsdale Road
Elmsford, NY 10523-3701
Phone: (914) 592-7720
Fax: (914) 592-8981
Website: http://www.cognizantcommunication.com
E-Mail: cogcomm@aol.com

A peer-reviewed quarterly in its 23rd year and indexed/abstracted in MEDLINE.

Alternative Medicine Review: A Journal of Clinical Therapeutics
Thorne Research, Inc.
P.O. Box 3200
Sandpoint, ID 83864
Phone: (208) 263-1337
Fax: (208) 265-2488
Website: www.acupuncturejournal.com

A peer-reviewed quarterly indexed/abstracted in MEDLINE.

American Journal of Acupuncture
1840 41st Avenue
Suite 102
Capitola, CA 95010
Phone: (831) 475-1700
Fax: (831) 475-1439

A quarterly peer-reviewed journal.

American Journal of Chinese Medicine
World Scientific Publishing Co., Inc.
1060 Main Street
River Edge, NJ 07661
Phone: (800) 227-7562 (orders)

AJCM's aims and scope are to "publish articles and essays related to traditional or ethnomedicine of all cultures."

European Journal of Oriental Medicine
63 Jeddo Rd.
London W12 9HQ
United Kingdom
Phone: 011 20-8749-1300

A quarterly research journal.

Guideposts: Acupuncture in Recovery
J&M Reports
7402 NE 58th Street
Vancouver, WA 98662-5207
Phone: (360) 254-0186
Fax: (360) 260-8620

A newsletter concerning acupuncture used to treat addiction, alcoholism, and mental health problems.

Journal of Alternative and Complementary Medicine: Research on Paradigm, Practice and Policy
Mary Ann Liebert, Publisher
2 Madison Avenue
Larchmont, NY 10538
Toll Free: (800) 654-3278
Phone: (914) 834-3100
Fax: (914) 834-3688
Website: http://www.liebertpub.com/
E-Mail: info@liebertpub.com

A quarterly journal abstracted/indexed in MEDLINE.

Journal of Chinese Medicine
22 Cromwell Road
Hove BN3 3EB
United Kingdom
Phone: 011 1273 748588
Fax: 011 1273 748588

A professional journal published three times a year.

Journal of Traditional Chinese Medicine
Co-sponsored by the China Association of Traditional Chinese
Medicine and Pharmacy and the China Academy of Traditional
Chinese Medicine
Distributed by the American Center of Chinese Medicine
3121 Park Avenue, Suite J
Soquel, CA 95073

A quarterly journal on clinical and theoretical research that is indexed/abstracted in MEDLINE.

Organizations

American Academy of Medical Acupuncture
Medical Acupuncture Research Organization
5820 Wilshire Boulevard
Suite 500
Los Angeles, CA 90036
Toll Free: (800) 521-2262
Phone: (323) 937-5514
Fax: (323) 937-0959
Website: http://www.medicalacupuncture.org

A professional association of medical doctors who practice acupuncture. The academy provides a referral list of doctors who practice acupuncture. It also provides general information about acupuncture, legislative representation, publications, meetings, and proficiency examinations.

American Association of Oriental Medicine
433 Front Street
Catasauqua, PA 18032
Toll Free: (888) 500-7999
Phone: (610) 266-1433
Fax: (610) 264-2768
Website: http://www.aaom.org
E-Mail: aaom1@aol.com

A nonprofit professional organization of acupuncturists and practitioners of Oriental medicine. The association determines standards of practice and education through the National Certification Commission for Acupuncture and Oriental Medicine. It also funds research and provides a list of acupuncturists and Oriental medicine practitioners by geographic area. The association provides articles and fact sheets, membership and licensing information, a list of acupuncture schools, and a list of state acupuncture associations.

British Medical Acupuncture Society
12 Marbury House, Higher Whitley
Warrington, Cheshire WA4 4WQ
United Kingdom
Phone: 01144 1925 730727
Fax: 01144 1925 730492
Website: http://www.medical-acupuncture.co.uk
E-mail: bmasadmin@aol.com

A group of doctors who practice acupuncture with more conventional treatments. The Society produces the journal *Acupuncture in Medicine*, published twice per year, covering original research and reviews.

Foundation for Traditional Chinese Medicine
122A Acomb Road
York YO2 4EY
United Kingdom
Phone: 011 44 1904 781630
Fax: 011 44 1904 782991
Website: http://www.ftcm.org.uk/index.asp

The Foundation funds the Acupuncture Research Resource Center and provides information about acupuncture research listed by condition, including migraine and lower back pain.

International Council of Medical Acupuncture and Related Techniques
Rue de l'Amazone 62
1060 Brussels
Belgium
Phone: 011 3225 393900
Fax: 011 3225 393692
Website: http://www.icmart.org

A nonprofit organization created in 1983 of more than 40 national acupuncture-related associations of medical doctors practicing acupuncture and/or related techniques.

National Acupuncture and Oriental Medicine Alliance
14637 Starr Road SE
Olalla, WA 98359
Phone: (253) 851-6896
Fax: (253) 851-6883
Website: http://www.acupuncturealliance.org

A professional society of state-licensed, registered, or certified acupuncturists, with membership open to consumers, schools, organizations, corporate sponsors, and health care providers. The Alliance lists thousands of acupuncturists across the country on its website and provides information about them to callers to their information and referral line. The Alliance requires documentation of state license or national board certification from all acupuncturists it lists.

National Acupuncture Detoxification Association
P.O. Box 1927
Vancouver, WA 98668-1927
Phone: (888) 765-6232
Fax: (805) 969-6051

A nonprofit organization that provides training and consultation for more than 500 drug and alcohol acupuncture treatment programs run by local agencies. The organization's clearinghouse provides a library of audiotapes, videotapes, and literature on using acupuncture to treat addiction and mental disorders.

National Acupuncture Foundation
P.O. Box 2271
Gig Harbor, WA 98335-4271
Phone: (253) 851-6538
Fax: (253) 851-6538

The Foundation publishes books, including the *Acupuncture and Oriental Medicine Law Book* and the *Clean Needle Technique Manual*. The Foundation filed the U.S. Food and Drug Administration needle reclassification petition of 1996.

Society for Acupuncture Research
6900 Wisconsin Avenue, Suite 700
Bethesda, MD 20815
Phone: (301) 571-0624
Fax: (301) 961-5340

A nonprofit organization that facilitates the scientific evaluation of acupuncture.

Training and Credentialing Organizations

Accreditation Commission for Acupuncture and Oriental Medicine
1010 Wayne Avenue
Suite 1270
Silver Spring, MD 20910
Phone: (301) 608-9680
Fax: (301) 608-9576

The Commission, established in 1982, evaluates professional master's degree and first professional master's-level certificate and diploma programs in acupuncture and Oriental medicine, with concentrations in both acupuncture and herbal therapy.

Council of Colleges of Acupuncture and Oriental Medicine
7501 Greenway Center Dr.
Suite 820
Greenbelt, MD 20770
Phone: (301) 313-0868
Fax: (301) 313-0869
Website: http://www.ccaom.org

This Council was formed in 1982 and has developed academic and clinical guidelines and core curriculum requirements for master's and doctoral programs in acupuncture as well as acupuncture and Oriental medicine.

NAFTA Acupuncture Commission
Standards Management, Inc.
14637 Starr Road SE
Olalla, WA 98359
Phone: (253) 851-6896
Fax: (253) 851-6883

This group of educators, acupuncturists, medical doctors, and naturopathic doctors meet to exchange information and discuss training standards of competence for the practice of acupuncture and Oriental medicine in North America, including Mexico and Canada.

National Certification Commission for Acupuncture and Oriental Medicine

11 Canal Center Plaza
Suite 300
Alexandria, VA 22314
Phone: (703) 548-9004
Fax: (703) 548-9079
Website: http://www.nccaom.org
E-mail: info@nccaom.org

This Commission was established in 1982 to implement nationally recognized standards of competence for the practice of acupuncture and Oriental medicine. It provides information and programs on certification standards for acupuncturists.

Online Resources

The Internet is one of the fastest ways to access health information, but much of this information is not controlled or reviewed by qualified health professionals. Approach information from the Internet with caution, as it may be misleading, incorrect, or even dangerous.

Acuall.org
Website: http://www.acuall.org

A site sponsored by the National Acupuncture and Oriental Medicine Alliance with general information on acupuncture and Oriental medicine, referrals to practitioners, legislative status, national issues, conferences and workshops, publications, and information for potential students.

Acupuncture.com
Website: http://www.acupuncture.com

Describes and summarizes acupuncture procedures, areas of research, and other pertinent information from multiple sources.

Health Info Library: Acupuncture
Website: http://www.americanwholehealth.com/library/acupuncture/tcm.htm

A site by the health care company American WholeHealth that provides acupuncture articles and research.

Medical Matrix
Website: http://www.medmatrix.org

A gateway to clinical medical resources, including numerous medical journals.

National Library of Medicine. Current Bibliographies in Medicine: Acupuncture
Website: http://www.nlm.nih.gov/pubs/cbm/acupuncture.html

Bibliographies to 2,302 scientific papers collected between January 1970 and October 1997.

Chapter 59

Clinical Psychophysiology, Biofeedback, and Neurofeedback

What Is Clinical Psychophysiology?

Clinical psychophysiologists (more familiarly known as biofeedback therapists) use sensitive electronic instruments, within a therapeutic relationship, to measure, amplify, and provide feedback on physiological responses going on within the human body. It is scientifically accepted that stress, environmental events, thoughts, and emotions all influence our ongoing patterns of physiological response.

Many people are unaware of the subtle ways in which our minds and bodies interact. It is, however, possible to observe and modify interactions between the two. Under the guidance of a trained and qualified practitioner, and using specialized electronic biofeedback instruments that monitor our internal physiology in real time, an

Information in this chapter is excerpted from "General Information Concerning Biofeedback: Clinical Psychophysiology and Biofeedback" by Donald C. E. Ferguson, Ph.D., MPH, and "Neurofeedback: Understanding Neurotherapy," by Donald C. E. Ferguson, Ph.D., MPH, and Elsie L. Ferguson, Ph.D., © 2000-2002 by Donald C. E. Ferguson, Ph.D., MPH. Reprinted with permission. Donald C. E. Ferguson, Ph.D., MPH is a Research Professor in the Department of Psychiatry at the Herbert School of Medicine, Uniformed Services University, Bethesda, MD, and a member of the board of Directors of the Mid-Atlantic Society for Biofeedback and Behavioral Medicine (MASBBM). Elsie L. Ferguson, Ph.D. is a Medical Psychologist and Clinical Psychophysiologist in private practice, Bethesda, MD. Complete information about MASBBM is included at the end of this chapter and can also be found on the Internet at www.biofeedack-bsdcmdva.org.

individual can be taught, and learn to apply self-regulation skills to influence and modify the way their body responds to events going on in their life in more healthful and efficient ways.

What Does "Biofeedback" Mean?

The word "biofeedback" was coined in late 1969 to describe laboratory procedures (developed in the 1940s) that trained research subjects to alter brain activity, blood pressure, muscle tension, heart rate, and other bodily functions not normally controlled voluntarily. Biofeedback is a training technique in which people are taught to improve their health and performance through using information and signals from their own bodies.

One commonly used device (an electromyograph or EMG), for example, picks up electrical signals from the muscles. It translates the signals into a form that people can see and hear. The EMG can display a light or activate a sound, tone, or music every time muscles become more tense. If one wants to relax tense muscles, one learns through practice, to slow down the change in the light's color or alter the tones heard. People soon learn to associate sensations from their muscles with actual levels of tension in them and to develop a new, healthier habit of keeping muscles only as tense as is necessary, and only for as long as necessary. In the case of muscle spasm, pain diminishes and disappears as muscles relax. After treatment, individuals are then trained to repeat this relaxation response voluntarily and at will without being attached to the sensors or the equipment. Scientists call this phenomenon generalization.

Other biological functions commonly measured and used in similar ways to help people learn to control their physical functioning are skin temperature (thermal biofeedback), heart rate, sweat gland activity (GSR [Galvanic Skin Response], SCL [Skin Conductive Level], or EDR [Electrodermal Response] biofeedback), and brain wave activity (EEG biofeedback or neurofeedback).

Biofeedback clinicians utilize complex computer-assisted biofeedback equipment, specialized software, video displays, and auditory (sound) signals in much the same way you rely on your bathroom scale to tell you how you are doing with your diet or the way your thermometer will feed back whether your medication is controlling a fever. Electronic biofeedback equipment, however, detects a person's internal bodily states and functions with far greater sensitivity and precision than any person without such equipment-mediated feedback can do alone. Both patients and therapists use the information produced by the equipment to gauge and direct the progress of treatment, and to learn and relearn more health-inducing and symptom-reducing modes of functioning.

Although most people initially viewed biofeedback with skepticism, researchers have repeatedly proven that most individuals can alter their involuntary, habitual responses by being "fed back" information visually and/or audibly when supplied with information about what is happening in their bodies from moment to moment.

What Kinds of Health Problems Can Clinical Psychophysiology/Biofeedback Help?

Physicians, psychologists, physical therapists, nurses, clinicians, social workers, and researchers who are specifically trained and experienced in the clinical use of biofeedback utilize biofeedback equipment and special training to assist individual patients in the treatment of stress-related illnesses and disorders, in rehabilitation, with neurological processing disorders, and in developing athletic and peak performance skills in both sports and occupational activities. Equipment alone does not do the training, but a combination of equipment and the training methods used by the qualified therapist in "coaching" the patient or client to use the information fed back, and to transfer that training to everyday life constitutes the regimen that is used to reduce or eliminate symptoms, promote healthy functioning, and very often to reduce or eliminate the need for medication or other supports. Habitual response modification forms the basis for what many patients or clients refer to as their "cure."

Stress-related disorders effectively treated with biofeedback include conditions such as headaches, high blood pressure (hypertension), anxiety disorders, diabetes, irritable bowel syndrome, motion sickness, chronic pain, myofascial pain, jaw pain, reduced peripheral blood flow (Raynaud's disease), and insomnia to name but a few. Biofeedback may be used alone, or in combination with medication. It is not an either/or treatment. A number of patients using biofeedback seek out this form of treatment because they are allergic to, intolerant of, or have adverse side effects from medications often used to treat their conditions. When administered by competent and experienced clinicians, there are no adverse physical side effects associated with biofeedback.

Clinical research and application of findings from many controlled studies have demonstrated biofeedback techniques to be safe, efficacious, non pharmacological, non-invasive procedures that are now widely used procedures to treat an ever lengthening list of conditions. A partial list of conditions related to pain and pain management which benefit from it includes:

- Migraine headaches
- Tension headaches
- Other types of chronic pain
- Disorders of the digestive system
- Raynaud's disease (a circulatory disorder that causes uncomfortably cold hands)
- Stress-related disorders and stress management

Neurofeedback and Neurotherapy

What Is Neurofeedback?

The use of biofeedback in treatment of many types of chronic pain is well established. Biofeedback has been found helpful and effective in chronic pain reduction when used alone, or in combination with physical, medical, surgical, pharmacologic, or rehabilitative regimens as part of pain reduction and pain management treatment programs. Use of neurofeedback for pain management and control is a more recent addition to chronic pain treatment regimens.

Neurofeedback is based on electroencephalography (EEG). Electroencephalography is a method used to gather information about ongoing brain function and brain wave patterns which are recorded on a moving paper chart. Diagnostic electroencephalography is used by neurologists and neurosurgeons for help in diagnosing brain abnormalities, tumors, seizure disorders, and other neurological conditions. Clinical electroencephalographers however are <u>not</u> neurofeedback specialists. Each comprises a different specialty with different purposes, and their training differs. Neurofeedback therapy is not an invasive procedure, and neurotherapists are thus not required to be (and seldom are) physicians.

The Development of Neurofeedback

For many years it was believed that brain waves were unmodifiable. In the late 1950s and early 60s researchers discovered animal and human brain wave patterns could be modified and re-trained. When done correctly, changes in physical, physiological, psychophysiological, and psychological functioning follow. After assessment, changing and modifying brain wave patterns towards more optimal patterns helps alleviate underlying problems and results in significant alteration, mitigation, improvement of function, and relieves symptoms of a number of medical conditions. Pain reduction is one outcome of a treatment regimen tailored to an individual with this problem.

Indications for the Use of Neurotherapy

Neurotherapy has been used successfully in treatment of a number of pain control, pain management, and chronic pain control treatment programs. Alone or in combination with other treatment methods, fibromyalgia, cancer pain, arthritis pain, muscle pain from tension states, several types of headache pain, and chronic pain conditions associated with a number of medical disorders give evidence of benefit from neurofeedback treatment. Some of these conditions benefit most from combinations of biofeedback and neurofeedback treatment since each method works with different aspects, components, or attributes of central nervous system (CNS) dysfunction or peripheral nervous system (PNS) dysfunction.

It is common to use *both* medication and neurotherapy simultaneously in pain reduction treatment. Treatment is often carried out in conjunction with a referring physician. In many, if not most cases the need for side-effect inducing medications can be gradually reduced, and in many cases eliminated entirely over time using this method. An additional benefit of neurotherapy, when properly administered, is that there are no negative or adverse side effects.

How Does Neurofeedback Treatment Work?

Electrical activity in the brain is monitored and measured by using externally attached electrodes to the scalp, in much the same way an electrocardiogram (EKG) uses externally attached electrodes to the chest. *No electrical stimulation is put into the head or the brain.* These are non-invasive techniques. Only detection, measurement, and active monitoring of brain waves takes place.

Patients voluntarily self-regulate brain wave modification though using visual information about their own ongoing brain activity presented to them on a computer screen. They see changes visually and hear tones indicating the direction of changes they are making while they are happening. Through monitoring, coaching, and the custom design of brain information presented on the screen, whose content is programmed by the therapist, patients are able to learn to modify components of their own brain's electrical activity patterns through their voluntary efforts in directions that are known to be beneficial.

At some point in treatment, which will vary with individuals, components of brain wave patterns become optimal, symptoms abate or disappear, relief is obtained, and the patient no longer needs neurofeedback treatment. A number of sessions, varying with the individual patient, are needed to achieve these effects. These modified optimal patterns persist for long periods after treatment, and relapse is rare. With conditions such as cancer pain, where the pain is caused by tissue pathology (such as a malignancy), neurofeedback often relieves or reduces pain, but will not reverse or change the tumor which causes the pain problem in the first place. In the case of those allergic or hypersensitive to pain medications, or who for their own reasons do not wish to take pain medication or "pills," neurofeedback can offer a non pharmacologic option.

Biofeedback and Neurofeedback Are Not Identical

Biofeedback concentrates on treatment using information fed back mostly from the body's periphery. Neurofeedback works with information directly measured from the brain itself. A different skill set and knowledge base is required to employ this treatment method. Knowledge and skills gained in using biofeedback are helpful to neurofeedback therapists, but do not take the place of the special body of knowledge and experience needed to practice neurofeedback therapy.

Pain patients are best served by seeking practitioners skilled and experienced in use of both biofeedback and neurofeedback methods. Each method offers benefits not shared by the other, though one or both may be useful in a pain reduction or pain control regimen.

Neurotherapy Is Not Psychotherapy

Neurofeedback is not a form of psychotherapy. It is not a "talking therapy." It is not behavior therapy. It is not cognitive therapy. It is a physiological—not a psychological—therapy. It is based on evidence that where the physical brain waves go much of the body will follow. Often feelings change too, but this is a beneficial side effect.

Many medical conditions give rise to psychological problems (somatopsychic conditions). The reverse can also be true. Psychological problems can give rise to physical problems as well (psychosomatic problems). It can be helpful in many cases to be treated by professionals skilled in neurofeedback, biofeedback, and some mental health discipline as well.

How Can I Identify Qualified Neurofeedback Practitioners?

State and regional associations are often of greatest help in finding suitable neurofeedback practitioners. Many associations maintain lists of qualified neurofeedback specialists and can identify those most competent to deal with the problem for which you seek help. You may wish to contact:

The Society for Neuronal Regulation (SNR): SNR (www.snr-jnt.org), a professional organization comprised of several hundred professionals involved in neurofeedback research and training, maintains a list of qualified member practitioners in the United States on its Web site (www.snr-jnt.org/index.htm).

The Mid-Atlantic Society for Biofeedback and Behavioral Medicine (MASBBM): MASBBM publishes a listing of qualified neurofeedback specialists on their web site (www.biofeedback-BSDCMDVA.org). MASBBM Officers ordinarily answer e-mail questions that do not require long complex responses.

The Biofeedback Network: The Biofeedback Network is another Web resource (www.biofeedback.net) which contains links to most existing State Biofeedback Societies in the United States and some countries abroad. Most provide point of contact information. Groups appearing are State Societies that often function as chapters of the National Association for Applied Psychophysiology and Biofeedback (AAPB). Additionally this site also provides links to other biofeedback related commercial Web sites.

About the Mid-Atlantic Society for Biofeedback and Behavioral Medicine

The Mid-Atlantic Society for Biofeedback and Behavioral Medicine (MASBBM), successor to the Biofeedback Society of Washington, D.C., Maryland, and Virginia, is a non-profit, professional, multi-disciplinary, regional organization of biofeedback and health care specialists dedicated to the improvement of practice, research, continuing education, and the advancement of knowledge in biofeedback, neurofeedback, and behavioral medicine. The MASBBM is an accredited regional affiliate of the Association for Applied Psychophysiology and Biofeedback. Executive Director (pro tem) and MASBBM contact: Jeanne Scammon, M.Ed., 15501 Straughn Avenue, Laurel, MD 20707.

Chapter 60

Hypnosis, Relaxation, and Massage Therapies

Hypnosis

Hypnosis can be used as a therapeutic tool for the control of pain.

Hypnotherapy can be used to counteract fear and anxiety that can heighten pain, complicate healing and slow labor in pregnant women. It can also help burn patients deal more effectively with pain.

What is hypnosis? Hypnosis is a sleep like state, induced by another person, in which the subject is in an altered state of consciousness and responds to the suggestions of the hypnotist. An hypnotic trance is when the subject is in a state of more awareness and focused concentration that allows the hypnotist to manipulate the patient.

Hypnosis is appropriate to use when you 1) find hypnosis appealing 2) if you have anxiety or fear, as long as the anxiety is not incapacitating or due to a psychiatric or medical condition requiring more extensive therapy 3) may benefit from avoiding or reducing drug therapy (e.g., a history of drug reactions, fear of /or physiological reason to avoid over sedation) 4) are likely to experience and need to cope with a prolonged interval of pain 5) your pain medications are not working effectively.

This chapter includes text from three documents: "Hypnosis" (Patient and Family Version) by Kathy Collins, edited by Deb Rickard RN; "Relaxation Therapy" (Patient and Family Version) by Chris Mentz RN, edited by: Ibtihal Almakhzoomy RN, BSN; and "Massage" (Patient and Family Version) by B. Michala Belongy RN, edited by Debra Wirth RN. These fact sheet are available online at http://www.nursing.uiowa.edu/sites/PedsPain/Nonpharm (accessed October 2001), © University of Iowa College of Nursing, reprinted with permission.

433

Hypnosis can involve a number of methods to help you understand more about your pain and become an active participant in helping your healthcare worker manage your pain. Ask your physician, nurse or other healthcare worker for information on hypnosis and how you can benefit.

Hypnosis should be considered as early as possible in pain management to allow you time to work with the hypnotist in finding the best type of hypnosis for you. This would include options such as self hypnosis or a hypnotic suggestion while in a hypnotic trance.

Hypnosis should only be administered by specially trained professionals. Ask your healthcare professional for a referral to a qualified therapist or contact a national organization.

Hypnosis is not contraindicated during pregnancy if performed by a qualified therapist.

References

Fine, Judylaine, *Conquering Back Pain*, 1987, Prentice Hall Press, New York.

Harris, Sally and Trulove, Susan, *Researchers Look at how Hypnosis Helps Control Pain*, www.technews.vt.edu/Archives/1996/Aug/96253.html

Rossi, Earnest Lawrence, *The Psychobiology of Mind-Body Healing: New Concepts of Therapeutic Hypnosis*, 1986, W.W. Norton & Company, New York.

The alternative advisor, 1997, Alexandria, Virginia: Time Life Books.

U.S. Department of Health and Human Services, *Acute Pain Management: Operative or Medical Procedures and Trauma*, February 1992.

U.S. Department of Health and Human Services, *Management of Cancer Pain*, March 1994.

Weitzenenhoffer, Andre M., *The Practice of Hypnotism*, 1989, John Wiley and Sons, New York.

Relaxation Therapy

What is relaxation therapy?

Relaxation therapy is a type of mind-body therapy used to promote health, decrease muscle tension, and recover from an illness.

How do you know this therapy works?

Research has shown there is a relationship between muscle tension, pain and anxiety. When a person is able to resolve muscle tension it directly affects pain and anxiety. The vice versa is true. Relaxation technique is rarely used alone but in combination with imagery and pain medications. However, relaxation methods can reduce your needs for certain medications. Keep your healthcare provider informed so he or she can make any necessary adjustments in dosage.

What does this therapy involve?

The relaxation exercise is a non-invasive intervention used by health professionals and families. A nurse or family member with little training can easily teach the exercises. Relaxation exercise results in the relaxation response. This response can slow breathing, lower blood pressure, lower amount of oxygen needed for your body, lower heart rate and increase brain waves.

What is involved in the exercise?

The relaxation exercise is a simple one to learn and use. There are different variations to the technique.

Deep Breathing and Relaxation

- Sit comfortably in a place with minimal distractions.

- Close your eyes and relax your muscles.

- Breathe naturally.

- As you exhale, silently repeat a word or phrase that has a meaning to you, "focus word". This can be an inspirational phrase such as "love", "peace", or prayer.

- Do not focus on any other thoughts that come to you.

- Concentrate for 10 to 20 minutes. Sit quietly for a moment before you get up.

- Practice this technique once or twice a day.

Another technique is called progressive muscle relaxation.

Progressive Muscle Relaxation

- This involves concentrating on each muscle group in the body one at a time.

- Move progressively from one end to the other.

- Inhale and clench your muscles for five seconds, then exhale and relax.

- Repeat for each area of your body until your entire body is relaxed.

Will it take away all of my pain?

This exercise will help to decrease pain, but is often used with other therapies and pain medications. Do not stop taking pain medications prescribed to you for pain.

Talk with your healthcare provider to find out more about this mind-body therapy.

References

Chiarmonte D. R. Mind-body therapies for primary care physicians. *Primary Care Clinics in Office Practice.* 24(4): 787-807, December 1997.

Soloman, R. Relaxation and the relief of cancer pain. *Nursing Clinics of North America.* 30(4): 697-709, December 1995.

Wallace K. G. Analysis of recent literature concerning relaxation and imagery interventions for pain. *Cancer Nursing.* 20(2): 79-87, April 1997.

Woodham A. & Peters D. *Encyclopedia of Healing Therapies,* 1997, DK publishing, Inc. New York, NY.

Massage

Pain control should be a high priority for two reasons. First, unrelieved pain causes unnecessary suffering. Second, the mental and physical effects of pain can result in additional problems such as a decrease in activity, appetite, sleep, and mood.

There are many drugs to help control pain, but also other methods that may allow the person suffering from pain to help himself

436

manage it better. Massage is one method that can do this, and it can also help the drugs work better. It may even decrease the need for pain relieving drugs, but should not be used as a complete replacement for them either. Massage as a therapy for pain should begin early, especially when used to treat aches and pains associated with decreased activity and movement.

Pain can be decreased by increasing stimulation to a specific area of the body. A massage for three to ten minutes can consist of massaging the whole body or just the feet, back, or hands. Common techniques include rapid stroking, kneading, and circular movements. Massage is also helpful with relaxation, helping one to distract from the pain. Long, smooth, slow strokes from the crown of the head to the lower back are used in relaxation.

Massage is safe for any patient, including those pregnant, with relatively no side effects. Some therapists offer specialized pregnancy massage. Massage therapy can be used for mild to moderate pain and may enhance other methods with severe pain. Not only does it help with pain control, but can reduce blood pressure and give the immune system a boost.

Massage therapists are certified through the American Massage Association and licensed in the state in which they practice. Listings of those licensed can be found in the yellow pages of the telephone directory.

References

Underwood, A. The magic of touch. *Newsweek*. April 6.1998.

U.S. Department of Health and Human Services. *Acute Pain Management: Operative or Medical Procedures and Trauma*. pg. 22, 1992.

U.S. Department of Health and Human Services. *Management of Cancer Pain*. Clinical practice number 9, pg. 8, 76-8, 1994.

Chapter 61

National Institutes of Health Endorses Alternative Therapies for Chronic Pain and Insomnia

Meditation, hypnosis, and biofeedback were among the alternative treatments endorsed by an independent 12-member panel convened October 16-18, 1995 to encourage wider acceptance of behavioral and relaxation therapies for treating chronic pain and insomnia.

The conference, *Integration of Behavioral and Relaxation Approaches Into the Treatment of Chronic Pain and Insomnia*, sponsored by the National Institutes of Health (NIH) National Center for Complementary and Alternative Medicine (NCCAM) and the NIH Office of Medical Applications and Research, emphasized broader use of alternative therapies in conjunction with conventional medical care for these disorders.

Millions of Americans are afflicted with chronic pain and insomnia—two conditions with both psychosocial and behavioral characteristics. The suffering and disability from these disorders result in a heavy burden for individual patients, their families, and their communities as well as the loss of billions of dollars to the Nation as a consequence of disability and lost productivity.

Conventional treatments for these conditions have principally focused on medical interventions such as drugs and surgery, which have

---

"NIH Panel Endorses Alternative Therapies for Chronic Pain and Insomnia," *CAM Newsletter*, National Center for Complementary and Alternative Medicine (NCCAM), December 1995. Despite the date of this document, readers seeking an explanation of the National Institutes of Health (NIH) perspective on complementary and alternative therapies will find the information useful.

had limited success. However, incorporation of behavioral and relaxation techniques have been used to enhance conventional treatments.

Led by panel chair, Julius Richmond, M.D., the John D. MacArthur Professor Emeritus of Health Policy Analysis at Harvard Medical School, the panel found strong evidence that relaxation approaches are effective in treating a variety of chronic pain conditions, such as low back pain, arthritis and headache.

Relaxation techniques involve the practice of two basic components: a repetitive focus on word, sound, prayer, phrase, or muscular activity, and neither fighting nor focusing on intruding thoughts. When performed properly, relaxation therapy can lower one's breathing rate, heart rate, and blood pressure.

The panel stated that there was evidence that hypnosis is effective in alleviating chronic pain associated with various cancers. Hypnosis can also be a part of the treatment program for irritable bowl syndrome, inflammatory conditions of the mouth, temporomandibular disorders, and tension headaches, the panel concluded.

After examining the data on biofeedback techniques, the panel determined that this therapy was effective in relieving chronic pain—citing tension headache in particular. Cognitive/behavioral techniques, which teach individuals to alter patterns of negative thoughts are also effective therapies, primarily in the treatment of low back pain and arthritis, the panel said.

The panel concluded that the relaxation and biofeedback therapies used for chronic pain were effective in alleviating some types of insomnia. However, they determined the most effective treatments for insomnia include sleep restriction, stimulus control, or a combination of a variety of sleep disorder therapies.

While behavioral and relaxation therapies have increasingly been used in conjunction with conventional medical care, the panel identified a number of barriers that to date have limited wider acceptance of these therapies. One of these barriers has been the emphasis on treating chronic pain and insomnia strictly as medical conditions without considering their psychosocial components. The panel recommended that health care practitioners adopt a biopsychosocial approach to disease that incorporates the patient's social and ethical experience of disease and expands the potential treatments available.

A second barrier identified by the panel is the patient's acceptance and willingness to participate in behavioral techniques, which can be time consuming and often must be practiced at home. The panel recommended patient education to promote increased understanding of the importance and potential health benefits and willingness to participate in these interventions.

The reluctance of insurance companies and other third party payers to reimburse for behavioral and relaxation interventions was identified by the panel as another barrier to wider use of alternative therapies. The panel encouraged insurance reimbursement of psychosocial therapy for chronic pain and insomnia as part of comprehensive medical services at rates comparable to standard medical care. Additionally, provision for these treatments should be included in expanding managed care programs.

The panel said that decisions will need to be made to identify practitioners best qualified to provide psychosocial and interventions in the most cost effective manner. The final conclusion was that a number of well-defined behavioral and relaxation interventions are now available, some of which are commonly used to treat chronic pain and insomnia. However, data are insufficient to conclude that one technique is more effective than another for a given condition. For any individual patient, however, one approach may be more appropriate than another.

This independent panel, comprised of doctors, nurses, epidemiologists and statisticians, presented their recommendations at the conclusion of a 3-day technology assessment conference. The complete statement of the panel's recommendations can be obtained by calling 1-800-NIH-OMAR.

Part Four

Living with Pain

Chapter 62

Action Guide for People with Pain

Pain Care Bill of Rights

As a person with pain, you have:

- The right to have your report of pain taken seriously and to be treated with dignity and respect by doctors, nurses, pharmacists and other healthcare professionals.

- The right to have your pain thoroughly assessed and promptly treated.

- The right to be informed by your doctor about what may be causing your pain, possible treatments, and the benefits, risks and costs of each.

- The right to participate actively in decisions about how to manage your pain.

- The right to have your pain reassessed regularly and your treatment adjusted if your pain has not been eased.

- The right to be referred to a pain specialist if your pain persists.

- The right to get clear and prompt answers to your questions, take time to make decisions, and refuse a particular type of treatment if you choose.

"Pain Action Guide and Pain Care Bill of Rights," American Pain Foundation, October 2000, available at www.painfoundation.org. © 2000 American Pain Foundation; reprinted with permission.

Although not always required by law, these are the rights you should expect, and if necessary demand, for your pain care.

Questions and Answers about Living with Pain

How serious is the pain problem?

Pain is a major healthcare crisis in the United States. More than 50 million Americans suffer from chronic pain caused by various diseases and disorders, and each year another 25 million experience acute pain as a result of injury or surgery.

Although most pain can be relieved or greatly eased with proper pain management, the tragedy is that most pain goes untreated, undertreated, or improperly treated. No one should have to suffer needlessly when the knowledge and skills are available today to manage most pain.

If left untreated, chronic pain can prevent you from having a full and meaningful life. Once your pain is under control, your body and mind will be less stressed. You'll be able to sleep better, focus on work, enjoy relationships with family and friends, and take part in social activities. If your pain has been caused by an injury or surgery, your recovery may be faster once your pain is managed.

Finding good pain care and taking control of your pain can be hard work. Learn all you can about pain and possible treatments. Be persistent, insist on your rights, and don't give up.

If most pain can be eased, why do so many people with pain suffer needlessly?

Many of us have beliefs about pain that are simply not true and prevent us from getting the relief we deserve. The truth is:

- **Pain is not something you "just have to live with."** Treatments are available to relieve or lessen most pain. If untreated, pain can make other health problems worse, slow recovery, and interfere with healing. Get help right away, and don't let anyone suggest that your pain is simply "in your head."

- **Not all doctors know how to treat pain.** Your doctor should give the same attention to your pain as to any other health problems. But many doctors have had little training in pain care. If your doctor is unable to deal with your pain effectively ask your doctor to consult with a specialist, or consider switching doctors.

- **Pain medications rarely cause addiction.** Morphine and similar pain medications, called opioids, can be highly effective for certain conditions. Unless you have a history of substance abuse, there is little risk of addiction when these medications are properly prescribed by a doctor and taken as directed. Physical dependence—which is *not* to be confused with addiction—occurs in the form of withdrawal symptoms if you stop taking these medications suddenly. This usually is not a problem if you go off your medications gradually.

- **Most side effects from opioid pain medications can be managed.** Nausea, drowsiness, itching, and most other side effects caused by morphine and similar opioid medications usually last only a few days. Constipation from these medications can usually be managed with laxatives, adequate fluid intake, and attention to diet. Ask your doctor to suggest ways that are best for you.

- **If you act quickly when pain starts, you can often prevent it from getting worse.** Take your medications when you first begin to experience pain. If your pain does get worse, talk with your doctor. Your doctor may safely prescribe higher doses or change the prescription. Non-drug therapies such as relaxation training and others can also help give you relief.

How do I talk with my doctor or nurse about pain?

- **Speak up! Tell your doctor or nurse that you're in pain.** It is *not* a sign of personal weakness to tell them about your pain. Pain is a common medical problem that requires urgent attention. So don't be embarrassed or afraid to talk about it.

- **Tell your doctor or nurse where it hurts.** Do you have pain in one place or several places? Does the pain seem to move around?

- **Describe how much your pain hurts.** On a scale from 0 to 10, zero means no pain at all and 10 means the worst pain you can imagine. In the past week, what was the highest level of pain you felt? When did you feel it? What were you doing at the time? When did it hurt the least? How bad does it hurt right now?

- **Describe what makes your pain better or worse.** Is the pain always there, or does it go away sometimes? Does the pain

447

get worse when you move in certain ways? Do other things make it better or worse?

- **Describe what your pain feels like.** Use specific words like sharp, stabbing, dull, aching, burning, shock-like, tingling, throbbing, deep, pressing, etc.

- **Explain how the pain affects your daily life.** Can you sleep? Work? Exercise? Are you able to do activities with family and friends? Can you concentrate on tasks? How is your mood? Are you sad? Irritable? Depressed? Do you feel unable to cope?

- **Tell your doctor or nurse about past treatments for pain.** Describe any medical treatments you've had such as medication or surgery, and mention other approaches you've tried. Have you done massage, yoga or meditation? Applied heat or cold to the painful areas? Exercised? Taken over-the-counter medications, or supplements such as vitamins, minerals, and herbal remedies? Tried other treatments? Explain what worked and what didn't.

Tip: Write down your questions for the doctor or nurse before an appointment. People often get nervous and forget to ask all their questions. Take notes so you can review them later. If possible, bring along a family member or friend to provide support, help take notes, and remind you of what was said.

How can I get the best results possible?

- **Take control.** It's your responsibility to tell your doctor you're in pain, take part in planning your treatment, follow your pain management plan, ask questions, and speak up if treatment isn't working. If necessary, seek other help. Be persistent until you find what works best for you.

- **Set goals.** Once you've found a doctor you trust, decide with your doctor on some realistic goals for things you most want to do again—for example, sleeping, working, exercising, enjoying sexual relations, etc. Begin working on the easiest goals first.

- **Work with your doctor or nurse to develop a pain management plan.** This might include a list of medications, when to take them, and possible side effects. It might include therapies other than medication. Make sure you understand the plan and carry it out fully. If you don't, you are less likely to get relief.

- **Keep a pain diary.** Write down information about your level of pain at different times, how you're feeling, and what activities you're able to do or not do. Keep a record of medications you're taking or any non-drug treatments. The diary will help you see what's working and measure progress. Bring your diary on visits to the doctor.

- **Ask your doctor or nurse about non-drug, non-surgical treatments.** These could include relaxation therapy, exercise, massage, acupuncture, meditation, application of cold or heat, behavioral therapy, and other techniques.

- **Ask your doctor or nurse about ways to relax and cope with pain.** The way you feel about your pain can actually affect the pain itself. Your pain may feel worse if you are stressed, depressed, or anxious.

- **If you have questions or concerns, speak up.** If you're worried about medications or other treatments, ask your doctor or nurse. If your treatment is not working, insist that your pain be reassessed and new treatments offered. Be polite, but be firm.

- **If you're going to have surgery, ask your doctor for a complete pain management plan beforehand.** Ask what medications you will receive before the operation to minimize pain later, and what will be available for pain relief afterwards.

- **If you're a patient in a hospital or other facility and you're in pain, speak up.** Ask a doctor or nurse for help. If you don't get help right away, ask again. If you still don't get help, ask to speak to the patient advocate or representative. Most likely the doctor or nurse will respond, but be sure to insist on effective pain care without delay.

- **Pace yourself.** Once you experience some degree of control over your pain, don't overdo it. Your body may be out of condition if you have been suffering pain for awhile. Take time to gradually build up to normal activity.

- **If you're not satisfied with your pain care, don't give up.** Does your doctor listen to you? Is your doctor able to assess and treat your pain? Are you getting adequate care? If after a reasonable time the answer is "no," find another doctor or pain care program.

Where can I find help?

If you want to learn from people in other organizations who understand particular types of pain:

- For chronic pain, contact the **American Chronic Pain Association** at www.theacpa.org or call (916) 632-0922.

- For cancer pain, contact **Cancer Care** at www.cancercare.org or call 1-800-813-HOPE, or contact your local **American Cancer Society** office.

- For a list of organizations that specialize in a particular disease or disorder, contact the **American Pain Foundation** at www.painfoundation.org or call (888) 615-PAIN.

If you want to find a pain specialist:

- Ask your regular doctor, if you have one, for a referral to a good pain specialist or pain clinic.

- Ask family members, friends and co-workers who have suffered from pain for a recommendation.

- Contact the largest local hospital or medical school in your area and ask if they have a pain team or know of a good local pain specialist or pain clinic.

- If you are under a managed care program, call your representative or caseworker and ask for their list of approved pain specialists.

- Call a local hospice, even though you may not need hospice care, and ask them to suggest doctors who are good at pain management.

Tip: Ask if the doctor belongs to any pain-related medical societies or has had special training or certification in pain medicine. Check the American Pain Foundation website or call us for information about professional organizations and certifying programs.

About the American Pain Foundation

The American Pain Foundation is an independent, nonprofit information, education and advocacy organization serving people with pain. Our mission is to improve the quality of life for people with pain by raising public awareness, providing practical information, promoting research, and advocating to remove barriers and increase access to effective pain management.

Our consumer friendly website has information about causes, treatment options, ways to find trained specialists and peer support, and how to cope with pain. It also links to over 200 carefully selected websites on pain and related topics.

Visit us at our website at: www.painfoundation.org

If you are unable to get access to the Internet and need more information, write to us at:

American Pain Foundation
201 N. Charles St., Suite 710
Baltimore, MD 21202

To order information by phone, leave a message on our toll-free information line at: (888) 615-PAIN (1-888-615-7246). Or send an e-mail to: info@painfoundation.org

Chapter 63

Keeping a Pain Diary

You are the only one who knows how much pain you are feeling. When your doctor asks you about the pain, you probably won't remember how hard some days were. You may not remember how bad the pain was. The diary is to help you describe what is happening to you while it is happening. It will be very helpful to your doctor to know when the pain was bad, what made you feel better, and what didn't make you feel better.

Don't worry about how much to write. You don't even have to write sentences. Just write the words that describe how you are feeling. Don't worry if you miss a day. Do it when you can. If thinking about your pain every day is too hard, put the diary away for a few days and go back to it when you are ready. This is your diary. Write when you can for as many days as you can and then stop.

Keep a small notebook or tape recorder with you all day and, during the course of the day, write down what you are feeling. The following questions might help you. Write the date and time every time you write in the diary. If writing is too painful, ask a family member or friend to do it for you or record the diary on a tape recorder.

1. **Where does it hurt?** List every place that hurts. Does the pain move? Does the pain feel different in different places?

"Keeping a Pain Diary," available at www.painfoundation.org. © 2001 American Pain Foundation; reprinted with permission.

2. **How does the pain feel?** The following words might be helpful: burning, stabbing, sharp, aching, throbbing, tingling, dull, pounding, or pressing.

3. **Did you have pain when you woke up or did it start later?**

4. **Does the pain change during the day?**

5. **What, if anything, makes the pain better or worse?**

6. **What medicines are you taking? Do they help—never, sometimes, always?** List all of the medicines your doctor gave you and all of the medicines you bought for yourself at the store.

7. **Have you stopped taking any medicines because they made you constipated, sleepy or sick, or for other reasons?**

8. **Do you do anything to help make the pain go away other than taking medicine such as getting a massage, or meditating, etc.?**

9. **Do you have trouble sleeping because of the pain?**

10. **Does the pain keep you from spending time with family or friends?**

11. **Do you skip meals because of the pain?**

12. **How has the pain changed your life?**

Chapter 64

Alcohol-Medication Interactions

Many medications can interact with alcohol, leading to increased risk of illness, injury, or death. For example, it is estimated that alcohol-medication interactions may be a factor in at least 25 percent of all emergency room admissions.[1] An unknown number of less serious interactions may go unrecognized or unrecorded. This *Alcohol Alert* notes some of the most significant alcohol-drug interactions. (Although alcohol can interact with illicit drugs as well, the term "drugs" is used here to refer exclusively to medications, whether prescription or nonprescription.)

How Common Are Alcohol-Drug Interactions?

More than 2,800 prescription drugs are available in the United States, and physicians write 14 billion prescriptions annually; in addition, approximately 2,000 medications are available without prescription.[2]

Approximately 70 percent of the adult population consumes alcohol at least occasionally, and 10 percent drink daily.[3] About 60 percent of men and 30 percent of women have had one or more adverse alcohol-related life events.[4] Together with the data on medication use,

National Institute on Alcohol Abuse and Alcoholism (NIAAA), *Alcohol Alert*, No. 27 PH 355, January 1995. Copies of the *Alcohol Alert* are available free of charge from the Scientific Communications Branch, Office of Scientific Affairs, NIAAA, Willco Building, Suite 409, 6000 Executive Boulevard, Bethesda, MD 20892-7003. Telephone: (301) 443-3860.

455

these statistics suggest that some concurrent use of alcohol and medications is inevitable.

The elderly may be especially likely to mix drugs and alcohol and are at particular risk for the adverse consequences of such combinations. Although persons age 65 and older constitute only 12 percent of the population, they consume 25 to 30 percent of all prescription medications.[5] The elderly are more likely to suffer medication side effects compared with younger persons, and these effects tend to be more severe with advancing age.[5] Among persons age 60 or older, 10 percent of those in the community—and 40 percent of those in nursing homes—fulfill criteria for alcohol abuse.[6]

How Alcohol and Drugs Interact

To exert its desired effect, a drug generally must travel through the bloodstream to its site of action, where it produces some change in an organ or tissue. The drug's effects then diminish as it is processed (metabolized) by enzymes and eliminated from the body. Alcohol behaves similarly, traveling through the bloodstream, acting upon the brain to cause intoxication, and finally being metabolized and eliminated, principally by the liver. The extent to which an administered dose of a drug reaches its site of action may be termed its availability. Alcohol can influence the effectiveness of a drug by altering its availability. Typical alcohol-drug interactions include the following:[7] First, an acute dose of alcohol (a single drink or several drinks over several hours) may inhibit a drug's metabolism by competing with the drug for the same set of metabolizing enzymes. This interaction prolongs and enhances the drug's availability, potentially increasing the patient's risk of experiencing harmful side effects from the drug. Second, in contrast, chronic (long-term) alcohol ingestion may activate drug-metabolizing enzymes, thus decreasing the drug's availability and diminishing its effects. After these enzymes have been activated, they remain so even in the absence of alcohol, affecting the metabolism of certain drugs for several weeks after cessation of drinking.[8] Thus, a recently abstinent chronic drinker may need higher doses of medications than those required by nondrinkers to achieve therapeutic levels of certain drugs. Third, enzymes activated by chronic alcohol consumption transform some drugs into toxic chemicals that can damage the liver or other organs. Fourth, alcohol can magnify the inhibitory effects of sedative and narcotic drugs at their sites of action in the brain. To add to the complexity of these interactions, some drugs affect the metabolism of alcohol, thus altering its potential for intoxication and the adverse effects associated with alcohol consumption.[7]

Some Specific Interactions

Note: The U.S. Government does not endorse or favor any specific commercial product (or commodity, service, or company). Trade or proprietary names appearing in this publication are used only because they are considered essential in the context of the studies reported herein.

Anesthetics: Anesthetics are administered prior to surgery to render a patient unconscious and insensitive to pain. Chronic alcohol consumption increases the dose of propofol (Diprivan) required to induce loss of consciousness.[9] Chronic alcohol consumption increases the risk of liver damage that may be caused by the anesthetic gases enflurane (Ethrane)[10] and halothane (Fluothane).[11]

Antibiotics: Antibiotics are used to treat infectious diseases. In combination with acute alcohol consumption, some antibiotics may cause nausea, vomiting, headache, and possibly convulsions; among these antibiotics are furazolidone (Furoxone), griseofulvin (Grisactin and others), metronidazole (Flagyl), and the antimalarial quinacrine (Atabrine).[7] Isoniazid and rifampin are used together to treat tuberculosis, a disease especially problematic among the elderly[12] and among homeless alcoholics.[13] Acute alcohol consumption decreases the availability of isoniazid in the bloodstream, whereas chronic alcohol use decreases the availability of rifampin. In each case, the effectiveness of the medication may be reduced.[7]

Anticoagulants: Warfarin (Coumadin) is prescribed to retard the blood's ability to clot. Acute alcohol consumption enhances warfarin's availability, increasing the patient's risk for life-threatening hemorrhages.[7] Chronic alcohol consumption reduces warfarin's availability, lessening the patient's protection from the consequences of blood-clotting disorders.[7]

Antidepressants: Alcoholism and depression are frequently associated,[14] leading to a high potential for alcohol-antidepressant interactions. Alcohol increases the sedative effect of tricyclic antidepressants such as amitriptyline (Elavil and others), impairing mental skills required for driving.[15] Acute alcohol consumption increases the

457

availability of some tricyclics, potentially increasing their sedative effects;[16] chronic alcohol consumption appears to increase the availability of some tricyclics and to decrease the availability of others.[17,18] The significance of these interactions is unclear. These chronic effects persist in recovering alcoholics.[17]

A chemical called tyramine, found in some beers and wine, interacts with some anti-depressants, such as monoamine oxidase inhibitors, to produce a dangerous rise in blood pressure.[7] As little as one standard drink may create a risk that this interaction will occur.

Antidiabetic medications: Oral hypoglycemic drugs are prescribed to help lower blood sugar levels in some patients with diabetes. Acute alcohol consumption prolongs, and chronic alcohol consumption decreases, the availability of tolbutamide (Orinase). Alcohol also interacts with some drugs of this class to produce symptoms of nausea and headache such as those described for metronidazole (see "Antibiotics").[7]

Antihistamines: Drugs such as diphenhydramine (Benadryl and others) are available without prescription to treat allergic symptoms and insomnia. Alcohol may intensify the sedation caused by some antihistamines.[15] These drugs may cause excessive dizziness and sedation in older persons; the effects of combining alcohol and antihistamines may therefore be especially significant in this population.[19]

Antipsychotic medications: Drugs such as chlorpromazine (Thorazine) are used to diminish psychotic symptoms such as delusions and hallucinations. Acute alcohol consumption increases the sedative effect of these drugs,[20] resulting in impaired coordination and potentially fatal breathing difficulties.[7] The combination of chronic alcohol ingestion and antipsychotic drugs may result in liver damage.[21]

Antiseizure medications: These drugs are prescribed mainly to treat epilepsy. Acute alcohol consumption increases the availability of phenytoin (Dilantin) and the risk of drug-related side effects. Chronic drinking may decrease phenytoin availability, significantly reducing the patient's protection against epileptic seizures, even during a period of abstinence.[8,22]

Antiulcer medications: The commonly prescribed antiulcer medications cimetidine (Tagamet) and ranitidine (Zantac) increase the availability of a low dose of alcohol under some circumstances.[23,24] The clinical significance of this finding is uncertain, since other studies have questioned such interaction at higher doses of alcohol.[25-27]

Cardiovascular medications: This class of drugs includes a wide variety of medications prescribed to treat ailments of the heart and circulatory system. Acute alcohol consumption interacts with some of these drugs to cause dizziness or fainting upon standing up. These drugs include nitroglycerin, used to treat angina, and reserpine, methyldopa (Aldomet), hydralazine (Apresoline and others), and guanethidine (Ismelin and others), used to treat high blood pressure. Chronic alcohol consumption decreases the availability of propranolol (Inderal), used to treat high blood pressure,[7] potentially reducing its therapeutic effect.

Narcotic pain relievers: These drugs are prescribed for moderate to severe pain. They include the opiates morphine, codeine, propoxyphene (Darvon), and meperidine (Demerol). The combination of opiates and alcohol enhances the sedative effect of both substances, increasing the risk of death from overdose.[28] A single dose of alcohol can increase the availability of propoxyphene,[29] potentially increasing its sedative side effects.

Nonnarcotic pain relievers: Aspirin and similar nonprescription pain relievers are most commonly used by the elderly.[5] Some of these drugs cause stomach bleeding and inhibit blood from clotting; alcohol can exacerbate these effects.[30] Older persons who mix alcoholic beverages with large doses of aspirin to self-medicate for pain are therefore at particularly high risk for episodes of gastric bleeding.[19] In addition, aspirin may increase the availability of alcohol,[31] heightening the effects of a given dose of alcohol.

Chronic alcohol ingestion activates enzymes that transform acetaminophen (Tylenol and others) into chemicals that can cause liver damage, even when acetaminophen is used in standard therapeutic amounts.[32,33] These effects may occur with as little as 2.6 grams of acetaminophen in persons consuming widely varying amounts of alcohol.[34]

Sedatives and hypnotics ("sleeping pills"): Benzodiazepines such as diazepam (Valium) are generally prescribed to treat anxiety and insomnia. Because of their greater safety margin, they have largely replaced the barbiturates, now used mostly in the emergency treatment of convulsions.[2]

459

Doses of benzodiazepines that are excessively sedating may cause severe drowsiness in the presence of alcohol,[35] increasing the risk of household and automotive accidents.[15,36] This may be especially true in older people, who demonstrate an increased response to these drugs.[5,19] Low doses of flurazepam (Dalmane) interact with low doses of alcohol to impair driving ability, even when alcohol is ingested the morning after taking Dalmane. Since alcoholics often suffer from anxiety and insomnia, and since many of them take morning drinks, this interaction may be dangerous.[37]

The benzodiazepine lorazepam (Ativan) is being increasingly used for its antianxiety and sedative effects. The combination of alcohol and lorazepam may result in depressed heart and breathing functions; therefore, lorazepam should not be administered to intoxicated patients.[38]

Acute alcohol consumption increases the availability of barbiturates, prolonging their sedative effect. Chronic alcohol consumption decreases barbiturate availability through enzyme activation.[2] In addition, acute or chronic alcohol consumption enhances the sedative effect of barbiturates at their site of action in the brain, sometimes leading to coma or fatal respiratory depression.[39]

Alcohol-Medication Interactions— A Commentary by NIAAA Director Enoch Gordis, M.D.

Individuals who drink alcoholic beverages should be aware that simultaneous use of alcohol and medications—both prescribed and over-the-counter—has the potential to cause problems. For example, even very small doses of alcohol probably should not be used with antihistamines and other medications with sedative effects. Individuals who drink larger amounts of alcohol may run into problems when commonly used medications (e.g., acetaminophen) are taken at the same time or even shortly after drinking has stopped. Elderly individuals should be especially careful of these potential problems due to their generally greater reliance on multiple medications and age-related changes in physiology.

References

1. Holder, H.D. *Effects of Alcohol, Alone and in Combination With Medications*. Walnut Creek, CA: Prevention Research Center, 1992.

2. Sands, B.F.; Knapp, C.M.; & Ciraulo, D.A. Medical conse-
    quences of alcohol-drug interactions. *Alcohol Health & Re-
    search World* 17(4):316-320, 1993.

3. Midanik, L.T., & Room, R. The epidemiology of alcohol con-
    sumption. *Alcohol Health & Research World* 16(3):183-190,
    1992.

4. American Psychiatric Association. *Diagnostic and Statistical
    Manual of Mental Disorders, Fourth Edition.* Washington,
    DC: the Association, 1994.

5. Gomberg, E.S.L. Drugs, alcohol, and aging. In: Kozlowski,
    L.T.; Annis, H.M.; Cappell, H.D.; Glaser, F.B.; Goodstadt,
    M.S.; Israel, Y.; Kalant, H.; Sellers, E.M.; & Vingilis, E.R. *Re-
    search Advances in Alcohol and Drug Problems.* Vol. 10. New
    York: Plenum Press, 1990. pp. 171-213.

6. Egbert, A.M. The older alcoholic: Recognizing the subtle clini-
    cal clues. *Geriatrics* 48(7):63-69, 1993.

7. Lieber, C.S. Interaction of ethanol with other drugs. In:
    Lieber, C.S., ed. *Medical and Nutritional Complications of Al-
    coholism: Mechanisms and Management.* New York: Plenum
    Press, 1992. pp. 165-183.

8. Guram, M.S.; Howden, C.W.; & Holt, S. Alcohol and drug in-
    teractions. *Practical Gastroenterology* 16(8):47, 50-54, 1992.

9. Fassoulaki, A.; Farinotti, R.; Servin, F.; & Desmonts, J.M.
    Chronic alcoholism increases the induction dose of propofol in
    humans. *Anesthesia and Analgesia* 77(3):553-556, 1993.

10. Tsutsumi, R.; Leo, M.A.; Kim, C.-i. ; Tsutsumi, M.; Lasker, J.;
    Lowe, N.; & Lieber, C.S. Interaction of ethanol with enflurane
    metabolism and toxicity: Role of P450IIE1. *Alcoholism: Clini-
    cal and Experimental Research* 14(2):174-179, 1990.

11. Ishii, H.; Takagi, T.; Okuno, F.; Ebihara, Y.; Tashiro, M.; &
    Tsuchiya, M. Halothane-induced hepatic necrosis in ethanol-
    pretreated rats. In: Lieber, C.S., ed. *Biological Approach to Al-
    coholism.* National Institute on Alcohol Abuse and Alcoholism
    Research Monograph No. 11. DHHS Pub. No. (ADM)83-1261.
    Washington, DC: Supt. of Docs., U.S. Govt. Print. Off., 1983.
    pp. 152-157.

12. Kelley, W.N., ed. *Textbook of Internal Medicine*. Philadelphia: Lippincott, 1989.

13. Jacobson, J.M. Alcoholism and tuberculosis. *Alcohol Health & Research World* 16(1):39-45, 1992.

14. Roy, A. ; DeJong, J.; Lamparski, D.; George, T.; & Linnoila, M. Depression among alcoholics. *Archives of General Psychiatry* 48(5):428-432, 1991.

15. Seppala, T.; Linnoila, M.; & Mattila, M.J. Drugs, alcohol and driving. *Drugs* 17:389-408, 1979.

16. Dorian, P.; Sellers, E.M.; Reed, K.L.; Warsh, J.J.; Hamilton, C.; Kaplan, H.L.; & Fan, T. Amitriptyline and ethanol: Pharmacokinetic and pharmacodynamic interaction. *European Journal of Clinical Pharmacology* 25(3):325-331, 1983.

17. Balant-Gorgia, A.E.; Gay, M.; Gex-Fabry, M.; & Balant, L.P. Persistent impairment of clomipramine demethylation in recently detoxified alcoholic patients. *Therapeutic Drug Monitoring* 14(2):119-124, 1992.

18. Rudorfer, M.V., & Potter, W.Z. Pharmacokinetics of antidepressants. In: Meltzer, H.Y., ed. *Psychopharmacology: The Third Generation of Progress*. New York: Raven Press, 1987. pp. 1353-1363.

19. Dufour, M.C.; Archer, L.; & Gordis, E. Alcohol and the elderly. *Clinics in Geriatric Medicine* 8(1):127-141, 1992.

20. Shoaf, S.E., & Linnoila, M. Interaction of ethanol and smoking on the pharmacokinetics and pharmacodynamics of psychotropic medications. *Psychopharmacology Bulletin* 27(4): 577-594, 1991.

21. Teschke, R. Effect of chronic alcohol pretreatment on the hepatotox-icity elicited by chlorpromazine, paracetamol, and dimethylnitrosamine. In: Lieber, C.S., ed. *Biological Approach to Alcoholism*. National Institute on Alcohol Abuse and Alcoholism Research Monograph No. 11. DHHS Pub. No. (ADM)83-1261. Washington, DC: Supt. of Docs., U.S. Govt. Print. Off., 1983. pp. 170-179.

22. Greenspan, K., & Smith, T.J. Perspectives on alcohol and medication interactions. *Journal of Alcohol and Drug Education* 36(3):103-107, 1991.

23. Caballeria, J.; Baraona, E.; Deulofeu, R.; Hernandez-Munoz, R.; Rodes, J.; & Lieber, C.S. Effects of H2-receptor antagonists on gastric alcohol dehydrogenase activity. *Digestive Diseases and Sciences* 36(12):1673-1679, 1991.

24. DiPadova, C.; Roine, R.; Frezza, M.; Gentry, R.T.; Baraona, E.; & Lieber, C.S. Effects of ranitidine on blood alcohol levels after ethanol ingestion: Comparison with other H2-receptor antagonists. *Journal of the American Medical Association* 267(1):83-86, 1992.

25. Fraser, A.G.; Hudson, M.; Sawyerr, A.M.; Smith, M.; Rosalki, S.B.; & Pounder, R.E. Ranitidine, cimetidine, famotidine have no effect on post-prandial absorption of ethanol 0.8 g/kg taken after an evening meal. *Alimentary Pharmacology and Therapeutics* 6(6):693-700, 1992.

26. Kendall, M.J.; Spannuth, F.; Walt, R.P; Gibson, G.J.; Hale, K.A.; Braithwaite, R.; & Langman, M.J.S. Lack of effect of H2-receptor antagonists on the pharmacokinetics of alcohol consumed after food at lunchtime. *British Journal of Clinical Pharmacology* 37:371-374, 1994.

27. Mallat, A.; Roudot-Thoraval, F.; Bergmann, J.F.; Trout, H.; Simonneau, G.; Dutreuil, C.; Blanc, L.E.; Dhumeaux, D.; & Delchier, J.C. Inhibition of gastric alcohol dehydrogenase activity by histamine H2-receptor antagonists has no influence on the pharmacokinetics of ethanol after a moderate dose. *British Journal of Clinical Pharmacology* 37(2):208-211, 1994.

28. Kissin, B. Interactions of ethyl alcohol and other drugs. In: Kissin, B., & Begleiter, H., eds. *The Biology of Alcoholism: Volume 3. Clinical Pathology.* New York: Plenum Press, 1974. pp. 109-162.

29. Girre, C.; Hirschhorn, M.; Bertaux, L.; Palombo, S.; Dellatolas, F.; Ngo, R.; Moreno, M.; & Fournier, P.E. Enhancement of propoxyphene bioavailability by ethanol: Relation to psychomotor and cognitive function in healthy volunteers. *European Journal of Clinical Pharmacology* 41(2):147-152, 1991.

30. Rees, W.D.W., & Turnberg, L.A. Reappraisal of the effects of aspirin on the stomach. *Lancet* 2:410-413, 1980.

31. Roine, R.; Gentry, R.T.; Hernandez-Munoz, R.; Baraona, E.; & Lieber, C.S. Aspirin increases blood alcohol concentrations in

humans after ingestion of ethanol. *Journal of the American Medical Association* 264(18):2406-2408, 1990.

32. Seeff, L.B.; Cuccherini, B.A.; Zimmerman, H.J.; Adler, E.; & Benjamin, S.B. Acetaminophen hepatotoxicity in alcoholics: A therapeutic misadventure. *Annals of Internal Medicine* 104(3):399-404, 1986.

33. Girre, C.; Hispard, E.; Palombo, S.; N'Guyen, C.; & Dally, S. Increased metabolism of acetaminophen in chronically alcoholic patients. *Alcoholism: Clinical and Experimental Research* 17(1):170-173, 1993.

34. Black, M. Acetaminophen hepatotoxicity. *Annual Review of Medicine* 35:577-593, 1984.

35. Girre, C.; Facy, F.; Lagier, G.; & Dally, S. Detection of blood benzodiazepines in injured people. Relationship with alcoholism. *Drug and Alcohol Dependence* 21(1):61-65, 1988.

36. Hollister, L.E. Interactions between alcohol and benzodiazepines. In: Galanter, M., ed. *Recent Developments in Alcoholism: Volume 8. Combined Alcohol and Other Drug Dependence.* New York: Plenum Press, 1990. pp. 233-239.

37. Linnoila, M.; Mattila, M.J.; & Kitchell, B.S. Drug interactions with alcohol. *Drugs* 18:299-311, 1979.

38. Medical Economics Data. *Physicians' Desk Reference.* Montvale, NJ: Medical Economics Data, 1993.

39. Forney, R.B., & Hughes, F.W. Meprobamate, ethanol or meprobamate-ethanol combinations on performance of human subjects under delayed autofeedback (DAF). *Journal of Psychology* 57:431-436, 1964.

Acknowledgment

The National Institute on Alcohol Abuse and Alcoholism wishes to acknowledge the valuable contributions of Charles S. Lieber, M.D., Director, Alcohol Research Center, Bronx VAMC, and professor, Mount Sinai School of Medicine, to the development of this *Alcohol Alert.*

Chapter 65

Painkillers and the Kidney (Analgesic Nephropathy)

An analgesic (AN-ul-JEE-zik) is any medicine intended to kill pain. Over-the-counter analgesics (medicines bought without a prescription) include aspirin, acetaminophen, ibuprofen, naproxen sodium, and others. These drugs present no danger for most people when taken in the recommended dosage. But some conditions make taking even these common painkillers dangerous for the kidneys. Also, taking one or a combination of these drugs regularly over a long period of time may increase the risk for kidney problems. Most drugs that can cause kidney damage are the ones that are excreted only through the kidneys.

Case reports have attributed incidents of acute kidney failure to the use of painkillers, including aspirin, ibuprofen, and naproxen. The patients in these reports had risk factors such as systemic lupus erythematosus, advanced age, chronic renal conditions, or a recent binge of alcohol consumption. These cases involved a single dose in some instances and never more than 10 days of analgesic use. Acute kidney failure requires emergency dialysis to clean the blood. But normal kidney function often returns after the emergency is over.

A different kind of problem can result from taking painkillers every day for several years. Analgesic nephropathy is a chronic kidney disease that gradually leads to end-stage renal disease and the permanent need for dialysis or a kidney transplant to restore renal function.

"Analgesic Nephropathy," National Institute of Diabetes and Digestive and Kidney Diseases (NIDDK), NIH Pub. No. 99-4573, 1998.

The painkillers that combine two or more analgesics (for example, aspirin and acetaminophen together) with caffeine or codeine are most likely to damage the kidneys. These mixtures are often sold as powders. Single analgesics (e.g., aspirin alone) have not been found to cause kidney damage.

Patients with conditions that put them at risk for acute kidney failure should check with their doctors before taking any medicine. People who take painkillers on a regular basis should check with their doctors to make sure they are not hurting their kidneys. The doctor may be able to recommend a safer alternative.

For More Information

American Kidney Fund
6110 Executive Boulevard
Suite 1010
Rockville, MD 20852
Phone: (800) 638-8299
website: http://www.akfinc.org

National Kidney Foundation
30 East 33rd Street
New York, NY 10016
Phone: (800) 622-9010
website: http://www.kidney.org

Additional Information on Analgesic Nephropathy

The National Kidney and Urologic Diseases Information Clearinghouse collects resource information on kidney and urologic diseases for the Combined Health Information Database (CHID). CHID is a database produced by health-related agencies of the Federal Government. This database (which is on the internet at http://chid.nih.gov) provides titles, abstracts, and availability information for health information and health education resources.

To provide you with the most up-to-date resources, information specialists at the clearinghouse created an automatic search of CHID. To obtain this information you may view the results of the automatic search on Analgesic Nephropathy.

Or, if you wish to perform your own search of the database, you may access the CHID Online website and search CHID yourself.

Chapter 66

Pain Relievers and Peptic Ulcers

A peptic ulcer is a sore that forms in the lining of the stomach or the duodenum (the beginning of the small intestine). An ulcer can cause a gnawing, burning pain in the upper abdomen; nausea; vomiting; loss of appetite; and weight loss. Most peptic ulcers are caused by infection with the bacterium *Helicobacter pylori* (*H. pylori*). But some peptic ulcers are caused by prolonged use of nonsteroidal anti-inflammatory drugs (NSAIDs) or pain relievers such as aspirin, ibuprofen, and naproxen sodium. NSAIDs cause ulcers by interfering with the stomach's ability to protect itself from acidic stomach juices.

Normally the stomach has three defenses against digestive juices: mucus that coats the stomach lining and shields it from stomach acid, the chemical bicarbonate that neutralizes stomach acid, and blood circulation to the stomach lining that aids in cell renewal and repair. NSAIDs hinder all of these protective mechanisms, and with the stomach's defenses down, digestive juices can damage the sensitive stomach lining and cause ulcers.

NSAID-induced ulcers usually heal once the person stops taking the medication. To help the healing process and relieve symptoms in the meantime, the doctor may recommend taking antacids to neutralize the acid and drugs called H2-blockers or proton-pump inhibitors to decrease the amount of acid the stomach produces.

"NSAIDs and Peptic Ulcers," National Institute of Diabetes and Digestive and Kidney Diseases (NIDDK), NIH Pub. No. 99-4644, 1998.

Medicines that protect the stomach lining also help with healing. Examples are bismuth subsalicylate, which coats the entire stomach lining, and sucralfate, which sticks to and covers the ulcer.

If a person with an NSAID ulcer also tests positive for *H. pylori*, he or she will be treated with antibiotics to kill the bacteria. Surgery may be necessary if an ulcer recurs or fails to heal, or if complications like bleeding, perforation, or obstruction develop.

Anyone taking NSAIDs who experiences symptoms of peptic ulcer should see a doctor for prompt treatment. Delaying diagnosis and treatment can lead to complications and the need for surgery.

Additional Information on NSAIDs and Peptic Ulcers

The National Digestive Diseases Information Clearinghouse collects resource information on digestive diseases for the Combined Health Information Database (CHID). CHID is a database produced by health-related agencies of the Federal Government. This database (which is available on the internet at http://chid.nih.gov) provides titles, abstracts, and availability information for health information and health education resources.

To provide you with the most up-to-date resources, information specialists at the clearinghouse created an automatic search of CHID. To obtain this information you may view the results of the automatic search on NSAIDs and Peptic Ulcers.

Or, if you wish to perform your own search of the database, you may access the CHID Online website and search CHID yourself.

Chapter 67

Harmful Effects of Medicines on the Digestive System

Many medicines taken by mouth may affect the digestive system. These medicines include prescription (those ordered by a doctor and dispensed by a pharmacist) and nonprescription or over-the-counter (OTC) products. A glossary at the end of this chapter describes some common prescription and nonprescription medicines discussed below that may affect the digestive system.

Although these medicines usually are safe and effective, harmful effects may occur in some people. OTC's typically do not cause serious side effects when taken as directed on the product's label. It is important to read the label to find out the ingredients, side effects, warnings, and when to consult a doctor.

Always talk with your doctor before taking a medicine for the first time and before adding any new medicines to those you already are taking. Tell the doctor about all other medicines (prescription and OTC's) you are taking. Certain medicines taken together may interact and cause harmful side effects. In addition, tell the doctor about any allergies or sensitivities to foods and medicines and about any medical conditions you may have such as diabetes, kidney disease, or liver disease.

"Harmful Effects of Medicines on the Adult Digestive System," National Institute of Diabetes and Digestive and Kidney Diseases (NIDDK), NIH Pub. No. 95-3421, February 1998. The U.S. Government does not endorse or favor any specific commercial product or company. Brand names appearing in this publication are used only because they are considered essential in the context of the information reported herein.

469

Be sure that you understand all directions for taking the medicine, including dose and schedule, possible interactions with food, alcohol, and other medicines, side effects, and warnings. If you are an older adult read all directions carefully and ask your doctor questions about the medicine. As you get older, you may be more susceptible to drug interactions that cause side effects.

People with a food intolerance such as gluten intolerance should make sure their medicines do not contain fillers or additives with gluten. Check with your doctor if you have any questions or concerns about your medicines. Follow the doctor's orders carefully, and immediately report any unusual symptoms or the warning signs described below.

The Esophagus

Irritation

Some people have difficulty swallowing medicines in tablet or capsule form. Tablets or capsules that stay in the esophagus may release chemicals that irritate the lining of the esophagus. The irritation may cause ulcers, bleeding, perforation (a hole or tear), and strictures (narrowing) of the esophagus. The risk of pill-induced injuries to the esophagus increases in persons with conditions involving the esophagus, such as strictures, scleroderma (hardening of the skin), achalasia (irregular muscle activity of the esophagus, which delays the passage of food), and stroke.

Some medicines can cause ulcers when they become lodged in the esophagus. These medicines include aspirin, several antibiotics such as tetracycline, quinidine, potassium chloride, vitamin C, and iron.

Warning Signs

- Pain when swallowing food or liquid.
- Feeling of a tablet or capsule "stuck" in the throat.
- Dull, aching pain in the chest or shoulder after taking medicines.

Precautions

- Swallow tablets or capsules while you are in an upright or sitting position.
- Before taking a tablet or capsule, swallow several sips of liquid to lubricate the throat, then swallow the tablet or capsule with at least a full glass (8 ounces) of liquid.

470

- Do not lie down immediately after taking medicines to ensure that the pills pass through the esophagus into the stomach.

- Tell your doctor if painful swallowing continues or if pills continue to stick in the throat.

Esophageal Reflux

The lower esophageal sphincter (LES) muscle is between the esophagus and the stomach. The muscle allows the passage of food into the stomach after swallowing. Certain medicines interfere with the action of the sphincter muscle, which increases the likelihood of backup or reflux of the highly acidic contents of the stomach into the esophagus.

Medicines that can cause esophageal reflux include nitrates, theophylline, calcium channel blockers, anticholinergics, and birth control pills.

Warning Signs

- Heartburn or indigestion.

- Sensation of food coming back up into the throat.

Precautions

- Avoid foods and beverages that may worsen reflux, including coffee, alcohol, chocolate, and fried or fatty foods.

- Cut down on, or preferably quit, smoking.

- Do not lie down immediately after eating.

The Stomach

Irritation

One of the most common drug-induced injuries is irritation of the lining of the stomach caused by nonsteroidal anti-inflammatory drugs (NSAIDs).

NSAIDs can irritate the stomach by weakening the ability of the lining to resist acid made in the stomach. Sometimes this irritation may lead to inflammation of the stomach lining (gastritis), ulcers, bleeding, or perforation of the lining.

In addition, you should be aware that stomach irritation may occur without having any of the symptoms below.

471

Older people are especially at risk for irritation from NSAIDs because they are more likely to regularly take pain medicines for arthritis and other chronic conditions. Also at risk are individuals with a history of peptic ulcers and related complications or gastritis. These individuals should tell their doctor about any of these previous conditions. Special medicines may be needed to protect the stomach lining.

Warning Signs

- Severe stomach cramps or pain or burning in the stomach or back.
- Black, tarry, or bloody stools.
- Bloody vomit.
- Severe heartburn or indigestion.
- Diarrhea.

Precautions

- Use coated tablets, which may lessen stomach irritation.
- Avoid drinking alcoholic beverages while taking medicines.
- Take medicines with a full glass of water or milk or with food, which may reduce irritation.

Delayed Emptying of the Stomach

Some medicines cause nerve and muscle activity to slow down in the stomach. This slowing down causes the contents of the stomach to empty at a slower rate than normal.

Drugs that may cause this delay include anticholinergics and drugs used to treat Parkinson's disease and depression.

Warning Signs

- Nausea.
- Bloating.
- Feeling of fullness.
- Vomiting of food eaten many hours earlier.
- Pain in midabdomen.
- Heartburn or indigestion.
- Sensation of food coming back up into the throat.

Precautions

- Eat frequent, small meals.
- Do not lie down for about 30 minutes after eating.
- Tell your doctor if symptoms continue. Your doctor may consider changing your dosage of the medicine or trying a new medicine.

The Intestine

Constipation

Constipation can be caused by a variety of medicines. These medicines affect the nerve and muscle activity in the large intestine (colon). This results in the slow and difficult passage of stool. Medicines also may bind intestinal liquid and make the stool hard.

Medicines that commonly cause constipation include antihypertensives, anticholinergics, cholestyramine, iron, and antacids that contain mostly aluminium.

Warning Sign

- Constipation that is severe or disabling or that lasts several weeks.

Precautions

- Drink plenty of fluids.
- Eat a well-balanced diet that includes whole grains, fruits, and vegetables.
- Exercise regularly.
- Take laxatives only under a doctor's supervision.

Diarrhea

Diarrhea is a common side effect of many medicines. Diarrhea is often caused by antibiotics, which affect the bacteria that live normally in the large intestine.

Antibiotic-induced changes in intestinal bacteria allow overgrowth of another bacteria, *Clostridium difficile* (*C. difficile*), which is the cause of a more serious antibiotic-induced diarrhea.

The presence of *C. difficile* can cause colitis, an inflammation of the intestine in which the bowel "weeps" excess water and mucus,

473

resulting in loose, watery stools. Almost any antibiotic may cause *C. difficile*-induced diarrhea, but the most common are ampicillin, clindamycin, and the cephalosporins. Antibiotic-induced colitis is treated with another antibiotic that acts on *C. difficile*.

Diarrhea also can be a side effect of drugs that do not cause colitis but that alter the movements or fluid content of the colon. Colchicine is a common cause of drug-induced diarrhea. Magnesium-containing antacids can have the effect of laxatives and cause diarrhea if over-used. In addition, the abuse of laxatives may result in damage to the nerves and muscles of the colon and cause diarrhea.

Warning Signs

- Blood, mucus, or pus in the stool.
- Pain in the lower abdomen.
- Fever.

Precaution

- If diarrhea lasts for several days, consult your doctor.

The Liver

The liver processes most medicines that enter the bloodstream and governs drug activity throughout the body. Once a drug enters the bloodstream, the liver converts the drug into chemicals the body can use and removes toxic chemicals that other organs cannot tolerate. During this process, these chemicals can attack and injure the liver.

Drug-induced liver injury can resemble the symptoms of any acute or chronic liver disease. The only way a doctor can diagnose drug-induced liver injury is by stopping use of the suspected drug and excluding other liver diseases through diagnostic tests. Rarely, long-term use of a medicine can cause chronic liver damage and scarring (cirrhosis).

Medicines that can cause severe liver injury include large doses of acetaminophen (and even in small doses when taken with alcohol), anticonvulsants such as phenytoin and valproic acid, the antihypertensive methyldopa, the tranquilizer chlorpromazine, antituberculins used to treat tuberculosis such as isoniazid and rifampin, and vitamins such as vitamin A and niacin.

Warning Signs (for liver injury)

- Severe fatigue.
- Abdominal pain and swelling.
- Jaundice (yellow eyes and skin, dark urine).
- Fever.
- Nausea or vomiting.

Precautions

- If you have ever had a liver disease or gallstones, you should discuss this with your doctor before taking any medicines that may affect the liver or the gallbladder.
- Take these medicines **only** in the prescribed or recommended doses.

Glossary of Medicines

The following glossary is a guide to medicines used to treat many medical conditions. The glossary does not include all medicines that may affect the digestive system. If a medicine you are taking is not listed here, check with your doctor.

Acetaminophen: Acetaminophen relieves fever and pain by blocking pain centers in the central nervous system. Examples of brand names include Tylenol, Panadol, and Datril.

Antacids: Antacids relieve heartburn, acid indigestion, sour stomach, and symptoms of peptic ulcer. They work by neutralizing stomach acid. Aluminum hydroxide antacids include Alu-Tab and Amphojel; calcium carbonate antacids include Tums, Alka Mints, and Rolaids Calcium Rich; magnesium antacids include Mylanta and Maalox.

Antibiotics: Antibiotics destroy or block the growth of bacteria that cause infection. Hundreds of antibiotics are available, including penicillins (Amoxil, Amcil, and Augmentin), clindamycin, cephalosporins (Keflex and Ceclor), tetracyclines (Minocin, Sumycin, and Vibramycin), quinolones (Cipro), and sulfa drugs (Bactrim).

Anticholinergics: This class of medicines affects the nerve cells or nerve fibers and includes drugs for depression, anxiety, and nervousness. Examples of anticholinergics include propantheline (Pro-banthine)

475

and dicyclomine (Bentyl). Examples of antidepressants include amitriptyline (Elavil and Endep), and nortriptyline (Aventyl and Pamelor). Medicines for relieving the symptoms of Parkinson's disease also are in this category. Examples include levodopa (Dopar) and carbidopa and levodopa combination (Sinemet).

Anticonvulsants: These medicines control epilepsy and other types of seizure disorders. They act by lessening overactive nerve impulses in the brain. Examples of this class of medicines include phenytoin (Dilantin) and valproic acid (Dalpro).

Antihypertensives: Antihypertensives lower high blood pressure. They act by relaxing blood vessels, which makes blood flow more easily. Examples of antihypertensives include methyldopa (Aldomet) and clonidine hydrochloride (Catapres).

Antituberculins: These drugs for tuberculosis limit the growth of bacteria or prevent tuberculosis from developing in people who have a positive tuberculin skin test. Brand names include INH, Dow-Isoniazid, Rifadin, and Rimactane.

Calcium channel blockers: These medicines for angina (chest pain) and high blood pressure affect the movement of calcium into the cells of the heart and blood vessels, relax blood vessels, and increase the flow of blood and oxygen to the heart. Examples of calcium channel blockers include diltiazem (Cardizem), nifedipine (Procardia), and verpamil (Isoptin).

Chlorpromazine: This tranquilizer relieves anxiety or agitation. Examples of brand names include Thorazine and Ormazine.

Colchicine: This medicine eases the inflammation from gout and prevents attacks from recurring.

Iron: Iron is a mineral the body needs to produce red blood cells. Iron supplements are used to treat iron deficiency or iron-deficiency anemia.

Laxatives: Many forms of laxatives are available for relieving constipation. Common brand names of laxatives include Phillips' Milk of Magnesia, Citroma, Epsom salts, Correctol, and ExLax.

Nitrates: These drugs for angina (chest pain) relax blood vessels and increase the flow of blood to the heart. Examples of generic and brand names include isosorbide dinitrate (Iso-Bid and Isonate) and nitroglycerin (Nitro-Bid and Nitrocap).

Nonsteroidal anti-inflammatory drugs (NSAIDs): These drugs block the body's production of prostaglandins, substances that mediate pain and inflammation. NSAIDs relieve the pain from chronic and acute inflammatory conditions, including arthritis and other rheumatic conditions, and pain associated with injuries, bursitis, tendinitis, and dental problems. NSAIDs also relieve pain associated with noninflammatory conditions. Generic and brand names of NSAIDs include aspirin (Bayer and Bufferin), ibuprofen (Advil, Nuprin, and Motrin), tometin (Tolectin), naproxen (Naprosyn), and piroxicam (Feldene).

Potassium chloride: Potassium is a vital element in the body. Potassium supplements help prevent and treat potassium deficiency in people taking diuretics.

Quinidine: This medicine often is used to correct irregular heartbeat. Brand names of quinidine include Quinalan and Quiniglute.

Theophylline: This medicine eases breathing difficulties associated with emphysema, bronchitis, and bronchial asthma. The medicine works by relaxing the muscles of the respiratory tract, which allows an easier flow of air into the lungs. Examples of brand names include Theo-Dur, Theophyl, and Bronkodyl.

Vitamins: Vitamins serve as nutritional supplements in people with poor diets, in people recovering from surgery, or in people with special health problems.

- **Niacin** helps the body break down food for energy and is used to treat niacin deficiency and to lower levels of fats and cholesterol.
- **Vitamin A** is necessary for normal growth and for healthy eyes and skin.
- **Vitamin C** is necessary for healthy function of cells.

Additional Readings

AARP Pharmacy Service Prescription Drug Handbook. Glenview, Illinois: Scott, Foreman and Company, 1988. General reference book for the public by the American Association of Retired Persons that provides information about medicines most frequently prescribed for persons over 50 years of age.

Advice for the Patient: Drug Information in Lay Language, USP DI, 12th edition. Rockville, Maryland: The United States Pharmacopeial

Convention, 1992. Guide for the patient that provides information about medicines by brand and generic names in sections on dosage forms, proper use directions, precautions, and side effects.

Drug Information for the Health Care Professional, USP DI, 12th edition. Rockville, Maryland: The United States Pharmacopeial Convention, 1992. Guide for health care professionals that provides information about medicines by brand and generic names in sections on pharmacology, indications, precautions, side effects, general dosing, dosage forms, and patient consultation.

Kimmey, MG. Gastroduodenal effects of nonsteroidal anti-inflammatory drugs. *Postgraduate Medicine*, 1989; 85(5): 65-71. General review article for primary care physicians.

Physicians' Desk Reference, 46th edition. Montvale, New Jersey: Medical Economics Company, Inc., 1992. Reference book for health care professionals that includes information about 2,800 pharmaceutical products in sections on pharmacology, indications, contraindications, precautions, adverse reactions, and dosage and administration.

Stehlin, D. How to take your medicine: nonsteroidal anti-inflammatory drugs. *FDA Consumer*, 1990; 24(5): 33-35. General review article for the public.

Additional Resources

National Council on Patient Information and Education
4915 St. Elmo Ave., Suite 505
Bethesda, MD 20814-6082
Phone: (301) 656-8565

Distributes resources to the public and health care professionals about prescription medicines.

The United States Pharmacopeial Convention, Inc.
12601 Twinbrook Parkway
Rockville, MD 20852
Phone: (301) 881-0666

Distributes information about drug use and drug standards to health professionals and the public.

Chapter 68

Chronic Pain and Depression

Which Comes First? Pain or Depression?

As early as 1684, Dr. Thomas Willis wrote of the sadness or long sorrow that accompanies many chronic illnesses.

Today, as noted by Depression.com, it is considered a two-way street. Chronic illnesses are depressing. And the depression they cause often exacerbates the illness.

Understanding Chronic Pain

Chronic pain. Intractable pain. Pain that never completely goes away. Difficult to measure. Often invisible.

Going from doctor to doctor to find the cause is exhausting and frustrating. Being told "It's all in your head."

Finding the cause, finally knowing the name of "The Intruder" as one of our readers put it (see below), still there may be no treatment that makes the pain cease and desist.

Friends and family, sympathetic at first, often tire of the burden of driving us to appointments, to surgeries, of hearing how much pain we're in today. Their love doesn't necessarily change (though it can) but they also feel a unique level of frustration.

People in chronic pain often find themselves alone in a world where only they and the pain exist, where no one else can understand. For those who live alone it can be a death curse. For others, the whole structure of the family may change. One partner may resent having to be the sole breadwinner, especially if they've always been taken care of. The one in chronic pain tries to be cheery, to be the same as before, to hang onto the love and life they've known, but chronic pain changes lives, period.

It seems that one loss piles on another and another until the burden has become so twisted and convoluted that it takes on a life of its own.

Spirits sink, gradually and almost immeasurable at first, then more and more. A spiral like water draining out a sink with a clogged pipe. Slowly but inevitably depression joins the pain.

And yet the question is begged: which came first, the pain or the depression?

Studies

Studies are showing overwhelmingly that chronic pain causes depression, not the other way around.

For example, a study recorded at Mediconsult.com used 254 chronic pain patients, whose pain had lasted at least six months.

Their statistics were:

- Average age: 40
- Employed: 33%
- Married: 66%
- Race: White 66%
- Receiving compensation: 33%
- Involved in litigation: 33%

Depression was evaluated according to the Beck Depression Inventory. Conceived by psychoanalyst Aaron Beck, this has been standard tool for 30 years. Patients rate the severity of 21 symptoms on a scale of 1 to 4.

For the 254 patients, the average score was 15.82 out of a possible 63, with the least depressed scoring 7 and the most depressed 50.

The strongest single predictor of depression was work status. Employment is heavily weighed in an adult's self-esteem and suddenly or gradually the chronic pain sufferer can no longer perform the duties the job demands.

Retirement comes early—but oh, what a retirement it is! There are no exotic vacations, no golf every morning because the person simply can't.

For those unemployed patients involved in litigation, it was a consolation which unfortunately wore off quickly once the process was confronted.

Among the employed, those pursuing litigation were most likely to be unhappy, due to the awkward position of suing their employer while still working.

Those less schooled were more vulnerable to depression.

The unmarried were less able to cope with their suffering than those who had a partner to lean on.

Ethnicity was found to bear no relation to stress.

This is perhaps the most interesting part of the test: "Comparisons of age and gender led to what are probably the most interesting results to come out of this survey. It was found that among women, depression declined with age, while among men it worsened. Thus, among those under 40, women were most affected, but among those older than this it was men who had the highest Beck scores. This is not at all a common finding in depression studies not looking at chronic pain sufferers. No obvious reason for this trend presents itself."

The degree and strength of the chronic pain, the number of surgical interventions, the number of drugs taken, and the common 1 to 10 measurement of pain—with 10 being suicidal—had no effect on level of depression.

Only the duration of the pain had an impact on the degree of depression, with the longest-suffering showing more depression.

The conclusion of the study showed that depressed chronic pain patients are less likely to respond to treatment for their pain. Since pain is harder to treat than depression, antidepressive therapy is often the best first step on the road to treating chronic pain.

Contributing to depression is the lack of adequate pain relief. More than four out of every ten people with moderate to severe chronic pain have yet to find adequate relief, saying their pain is out of control, according to a new survey by the American Pain Society, the American Academy of Pain Medicine and Janssen Pharmaceutica.

According to this survey, "Many Americans with chronic pain are suffering too much for too long and need more aggressive treatment," says Russell Portenoy, MD, president of the American Pain Society and chairman of the Department of Pain Medicine and Palliative Care at the Beth Israel Medical Center in New York City. "This survey suggests that there are millions of people living with severe uncontrolled pain. This is a great tragedy. Although not everyone can be helped, it is very likely that most of these patients could benefit if provided with state-of-the-art therapies and improved access to pain specialists when needed."

"This survey shows the stigma associated with opioid drugs. Although these drugs can clearly benefit some patients with chronic pain, patients, caregivers and physicians overestimate the risks and fail to use them appropriately," observes Dr. Portenoy. "Many patients suffer needlessly because of an inappropriate level of concern about long-term reliance on medication in general, and about addiction caused by strong pain medications such as opioids specifically. The input of pain specialists may be helpful when deciding on the best drug therapy for patients with severe chronic pain."

Depression.com also addresses the problem of depression in patients with chronic pain. Interestingly, they refer to depression specialist Arthur Rifkin, M.D., a psychiatrist at Albert Einstein Medical Center in New York, who says "the most common misconception about depression and chronic illness is that it's understandable to become depressed when faced with a chronic illness. It is understandable—but only during the initial adjustment period that should not last for more than a few months. Beyond that, persistent depression should be treated as a separate illness."

Depression.com says that any chronic condition can trigger depression, but the risk increases in direct proportion to the severity of the condition.

A broken leg that makes you miss a few ball games is a drag, but an accident that leaves you paraplegic can be severely depressing. Likewise depression increases with chronic diseases.

Chapter 69

Anger: Helpful or Harmful?

In 1894, Psychologist G. Stanley Hall completed the first modern, scientific effort to study anger. He asked 2,184 people to complete questionnaires in which they recalled an incident that made them angry and then to compare their reactions to a list of symptoms. Surprisingly, Hall found that while some people reported that the physical experience of the expression of their anger made them feel good, others reported that it made them feel sick. While many causes of anger were identified, the one that was identified most frequently and with the greatest passion was: Injustice.

Chronic pain patients often ask themselves, "Why me?" The loss and suffering that can follow chronic pain into your life can leave you feeling angry, frustrated, fearful, and overwhelmed with a sense of injustice. Anger can be experienced and acted on in a wide variety of ways, ranging from feelings, thoughts, or beliefs that leave you feeling uncomfortable to impulsive, destructive, violent episodes of behavior that can be harmful or fatal to yourself or to others. The feeling of anger is not in itself a problem. It is how you think about the events that cause your anger and how these thoughts influence your choices and behaviors that determines whether anger is helpful or harmful to you. Anger is a mind, body, and behavior experience. How you deal with anger as an adult is determined in part by the coping skills you have acquired over the years to deal with conflict and stress and whether the way you have expressed anger in the past has helped you get the result you wanted. Anger, for chronic pain patients can be a double-edged sword. Long after the cause of the anger has been resolved or forgotten, the physical impact of pain flare-up that anger can cause lingers. If you experience residual emotional or physical effects from anger, it may be time to take a look at experiencing anger in a more constructive way.

Why Am I Angry?

Anger, a powerful emotion, is one of the most common feelings experienced by people with chronic pain. If you are unable to express your anger, you may be viewed as depressed. Anger and depression are thought to be expressions of powerlessness, hopelessness, and insecurity. (Barbara Headley, MS, National Chronic Pain Outreach Association, 1989). Anger is a natural response to many life events and can be a useful emotion when it leads you to problem-solve difficult situations and put a positive plan of action into place. You may find it hard to identify the reasons for your anger. There are likely several reasons and common contributing factors are:

- Anger that your pain has caused you loss of physical functioning resulting in a decreased ability to work and a decreased ability to interact with family and friends. You may fear loss of your job or rejection by your family.

- Anger at financial losses.

- Anger at feeling that you are doing everything that is asked of you by healthcare providers and you still have pain.

- Anger at an uncertain future and the loss of order and predictability in your life.

- Anger at the role changes that occur within your family and your fear that you may be a burden to your loved ones.

- Anger at your fear that you will never be able to get on with your life or that your pain will become uncontrollable.

- Anger at the person(s) you feel are responsible for your pain—including yourself.

- Anger at the time demands that medical appointments and therapies place on you.

- Anger at yourself for thinking that you are not coping well.

What Can I Do?

Sorting out your anger and starting to let go of it are likely to be two of the most difficult things you have tried to do.

- Take time to sort out what you are feeling. Are you feeling anger or is it frustration, disappointment, sadness, fear, or anxiety? You may be surprised to learn that you are not really experiencing anger, but some other emotion that your anger is hiding.

- Write down all the issues you are angry about and then cross out the ones that you have no control to change.

- Think about the things in your life that you can change and work toward accomplishing these changes. This will increase your sense of control over your life.

- Try creating positive expectations for your day and take a look at how your attitude toward daily events influences your emotions and the amount of pain you feel.

Chapter 70

Anxiety and Its Effect on Pain Perception

Anxiety in particular can be something that makes pain worse in children (and adults for that matter). Children who are injured, ill or chronically ill often become anxious about doctors, nurses, doctors offices, hospitals, labs—you name it. One of the biggest problems can be that children are not given explanations that they understand to help them be more calm. Other times the things that health professionals must do—hurt—there is no other way to say it. Having a plan to help a child deal with being afraid can be very helpful. Always share with those taking care of your child what s/he does to not be afraid.

What factors contribute to anxiety when an individual is hospitalized?

For some, hospitalization means the worsening of a pre-existing illness. For others, hospitalization is their first encounter with a serious illness. Loss of health affects how people view themselves. If the illness requires surgery there will be a reaction to a change in body image. If a diagnosis has not been confirmed prior to admission, fear of the unknown can escalate anxiety to severe levels. In other cases, the diagnosis may be made, but the course of treatment is uncertain

"Anxiety and Its Effect on Pain Perception" Patient and family version, by Carol Kline, edited by Allison Deike, RN, an undated fact sheet available online at http://www.nursing.uiowa.edu/sites/PedsPain/GenePain/anxnt.htm (accessed October 2001), © University of Iowa College of Nursing, reprinted with permission.

or questionable. For many people the ultimate fear is the fear of/death, especially when surgery is indicated. The focus of one's health shifts from independence to dependence. The individual may be separated from their family and any readily available support systems.

What happens when a person is in pain?

Pain is an ancient warning system of the body. Acute pain is the result of recent tissue damage. Most people become anxious when they are in pain. Waiting for medication to relieve the pain, especially when the medication schedule is rigid, tends to increase anxiety and subsequently increases pain. Pain and anxiety are closely entwined, and both need to be treated.

How does your body react to anxiety?

When you feel anxious, your body becomes tense. This muscle tension can increase your pain. The increased pain can make you feel helpless because it may limit your abilities. This can cause you to become depressed. A cycle of stress, pain, limited abilities and depression may develop. Recognizing how your body reacts physically and emotionally to stress will enable you to break its destructive cycle.

What are the physical changes that occur as a result of anxiety?

During stressful times the body quickly releases chemicals into your bloodstream. This sets in motion a series of physical changes called the fight-or-flight response. These changes include a faster heart rate, rapid breathing, high blood pressure, and increased muscle tension. Stress-related tension can build up and take a toll on your body. You may experience headaches, develop an upset stomach, or a disease flare up. Stress impacts the body's immune system leading to prolonged illness and fatigue.

What are the emotional responses to anxiety?

Common emotional reactions to stress are anger, fear, helplessness, loss of control, annoyance, and frustration. You may also have difficulty concentrating and making decisions. People tend to withdraw into themselves. This can result in strained relations with family and friends. Appetite and sleep will be decreased.

What can one do to gain control of their health and ensure optimal pain management?

Have all procedures and tests explained to you in a way you understand. If you are feeling overwhelmed write things down. Ask a lot of questions. If you're not getting answers to your questions insist someone be notified who can answer them. Reserve and exercise the right to refuse any procedure that makes you too uncomfortable. Ask for your pain medication. If your pain is not being brought under control ask that another medication be considered. Let your medical team know you want this alternate medication started without delay so that your pain will continue to be managed. Also don't forget, you have the right to refuse any procedure with which you are not comfortable.

What skills can be learned to reduce the effects of anxiety on your body?

Learning how to relax is one of the most important ways to cope with anxiety. It is more than simply sitting back and being quiet. It is an active process involving methods designed to calm your body and mind. These techniques will be more helpful if they are practiced before you are in pain rather then waiting until you are in pain to apply them. Relaxation skills to work at developing could include deep breathing, progressive muscle relaxation, guided imagery, visualization, distraction, and positive self-talk.

Resources

Campbell, J. (July 5, 1995). Making sense of ... pain management. *Nursing Times*. 91(27); 34-36.

Stress Management Foundation. (August, 1995). *Managing Your Stress*. Atlanta, GA.

Varcarolis, E. (1994). *Foundations of Psychiatric-Mental Health Nursing*. Philadelphia: W.B. Saunders Company. p. 750-752.

Chapter 71

Interpersonal Relationships and Pain

Successful relationships take a lot of effort. The factors that influence relationships are constantly changing, creating an ebb and flow to the patterns of interaction that exist. Changes in relationships that you seek or that are of benefit to you can alter your relationships with friends, family, and co-workers in a positive and fulfilling way. They often increase your sense of stability and help define your role within the context of the relationship. The end result is that your relationships feel safe and secure allowing you to relax and be comfortable within them. Changes that happen in relationships because of events or situations that occur over which you may have limited control, such as chronic pain, are far more difficult to navigate and your emotional and physical response to these events will determine what you bring to or take away from your interactions with others.

Pain is a powerful mediator of relationships. It challenges past effective patterns of interacting with people and may leave you feeling isolated, angry, depressed, or fearful. Individuals with chronic pain often report that in relationships they feel:

- Others think they are faking and don't believe their pain is real.

- They are viewed as lazy or as a failure and are seen as not trying to get better.

- Others don't understand their pain and ask too much of them.

- They need to hide their pain so they won't be rejected by people or lose their job.

- They are judged as drug-seekers.

- Their concerns and fears are unheard by family, friends, and care-providers.

The impact of pain on your relationships can be reduced if you are willing to make the effort to take a look at the dynamics of the relationships you are in and to be open to changes in expectations and roles. It is important to:

- **Recognize** that some of the stress on your relationship is directly related to your pain and how you think about and respond to pain on a daily basis. You will need to be able to be honest with yourself about what you bring into your relationships that changes the dynamics during periods of pain flare-up. How much of what you say and do is your "pain talking"?

- **Recognize** that expectations, roles, and responsibilities within family, job, and social systems may need to change to accommodate to your taking an active approach in managing your pain.

- **Recognize** that clear and honest communication about your pain will help others to understand what your needs are. Don't assume others know what you are experiencing or what you need.

- **Recognize** the need to be honest with yourself about difficult patterns of interacting within relationships that existed prior to the onset of your pain. Don't blame your pain for all the problems you experience in relationships.

- **Recognize** the need to communicate openly with family, friends, and employers about what your needs, expectations and limitations are. Don't be afraid to share with others your emotional response to things that are changing in your life.

- **Recognize** the need to take action in changing the pattern of relationships that are not adding to the quality of your life. Be certain that those around you know what you are thinking and feeling and what changes you are hoping to achieve.

It is possible to improve relationships by increasing your awareness of your expectations, thoughts, and feelings and using this information to help guide the choices you make in determining how you will interact with others. While pain can interrupt past patterns of interacting effectively with others, it does not need to set you on a collision course with those around you or leave you feeling isolated, angry or alone. Take time to identify if your pain is "talking" in your relationships and then think about ways to silence the negative impact it can have. Creating positive change in relationships takes time, but the result is well worth the effort.

I feel the capacity to care is the thing which gives life its deepest significance.   —Pablo Casals

Chapter 72

Sexual Expression and Chronic Pain

Sex: The Unspoken Pleasure

Talking about sex is difficult for most people. Often patients don't volunteer information about their sexual functioning when they visit their doctor and treating professionals are hesitant to ask for this information fearing that they will add to the discomfort of their patients.

Being sexually active is a vital part of life. Dr. Edward Abraham states in his book, *Freedom From Back Pain,* "All people, including those with chronic pain, need to be caressed, loved, and held; and sexual expression is one of our most basic needs. Sex is great exercise—releasing muscular tension, toning muscles, and relaxing the nervous system. In addition, touch is a stronger sensation than pain with the ability to calm and soothe."

Communication with your partner is a key factor in how to stay sexually active and optimize your pleasure following the onset of chronic pain. Changed levels of sexual activity as well as alternative ways to give and receive pleasure may have to be explored within the safety of your relationship. This takes an enormous amount of trust and a willingness to look at your sexual practices in a different way.

Factors that block sexual expression in chronic pain patients have been identified as:

- lack of confidence
- fatigue
- stress
- poor communication
- poor body image
- loss of muscle tone
- loss of range of motion
- depression
- fear of pain or reinjury
- frustration and anger
- isolation
- medication

It is not uncommon for people to feel uncomfortable asking their partners to change their sexual practices. That is why trust and honest communication are essential. Ways to give and receive pleasure include:

- gentle words
- touching
- kissing
- massage
- holding hands
- shared baths / showers
- oral sex
- masturbation
- intercourse

Remember to think about all of your body senses in your exploration for ways to maintain a healthy sex life. Don't feel as though all sexual activity must lead to orgasm. Focus on the process of communication, sharing, loving, and mutual pleasure.

How you think about yourself and your partner will have a direct impact on the benefits of sex for you. Talk openly about your likes and dislikes. Share with your partner any concerns you have about pain or injury. Make time in your schedule for sexual encounters and be sensitive to both of your current physical and emotional needs. Talk with your physician about any physical concerns or problems you may have with sexual functioning to rule out physical cause. If available, talk with your physical therapist about positions that are more likely to allow you to express yourself sexually without pain flare-up. Finally, talk with a psychologist if you have fears of pain or reinjury that keep you from engaging in sex.

Most importantly, relax—sex is supposed to be fun. It is not about performance, but about mutual sharing. Be creative in your approach to achieving sexual satisfaction in your life.

A quote from Dr. Abraham's book is a good guide to reclaiming your sex life: "...the fear of injury during sex had a disastrous effect on my sex life for years. The solution is not to read a manual about sex, or try to hide from it, but to talk about it openly with your partner. And once you've discussed what *you can't do,* talk a lot about all the wonderful pleasure *you can have*. Then stop talking and start doing."

Improving Communication

- Be clear about what you want to get across.

- Be open and direct.

- Allow the other person time to react and express themselves.

- Let your thoughts guide what you say rather than your emotions.

- Take responsibility for what you are feeling and saying.

- Be conscious that you have a choice about what you will say and how you will say it.

- Let others know your reaction to what they are saying.

- Don't feel that you have to convince the other person to see things your way.

- Be willing to disagree.

- Be willing to listen.

Chapter 73

Sleep and Chronic Pain

Chronic pain and poor sleep seem to go together. In fact, more than half of chronic pain sufferers have trouble falling asleep or staying asleep. Lack of sleep leads to fatigue, irritability, stress and tension, which make it harder to cope with pain.

Chronic pain makes it more difficult to obtain truly restful sleep. Finding a comfortable position for falling asleep is a challenge for many. It may be difficult to relax and let go of worrisome thoughts about medical, financial, or other issues. Distress about inability to sleep can make falling asleep even more difficult. Movement during the night can result in increased pain that disrupts sleep.

The depression that often accompanies chronic pain and disability frequently results in sleep difficulty. The most common sleep disturbance associated with depression is the tendency to awaken very early in early morning and be unable to fall back asleep.

Sleep disturbance can even be a byproduct of inefficient pain coping strategies such as resting in bed excessively, organizing daily activities around the bedroom, and sleeping late in the morning or napping throughout the day to make up for sleepless nights. These strategies have long-term detrimental effects on sleep patterns.

Scientists are studying the chemical basis for the connection between sleep and pain. Some researchers have found that lack of sleep

From "Sleep Improvement Strategies for Persons with Chronic Pain," by Richard L. Wanlass, Ph.D. and Ronn Johnson, Ed.M. Department of Physical Medicine and Rehabilitation, University of California, Davis. © 1999. Reprinted with permission of the authors and the regents of the University of California.

is associated with release of a pain-causing chemical, substance P, while deep sleep is associated with the release of a pain-stopping chemical, somatostatin.

Thus, a disturbed sleep pattern can be one of the most disabling consequences of chronic pain and may actually worsen pain. Fortunately, there are five proven strategies to help you increase your restful nighttime sleep.

1. Provide a Proper Environment for Sleep

Many people treat their bedroom as if it were a TV room, study, or workshop instead of a special place for the mind to associate with sleep. The following steps can help to remedy this problem:

- Set your bedroom aside as a special place for sleep and physical intimacy.

- Clear your bedroom of clutter—move out piles of paperwork and dirty dishes, and consider relocating televisions, radios, and CD players. A cluttered bedroom decreases your chance to enjoy a restful night's sleep. Relocate all non-essential activities and objects.

- Treat your bedroom like a sanctuary. You might consider soothing color schemes. Lining your drapes to block out unwanted light and street noises may help. Foam earplugs can be useful.

- Keep your bedroom temperature cool.

2. Watch What You Consume

Your eating and drinking habits affect your ability to sleep restfully. Here are some suggestions:

- Consume no meals within two hours of bedtime.

- Avoid stimulants in the afternoon and evening. Stimulants include caffeinated drinks such as coffee, tea, and cola. If you take herbs or over-the-counter medicines, consult with your pharmacist about whether they have stimulant properties.

- Use no alcohol within three hours before going to bed. Alcohol may help you fall asleep, but it reduces sleep quality (deep, restful sleep) and causes havoc with sleep maintenance (sleeping through the night).

- A light snack of carbohydrates and milk right before bed helps reduce the time it takes to fall asleep by encouraging the production of the chemical tryptophan.

- Sleeping pills (e.g., benzodiazepines) prescribed by your physician as a sleep aid generally are useful only for a short term. Like alcohol, these reduce time it takes to fall sleep, but may suppress truly deep, restful sleep. Also like alcohol, there can be problems with tolerance and dependence.

- Sometimes sedating antidepressants are prescribed instead of sleeping pills to avoid some of these problems. Discuss this with your physician.

- You may also wish to consult with your physician regarding the possible benefit of melatonin or other over-the-counter sleep aids.

3. Slow Down Before You Lie Down

Certain activities can affect the time it takes to fall asleep. Research supports the following guidelines:

- Do not exercise within 3 to 4 hours before bed.

- However, morning walks of 30 minutes or longer in the sunlight are especially good at resetting your internal clock for sleep and wakefulness.

- Take a warm bath prior to going to bed.

- Perform peaceful, pre-bedtime rituals or engage in calming activities, such as reading or listening to relaxing music.

4. Relax in Bed

As stated earlier, treat your bedroom like a sanctuary reserved for sleep and physical intimacy. This means television watching, reading, studying, office work, etc. should be done elsewhere. Positive activities to do in bed to help you fall asleep include:

- Adopt a relaxed mental attitude. Don't *work* at falling asleep. This only increases your anxiety and sets you up for becoming discouraged over failure. Enjoy the process. Get comfortable and relax.

501

- Relax your muscles progressively from your feet all the way up to your head. It helps first to practice this technique in the daytime until you become skilled at relaxing. Audiotapes are available to help you learn to relax.

- Visualize soothing imagery, such as a mountain lake or beach.

- Practice slow, rhythmic breathing from the diaphragm. You will know you are doing this correctly if your abdomen rises each time you inhale and falls back down when you exhale. Each time you exhale, think a calming word such as "relax", or picture a calming image. If distracting thoughts come into your mind, just let them drift away and return to your calming word or image. Remind yourself that, even if you do not fall asleep, you are obtaining valuable rest through this meditative breathing activity.

- Postpone worrisome thoughts. Keep a note pad on your night stand, and if a thought refuses to go away, write it down and promise yourself to deal with it the next day—and keep your promise.

- Use support pillows. A pillow under the knees may reduce lower back pain, and support for the neck muscles may reduce neck pain or headaches. Consult your physician or physical therapist for the strategic use of support pillows.

5. Restrict Your Time in Bed

Research demonstrates that, at a certain point, sleep quality is inversely related to time spent in bed. The following restrictions have proven to be helpful in regaining control over your sleep quality:

- Go to bed only when sleepy.

- If you do not fall asleep within 20 minutes, get out of bed, leave your bedroom, and do something relaxing until you become sleepy again.

- Limit your time in bed to 7 hours or less.

- Arise at about the same time every morning, even on weekends.

- It is generally best to avoid naps during the daytime.

502

- However, very brief naps may be permitted, if necessary, to restore alertness. Naps longer than 30 minutes hinder recovery of the normal sleep cycle, and they often leave one feeling groggy and disoriented.

- If you do nap regularly, it is best to nap at approximately the same time each day. Afternoon naps are usually best, since the body has a natural tendency to be drowsy between 2 pm and 4 pm.

What to Do If Nightmares Disrupt Your Sleep

Should recurring nightmares disrupt your sleep, the following steps have proven effective in reducing them:

- Write down your nightmare and relax while recalling it as vividly as possible.

- Change the ending of the nightmare to something pleasant.

503

Chapter 74

Chronic Pain: Financial Issues

Chronic pain can affect all areas of your life including your finances. The following are some practical financial tips to cope with the financial issues that often go hand-in-hand with a chronic illness.

If you are using an HMO or PPO insurance type of plan to pay for your pain treatment, the following information may be helpful to you:

1. Find out what pain management services are provided under your current insurance plan. Note: many HMO/PPO plans may not address pain issues directly and some do not provide coverage.

2. Find out what medications are covered by your insurance. Many insurance plans have a list of medications that they will pay for (this is called a formulary). Often times the insurance plan does not have several of the medications used to treat pain on their formulary. In that case, your physician will need to write a special appeal letter to see if the medication can be covered.

    Many types of pain are treated with medications used to treat other conditions, (called adjuvant medication). Sometimes insurance companies won't pay for a medication that is used for a different use (for example, Tegretol is used mainly to treat

"Financial Issues," available at www.painfoundation.org. © 2001 American Pain Foundation; reprinted with permission.

seizures but can also be helpful for certain pain conditions). In that case, your physician will need to write a special appeal letter to see if the medication can be covered.

3. If your primary care doctor refers you to a specialist or for treatment somewhere outside his/her office, always check with both your insurance company and the specialist that you are being referred to to ensure that they are a part of your insurance plan. Note: if the physician/nurse is not a part of your plan it will usually cost you more out of pocket.

4. Many HMO/PPO plans require you to have a referral from your primary care doctor in order to see a specialist. ALWAYS get a copy of the referral or the referral number and keep it in your records. This is your proof to the insurance company that you had the referral.

5. Many HMO/PPO plans also require you to have pre-authorization for the service. This is something that is in addition to the primary care referral. The insurance company issues pre-authorization. You may want to check with the insurance company prior to seeing the specialist to make sure that your visit(s) are pre-authorized.

6. The day before you see a specialist you may want to call his/her office and make sure that they have received both the referral from the primary care physician and pre-authorization for the visit. This will protect you from going to a visit where you will have to pay for services that your insurance won't cover.

7. Most insurance companies have a customer service department. Call them should you have any questions regarding what is a covered benefit or why a service is not being covered. If you don't receive answers to your questions by talking with the person who answers the phone, ask to speak to a supervisor. You are a consumer of your health care and you deserve excellent service.

8. If you believe that you have received an incorrect bill, always notify the insurance company as well as the doctor, hospital or clinic that sent you the bill. Don't be afraid to ask questions until you receive the answers that you need.

9. If you have problems that are not resolved to your satisfaction, you can call the customer service department at the insurance company and ask for a supervisor. If that does not provide the results you are looking for you can call your state insurance commissioner.

If your pain is the result of a work injury or a personal injury such as a car accident, the following information may be helpful to you:

1. File an injury report form with your employer or your car insurance carrier as soon as possible.

2. Find out your case number. Write this number on a piece of paper with the date, time, and location of your injury (most everyone you visit will ask for this information).

3. Find out if you have a case manager assigned to your case. If you do, write down his/her name and phone number on the same paper as the other information listed in tip #2.

4. Find out what your rights and responsibilities are under the laws in your state. You may be entitled to compensation for the time you are off work, the time it takes you to see your health care professionals as well as other expenses.

5. If you have a case manager it is helpful to inform him/her of appointments with your health care professionals or even have them coordinate the appointments for you. In addition, it is helpful if they know what treatments and medications have been recommended so that they can facilitate payment for those items.

6. If you are having difficulty reaching your case manager or if you are having difficulties with reimbursement or payments it may be necessary to talk to a supervisor at the insurance company. You should have your questions and concerns addressed to your satisfaction. If that does not occur even after talking with a supervisor you may find assistance by contacting your state insurance commissioner.

7. If you continue to experience difficulties or if you have questions regarding your rights and responsibilities under the law it may be helpful to contact a personal injury attorney.

General Information

If you feel as if you are in over your head and overwhelmed with your financial obligations your stress level will go up and it is common for anxiety and depression to follow. Get some assistance with financial planning. There are several free consumer credit counseling agencies/groups.

Chapter 75

Physical Pain and Suicide

Background

Contrary to what many believe, the vast majority of individuals who are terminally ill or facing severe pain or disability are not suicidal. Moreover, terminally ill patients who do desire suicide or euthanasia often suffer from a treatable mental disorder, most commonly depression. When these patients receive appropriate treatment for depression, they usually abandon the wish to commit suicide.

Uncontrolled pain, particularly when accompanied by feelings of hopelessness and untreated depression, is a significant contributing factor for suicide and suicidal ideation. Medications and pain relief techniques now make it possible to treat pain effectively for most patients.

Despite the fact that effective treatments are available, severely and terminally ill patients generally do not receive adequate relief from pain. Studies report that over 50 percent of cancer patients suffer from unrelieved pain, even though patients with cancer are more likely than other patients to receive pain treatment.

Excerpted from "Preface: Executive Summary," "Chapter 1: The Epidemiology of Suicide," and "Chapter 2: Suicide in Special Patient Populations" from *When Death Is Sought: Assisted Suicide and Euthanasia in the Medical Context*, a report of the Task Force on Life and Law, convened in 1984, revised March 1999, © New York State Department of Health; reprinted with permission. The full report is available online beginning at http://www.health.state.ny.us/nysdoh/consumer/provider/death.htm.

Numerous barriers contribute to the pervasive inadequacy of pain relief and palliative care in current clinical practice, including a lack of professional knowledge and training, unjustified fears about physical and psychological dependence, poor pain assessment, pharmacy practices, and the reluctance of patients and their families to seek pain relief.

Suicide in the General Population

Suicide is generally described as the intentional taking of one's own life. For the individual who commits suicide, the act usually represents a solution to a problem or life circumstance that the individual fears will only become worse. Believing that their suffering will continue or intensify, suicidal individuals can envision no option but death. As articulated by a prominent suicidologist, the common stimulus to suicide is intolerable psychological pain. Suicide represents an escape or release from that pain.

Contrary to popular opinion, suicide is not usually a reaction to an acute problem or crisis in one's life or even to a terminal illness. Single events do not cause someone to commit suicide. Instead, certain personal characteristics are associated with a higher risk of attempting or committing suicide. The way in which an individual copes with problems over the course of his or her life usually indicates whether the person is emotionally predisposed to suicide. Studies that examine the psychological background of individuals who kill themselves show that 95 percent have a diagnosable mental disorder at the time of death. Depression, accompanied by symptoms of hopelessness and helplessness, is the most prevalent condition among individuals who commit suicide. This is especially true of the elderly, who are more likely than the young to commit suicide during an acute depressive episode.

Individuals who commit suicide generally have no history of mental health treatment, although they often evidence a major psychiatric illness at the time of death. The primary risk factors for completed suicides are major depression, substance abuse, severe personality disorders, male gender, older age, living alone, physical illness, and previous suicide attempts. For terminally ill patients with cancer and AIDS, several additional risk factors are also present.

Another significant predictor of suicide is a feeling of hopelessness or helplessness, a principal symptom of depression. Hopelessness is the common factor that links depression and suicide in the general population. In fact, hopelessness is a better predictor of completed suicide than depression alone. Feelings of hopelessness and helplessness interact with the perception of psychological pain and the individual's sense that his or her current suffering is inescapable.

Chronic Illness and Suicide

Individuals with serious chronic and terminal illness face an increased risk of suicide—some studies suggest that the risk for cancer patients is about twice that of the general population. Some experts, however, have observed that many terminally ill patients experience a phenomenon called "cancer cures psychoneuroses." This phenomenon occurs when patients become aware that they have cancer or another progressive terminal illness, and the process of facing and mastering their fear of death dissolves many other anxieties or neuroses. As explained by one psychiatrist, "As one's focus turns from the trivial diversions of life, a fuller appreciation of the elemental factors in existence may emerge."

Thus, some terminally ill patients may exhibit lower psychological stress than might be expected. Apart from circumstances where patients are depressed, terminally ill individuals are often resilient, and fight for life throughout their illness. Studies indicate that for many patients with severe pain, disfigurement, or disability, the vast majority do not desire suicide. In one study of terminally ill patients, of those who expressed a wish to die, all met diagnostic criteria for major depression. Like other suicidal individuals, patients who desire suicide or an early death during a terminal illness are usually suffering from a treatable mental illness, most commonly depression.

Patients with advanced disease or terminal illness frequently experience many psychological symptoms, including anxiety, fatigue, and lack of concentration. Terminally ill patients may also develop major depression or severe depressive symptoms. Although it is normal and expected that terminally ill patients "feel sadness for the anticipated loss of health, life and all it means, and loss of a future with all that it might hold," most patients call upon their coping mechanisms to manage these feelings. (Statement by Jimmie C. Holland, Chief, Psychiatry Services, Memorial Sloan-Kettering Cancer Center, "Letter to the Task Force on Life and the Law," August 16, 1993.) It is a myth, however, that severe clinical depression is a normal and expected component of terminal illness.

Pain and Suffering

For some patients, uncontrolled pain is an important contributing factor for suicide and suicidal ideation. Patients with uncontrolled pain may see death as the only escape from the pain they are experiencing. However, pain is usually not an independent risk factor. The significant variable in the relationship between pain and suicide is the interaction between pain and feelings of hopelessness and depression. As stated by one psychiatrist: "Pain plays an important role in vulnerability to suicide; however, associated psychological distress and mood disturbance seem to be essential co-factors in raising the risk of cancer suicide." (Breitbart, W. "Suicide Risk and Pain," in *Advances in Pain Research and Therapy*, ed. K.M. Foley et al., New York: Raven Press, 1990.)

Suffering represents a more global phenomenon of psychic distress. While suffering is often associated with pain, it also occurs independently. Different kinds of physical symptoms, such as difficulty breathing, can lead to suffering. Suffering may also arise from diverse social factors such as isolation, loss, and despair.

Even more so than with pain, an individual's experience of suffering reflects his or her unique psychological and personal characteristics. Suffering is in effect the experience of severe psychological pain, arising from medical or personal causes. Because the experience of suffering is subjective, people are often unaware of the causes or extent of another person's suffering. Ultimately, suffering is a distinctly human, not a medical, condition.

Patients with Cancer

Cancer patients face approximately twice the risk of suicide than the general population does, although few commit suicide. The risk of suicide is greatest for patients in the later stages of the disease; 16 percent to 20 percent of these patients experience suicidal ideation. In contrast, studies have found that few ambulatory cancer patients express thoughts of suicide. Despite the low rates of suicidal ideation reported by studies, health care professionals who care for cancer patients believe that suicidal thinking is prevalent among these patients.

Almost all patients who receive a cancer diagnosis, even when the prognosis is good, carry a "secret," rarely acknowledged, thought that says "I won't die in pain with advanced cancer—I'll kill myself first." They often have a hidden supply of drugs which is usually kept for this purpose. For most patients, the time never comes to take the pills and life becomes dearer as death approaches.

For cancer patients, pain, depression, and psychiatric disorders are closely linked. Uncontrolled or poorly controlled pain can increase a patient's feelings of hopelessness and helplessness. One study of cancer patients showed that 47 percent of patients had a psychiatric disorder (of whom 68 percent had reactive anxiety or depression). The incidence of psychiatric disorders—in particular anxiety and depression—was higher in patients with pain.

Treating cancer patients for depression and pain reduces levels of suicidal ideation. Allowing patients to discuss suicidal thoughts may also decrease the risk of suicide. A discussion can help patients feel a sense of control over their death. Treatment for depression can also eliminate a patient's wish to die. One study of cancer patients at a major hospital found that nine percent of psychiatric consultations concerned acutely suicidal patients. Virtually all these patients had a previously undiagnosed psychiatric disorder. Treatment for depression resulted in the cessation of suicidal ideation for 90 percent of these patients. Like the common myth that it is reasonable for terminally ill patients to be suicidal, these data argue against the common misperception that cancer patients appropriately suffer from severe clinical depression.

Patients with AIDS

Individuals with AIDS are far more likely to be suicidal than the general population. Organic mental disorders such as delirium and dementia are important risk factors for suicide as AIDS progresses. Clinicians have had success in treating delirium and reducing the levels of suicidal ideation among AIDS patients. Depression is also a key factor. In one study in New York city of 12 patients with AIDS who committed suicide, 50 percent were significantly depressed. Pre-existing personality disorders and history of suicidal attempts or expression of suicidal thoughts can also heighten the risk of suicide. Given the relatively recent appearance of AIDS and the changing population of individuals with AIDS (most of the earliest studies focused primarily on gay men), continued research must be conducted to understand more fully the nature of suicide within this patient population.

Patients with AIDS exhibit a range of pain symptoms similar to that of patients with cancer. Studies have found that more than half of patients with advanced AIDS experience significant pain. Pain may arise from AIDS and related infections. AIDS therapy, including antiviral agents, also causes side effects and discomfort. Common types of pain arising from the disease and treatment include abdominal pain, headache, joint pain, and peripheral neuropathy, which may produce sensations of burning, numbness, or pins and needles. Other physical symptoms include gastrointestinal manifestations such as oral infections, difficulty swallowing, and diarrhea.

The Elderly

Older age and physical illness are two risk factors for suicide. Facing deteriorating health and increasing age, the elderly are at a greater risk of suicide than any other age group. Risk factors for suicide, such as depression, alcoholism, physical illness, and organic mental dysfunction, which impair judgment and the ability to generate alternative options, contribute to the increased rates of suicide among the elderly. Unlike younger suicidal individuals for whom a history of suicide attempts, substance abuse, and mental illness play a major role, for the elderly social isolation and physical disability are more important variables. Some data suggest that when older individuals commit suicide, they are more likely to suffer from a mood disorder than are younger individuals who commit suicide. Available clinical data estimate that a majority of elderly persons who commit suicide suffer from depressive episodes.

A recent study of the treatment of depressed elderly nursing home residents confirmed that inadequate diagnosis and treatment for depression was pervasive. The elderly are also at risk for both the undertreatment and overtreatment of pain. Cognitive impairment can make it difficult for elderly patients to express their feelings of pain adequately. Thus, pain is often overlooked by health care providers. Elderly patients may also be overtreated for pain resulting from the physiological changes that take place as individuals age. Because the elderly have a decreased ability to metabolize certain medications, they are more sensitive to analgesic effects of opioid drugs. As a result, they experience higher peaks and a longer duration of pain relief from the medication than younger patients. Finally, side effects of pain medication, such as constipation, urinary retention and respiratory depression, are also more common among elderly patients.

Assisted Suicide and Euthanasia

Statement from the New York Task Force on Life and the Law

Assisted suicide and euthanasia would carry us into new terrain. American society has never sanctioned assisted suicide or mercy killing.

We believe that the practices would be profoundly dangerous for large segments of the population, especially in light of the widespread failure of American medicine to treat pain adequately or to diagnose and treat depression in many cases. The risks would extend to all individuals who are ill. They would be most severe for those whose autonomy and well-being are already compromised by poverty, lack of access to good medical care, or membership in a stigmatized social group. The risks of legalizing assisted suicide and euthanasia for these individuals, in a health care system and society that cannot effectively protect against the impact of inadequate resources and ingrained social disadvantage, are likely to be extraordinary.

Part Five

Pain Research

Chapter 76

The Need for Pain Research

There are more than 50 million Americans who experience chronic pain and more than half of dying patients experience moderate to severe pain during the last days of their life. Pain is a frequent cause for clinical visits with approximately 45% of the population seeking medical help for pain at some point in their lives. Pain is found across the lifespan and it has been estimated that four out of every ten people with moderate or severe pain do not get adequate relief.

Pain is personal and subjective, is affected by mood and psychosocial factors, and demonstrates tremendous individual variation. Depression commonly complicates pain and adds to the disability and impairment found in disorders with chronic pain. Pain in combination with depression is a risk factor for suicide. Pain interferes with quality of life, sleep and productivity, and pain increases utilization of health care resources. However, many health care providers do not have the background to effectively treat pain.

Pain is frequently undertreated by health care providers. For example, a survey of several hundred ambulatory AIDS patients found that fewer than 8% of patients reporting "severe" pain were prescribed a strong opioid such as morphine, despite published guidelines. Adjuvant analgesic drugs (e.g., antidepressants) were also prescribed to only a small fraction of these patients. Opioid analgesics are the accepted treatment for acute pain, cancer pain and pain at the end of

Excerpted from "NIH Guide: The Management of Chronic Pain," National Institutes of Health (NIH), Program Announcement, Release Date July 2, 2001.

life, and recently have been recommended for chronic, nonmalignant pain. Patients can be treated with this therapy without developing tolerance, addiction or toxicity. Nevertheless, health care providers continue to fear these adverse outcomes, and believe that opioid use may result in a downhill spiral of further disability, depression and pain, in spite of contrary evidence. A further barrier to chronic opioid therapy is the lack of a good objective measure to determine whether a person requesting increased opioid dosage is abusing opioids or is receiving insufficient benefit from therapy. This second scenario is so common in certain conditions (e.g., cancer, sickle cell disease) that the term "pseudo addiction," has been used to describe the patient who is demonstrating drug-seeking behavior because his or her pain is undertreated.

In addition to health care provider barriers, there are patient and family barriers to effective pain relief. Patients may underuse effective pharmacological treatments because of a stoic or fatalistic attitude, and/or a belief that complaining of pain makes one a "bad" patient. Patients with cancer may believe that cancer pain cannot be alleviated; they may fear that pain indicates disease progression and/or they may fear that current usage will lead to future ineffectiveness. Patients who are treated with opioids may have additional fears of dependence, addiction and tolerance, and fear of injections. Thus, underusage may also be due to the stigma of using opioids. Research is needed to determine the relationship between patient-related barriers and pain management and to determine whether the patient barriers are a cause or result of inadequate treatment.

Pain and pain management in infants is another area of research need. Premature infants often undergo painful medical and surgical procedures and may be in ongoing pain as a result. Until recently it was believed that infants are insensitive to pain because of their immature nervous systems. Recent research demonstrates that infants do feel pain and a recent study on an animal model demonstrated that the pain experienced as a neonate resulted in greater sensitivity to pain as an adult. Thus, painful procedures in infancy may lead to permanent changes in the pain threshold. Effective pain interventions are needed for premature infants who are now surviving due to medical and technical advances.

Individuals with certain demographic characteristics or medical conditions are likely to experience less effective pain management and report higher pain levels than others. Older patients are often undertreated, especially the cognitively impaired. Women may experience further undertreatment as they are over represented in certain conditions associated with pain such as fibromyalgia and temporomandibular joint disorders. In addition, individuals with less education or lower incomes, minority patients, patients with a history of injection drug use, and patients with AIDS are at risk for receiving suboptimal pain treatment. The specific barriers to the undertreatment and underuseage of pain medication and non-pharmacological regimens need to be identified in these underserved populations.

Similarly, chronic pain is frequently undertreated in those who are unable to verbalize their pain (e.g., premature infants, cognitively impaired individuals). Assessment of chronic pain in nonverbal populations is difficult. Sympathetic arousal is frequently found in acute pain, but is not commonly found in patients with chronic pain and therefore a patient may not look as if s/he is in pain. The cues suggesting pain in nonverbal patients can be identified by those who are familiar with the patient and who can detect changes in behavior. However, in any health care facility and particularly the long-term care facility, the staff turnover and different patient assignments are barriers to the assessment of pain in nonverbal patients. Some cognitively impaired elders can report pain reliably in response to simple questions. However, pain needs to be assessed in order to be treated. The Department of Veterans Affairs and other health care institutions have institutionalized the assessment of pain as a fifth vital sign, similar to other vital signs like blood pressure, pulse, temperature and respiratory rate. Other innovative systematic approaches to pain management are needed. Educational training is not sufficient for instituting changes in pain management; further research on other institutional changes is needed to support pain management interventions in the practice setting.

Non-pharmacological treatments have been found to be effective in managing chronic pain either alone or in combination with pharmacological therapy. These treatments include relaxation training, cognitive behavioral interventions, family support, biofeedback, and improving self-efficacy. Further research is needed to refine the most effective treatment strategies for specific conditions and to determine the most effective treatment strategies for underserved populations. This research should include investigation of innovative complementary and alternative therapies for the effective treatment of chronic pain such as acupuncture, spinal manipulation and botanical products. A recent report concluded that there is little research on the management of cancer pain. The report recommended that further research is needed to determine the best combinations of pharmacological and non-pharmacological regimens in long-term cancer patients and in children with cancer pain. In addition, further research is needed to determine the impact of ethnicity, race, gender, age, psychosocial context and culture on cancer pain.

Chapter 77

Complementary and Alternative Medicine: Research Challenges

"CAM research is making inroads fastest in the area of pain management," says Richard L. Nahin, Ph.D., M.P.H., director of the National Center for Complementary and Alternative Medicine's (NCCAM) Division of Extramural Research, Training, and Review. The NCCAM has committed considerable support to research studying CAM therapies to relieve pain.

Responding to a Public Need

"Pain is a widespread public health problem," says Christine Goertz, D.C., Ph.D., a program officer for the Division. "We're looking at alternative medicine because there is so much consumer interest in it, and managing pain is of primary importance to the public."

Take chronic back pain, for example. "Acupuncture, chiropractic, and massage all are being sought by people with chronic back pain because conventional medicine often provides no long-term solution," says Dr. Nahin. Drugs have not been effective in treating back pain, or they have side effects that some people cannot tolerate.

In addition, a growing number of conventional practitioners (physicians, registered nurses, physical therapists, etc.) are interested in alternative treatments for pain, "because their patients need and

"Studying Pain Management: CAM Research Challenges," *CAM Newsletter*, National Center for Complementary and Alternative Medicine (NCCAM), Summer 2000.

demand them," says Dr. Nahin. "Practitioners and their patients are more willing to try different types of treatments."

Responding to these critical needs, the NCCAM funds several randomized clinical trials of CAM treatments for managing pain. For example, NCCAM-funded trials in Boston, Massachusetts, and Seattle, Washington, are comparing CAM treatments with standard medical therapy for back pain.

Other pain management research projects funded by the NCCAM include studies of acupuncture for osteoarthritis, fibromyalgia, dental pain, and carpal tunnel syndrome; chiropractic for chronic pelvic pain in women; and relaxation, guided imagery, and chamomile tea for abdominal pain in children.

Dr. Goertz points out that both CAM and conventional medicine practitioners are interested in this research. "They're excited by opportunities to access National Institutes of Health (NIH) funding for the first time" to begin clinical research on CAM treatments. However, the research has its challenges.

Producing a Placebo

"Alternative medicine does not always fit in a box," says Dr. Goertz, referring to chiropractic, acupuncture, massage, and other CAM therapies that require physical intervention. A randomized, controlled trial requires that one group of patients receives a placebo (a presumably pharmaceutically inactive or "fake" treatment), and it is difficult to devise a hands-on treatment that mimics acupuncture, for example.

For chiropractic and osteopathic manipulation, "there's a lot of discussion about sham manipulation," according to Dr. Goertz, a chiropractor herself. "Some chiropractic researchers have tried massage or thrust [manual force] that they believe is not strong enough to produce an effect," says Dr. Goertz.

In a research setting, attempts have been made to include patients who have never had real treatment by a chiropractic or acupuncturist so they do not know the difference between real and sham chiropractic or acupuncture procedures, and that poses another challenge. "It's more and more difficult to find patients who are naive to alternative therapies," says Dr. Goertz. "The subject pool gets smaller as time goes on."

When used, sham treatment provides some other information as well. For example, "the amount of attention from a CAM practitioner you get as a patient usually exceeds the attention you would get from a conventional doctor," says Marguerite Evans, M.S., R.D., another program officer for the Division. Even patients in the control group (the comparison or placebo group) receive a comparable amount of the practitioner's time as well as physical contact, which may have an effect on the patient.

Standardizing Holistic Treatments

Another challenge to research is the individualized, holistic nature of CAM treatment itself. To yield good, consistent data, studies must ensure that all treatment is the same (standardized). "One thing to be mindful of is the extent to which standardizing a protocol takes away some therapeutic benefit," says Dr. Goertz.

Ms. Evans points out how this concern multiplies with larger, multicenter trials. "You have to train a number of people to do the CAM intervention the same way to all patients at all centers, and train several people to collect the data in a standard fashion. This is common to any trial," she notes.

Measuring Outcomes

Yet another challenge lies in measuring the results of studies to ease pain. Although a number of reliable tools to measure pain have been validated by research, such as patient questionnaires, "it is hard to measure pain, and you rely mostly on patient perceptions," says Dr. Goertz.

From a research point of view, "you want to see a double-blind, placebo-controlled trial with a physiologic mechanism or other outcome measure," she says. Studies of pain so far cannot show the kind of concrete outcome data as, for example, studies that can demonstrate how insulin reduces high blood sugar levels in diabetics.

Facilitating Research

Chiropractic and acupuncture have been used in the United States for many years, so it is not surprising that a significant proportion of NCCAM-funded studies, especially those for pain, focus on chiropractic, acupuncture, or both. CAM practitioners have been interested in conducting research for some time, but funding has been limited.

According to Dr. Goertz, the availability of NCCAM research funds will not only enable CAM practitioners to undertake large, well-designed, rigorously controlled trials, but it also will encourage researchers from more mainstream fields to take part in such studies. "This, along with consumer interest, will cause a boom in CAM research," Dr. Goertz predicts.

Chapter 78

Glucosamine/Chondroitin Arthritis Intervention Trial (GAIT)

Questions and Answers

What is the National Institutes of Health (NIH) Glucosamine/Chondroitin Arthritis Intervention Trial (GAIT)?

GAIT is the first multicenter clinical trial in the United States to test the effects of the dietary supplements glucosamine and chondroitin for treatment of knee osteoarthritis. The study will test whether glucosamine and chondroitin used separately or in combination are effective in reducing pain and improving functional ability in patients with knee osteoarthritis. GAIT includes an additional study (or sub-study) that will assess whether glucosamine and chondroitin can reduce or halt the progression of knee osteoarthritis.

The University of Utah School of Medicine was awarded a contract to coordinate this study, which will be conducted at thirteen research centers across the U.S. The National Center for Complementary and Alternative Medicine (NCCAM) and the National Institute of Arthritis and Musculoskeletal and Skin Diseases (NIAMS) are two components

This chapter includes text from "Questions and Answers: NIH Glucosamine/Chondroitin Arthritis Intervention Trial (GAIT)," an undated fact sheet produced by the National Center for Complementary and Alternate Medicine (NCCAM), and "NIAMS-Funded Analysis of Glucosamine/Chondroitin Sulfate Trials," National Institute of Arthritis and Musculoskeletal and Skin Diseases (NIAMS), March 20, 2000.

of the National Institutes of Health (NIH) that are responsible for initiating this study.

What is the purpose of the study?

Results of previous studies in the medical literature have yielded conflicting results on the effectiveness of glucosamine and chondroitin as treatments for osteoarthritis. This study will test the short-term (6 months) effectiveness of glucosamine and chondroitin in reducing pain and improving function in a large number of patients with knee osteoarthritis.

The study will also evaluate the impact of glucosamine and chondroitin on progression of knee osteoarthritis following an additional 18 month treatment regimen.

What prompted the NIH to study glucosamine and chondroitin for osteoarthritis?

On January 27, 1998, the NCCAM held a meeting to discuss the need, rationale, and feasibility of conducting a Phase III study (a human study involving over 1,000 patients to test the efficacy, safety, and side effects of a substance(s) of glucosamine and chondroitin for the treatment of knee osteoarthritis. Meeting participants included experts in osteoarthritis, alternative medicine, biostatistics and family practice, and staff of the NIH and the U.S. Food and Drug Administration. The group determined that there is a real and urgent public health need to test these agents in a rigorous way, and that current scientific data support short-term testing of glucosamine and chondroitin for pain control and functional improvement of osteoarthritis.

What is the basic design of the study?

In this study, patients will be randomly assigned to receive either (1) glucosamine alone, (2) chondroitin alone, (3) glucosamine and chondroitin in combination, (4) celecoxib (brand name Celebrex®), or (5) a placebo (an inactive substance that looks like the study substance). Glucosamine and chondroitin and their combination will be compared to a placebo to verify that these substances significantly improve joint pain and flexibility. Celecoxib, which is an established effective conventional treatment for osteoarthritis, will also be compared to placebo to validate the study design. To reduce the chance of biased results, double-blind research procedures will be used to ensure that neither the researchers nor the patients will know to which of the five treatment groups the patients belong.

In the main or primary study, each patient will be treated for 24 weeks. During this time, patients will be evaluated at 4, 8, 16, and 24 week intervals and closely monitored for improvement of their symptoms as well as for any possible adverse reactions to the agents. Medical evaluations and x rays will be used to document each patient's diagnosis. The primary outcome will be measured as improvement in pain. Improvement in function will be included as a secondary outcome. All patients will have the option to use acetaminophen (e.g., Tylenol®) as required to control severe pain from osteoarthritis throughout the clinical trial.

In the sub-study, which will evaluate the progression of knee osteoarthritis, about one-half of the patients enrolled in GAIT will receive blinded treatment for an additional eighteen months. As in the primary study, patients will not know to which treatment group they are assigned. Researchers will compare x-rays taken at the beginning of the study and after one and two years of treatment. Then they will compare and evaluate x rays from all sub-study participants to identify changes in the knee joints as a result of treatment.

How many patients are needed and when will the study begin?

A total of 1,588 people will be recruited for the study.

Who will be eligible to participate in the study?

Patients with knee pain and x-ray evidence of osteoarthritis are encouraged to consider participation in the study. People who are interested in the study must not have used glucosamine for 3 months and chondroitin for 6 months prior to entering the study.

Where will the study be conducted and how can I sign up?

The University of Utah School of Medicine, Salt Lake City, UT, will serve as the coordinating study center and oversee the research and patient recruitment efforts of the thirteen study centers. People interested in the study can contact the coordinators at any of the thirteen centers listed below.

University of Alabama at Birmingham, Birmingham AL
Phone: (205) 934-9851

Cedars-Sinai Medical Center, Los Angeles, CA
Phone: (310) 358-5757

University of California, San Francisco, San Francisco, CA
Phone: (415) 206-8644

Indiana University, Indianapolis, IN
Phone: (317) 278-0555

Arthritis Research Center Foundation, Wichita, KS
Phone: (316) 263-2125

Hospital For Joint Diseases, New York, NY
Phone: (212) 598-6650

Case Western Reserve University, Cleveland, OH
Phone: (216) 844-6016

University of Pennsylvania, Philadelphia, PA
Phone: (215) 823-5979

Arthritis Consultation Center at Presbyterian Hospital of Dallas,
Dallas, TX
Phone: (214) 345-8067

University of Pittsburgh, Pittsburgh, PA
Phone: (412) 692-4269

University of Utah, Salt Lake City, UT
Phone: (801) 581-4911

Virginia Mason Research Center, Seattle, WA
Phone: (206) 223-6836

University of Nebraska Medical Center, Omaha, NE
Phone: (402) 559-3359

What is osteoarthritis?

Osteoarthritis, also called degenerative joint disease, is caused by the breakdown of cartilage, which is the connective tissue that cushions the ends of bones within the joint. It is characterized by pain, joint damage, and limited motion. The disease generally occurs late in life, and most commonly affects the hands and large weight-bearing joints. Although the disease can impact several joints, the knees are often affected. Age, female gender, and obesity are risk factors for this condition.

What are glucosamine and chondroitin?

Glucosamine and chondroitin are natural substances found in and around the cells of cartilage. Researchers believe these substances may help in the repair and maintenance of cartilage. In addition, researchers believe that glucosamine inhibits inflammation and stimulates cartilage cell growth, while chondroitin provides cartilage with strength and resilience. Currently, glucosamine and chondroitin are classified as dietary supplements.

What is a dietary supplement?

A dietary supplement is a product (other than tobacco) intended to supplement the diet, which bears or contains one or more of the following dietary ingredients: a vitamin, mineral, amino acid, herb or other botanical; is intended for ingestion in the form of a capsule, powder, softgel or gelcap; and is not represented as a conventional food or as a sole item of a meal or the diet (as defined by the U.S. Dietary Supplement Health and Education Act, Oct. 25, 1994).

What is Celecoxib?

Celecoxib (brand name Celebrex®) is a new type of nonsteroidal anti-inflammatory drug (NSAID), called a Cox-2 inhibitor. Like traditional NSAIDS, celecoxib blocks the Cox-2 enzyme in the body that stimulates inflammation. Unlike traditional NSAIDS, however, celecoxib does not block the action of Cox-1 enzyme, which is known to protect the stomach lining. As a result, celecoxib reduces joint pain and inflammation with reduced risk of gastrointestinal ulceration and bleeding.

Resources for Further Information

For information on complementary and alternative medicine, including research activities, conferences and events, contact:

National Center for Complementary and Alternative Medicine
Clearinghouse
P.O. Box 8218
Silver Spring, Maryland 20907-8218
Phone: (888) 644-6226
website: www.nccam.nih.gov

For information on rheumatic diseases such as osteoarthritis and diseases of the musculoskeletal and skin systems, contact:

National Institute of Arthritis and Musculoskeletal and Skin Diseases
Information Clearinghouse
NIAMS/National Institutes of Health
1 AMS Circle
Bethesda, Maryland 20892-3675
Phone: (301) 495-4484
website: www.niams.nih.gov

For information on dietary supplement labeling requirements and safety monitoring, order the FDA Guide to Dietary Supplements from the U.S. Food and Drug Administration, Center for Food Safety and Applied Nutrition at:

Phone: (800) FDA-4010
website: www.fda.gov/CFSAN

Glucosamine/Chondroitin Sulfate Trials

A systematic analysis of clinical trials on glucosamine and chondroitin sulfate for treating osteoarthritis (OA) has shown that these compounds may have some efficacy against the symptoms of this most common form of arthritis, in spite of problems with trial methodologies and possible biases. The study, by Timothy E. McAlindon, D.M., and colleagues at the Boston University School of Medicine, published in the March 15, 2000, issue of the *Journal of the American Medical Association (JAMA)*,[1] recommends that additional, rigorous, independent studies be done of these compounds to determine their true efficacy and usefulness.

"About 21 million adults in the United States have OA," says Stephen I. Katz, M.D., Ph.D., director of the National Institute of Arthritis and Musculoskeletal and Skin Diseases (NIAMS), which funded this study and has helped launch a major clinical trial on the compounds in OA, along with the National Center for Complementary and Alternative Medicine (NCCAM), both parts of the federal government's National Institutes of Health (NIH). "Effective treatments are key to improving the quality of life of Americans affected by this common disorder."

The Boston researchers point out that glucosamine and chondroitin sulfate have received significant media attention and have been used in Europe for OA for over 10 years. The researchers say that physicians in the United States and the United Kingdom have been skeptical about these products, probably because of well-founded concerns about the quality of scientific trials conducted to test them. Glucosamine and chondroitin sulfate, which are sold in the United States as dietary supplements, are natural substances found in and around the cells of cartilage. Researchers believe these substances may help in the repair and maintenance of cartilage.

The Boston University team located 37 studies of the compounds in osteoarthritis by a thorough review of the scientific literature going back more than three decades. Of these, 15 trials published between 1980 and 1998 met their criteria: double-blind, randomized placebo-controlled trials that lasted four or more weeks, tested glucosamine or chondroitin for osteoarthritis of the knee or hip, and reported data that the team could extract on the effect of treatment on OA symptoms. Six of the 15 trials involved glucosamine and nine used chondroitin. The team used only trials of four or more weeks duration because of evidence that it may take several weeks for the compounds to have a therapeutic benefit. Only one of the 15 trials was completely independent of manufacturer support.

The team's analysis of the trials had two key facets: a quality assessment to evaluate each of the clinical trials and a meta-analysis, which enabled them to integrate the data from different trials. The trials studied had many methodological flaws and biases, including those that tended to inflate the benefits of the compounds. The team was also concerned that trials having small or negative effects might not have been published, but after contacting study authors and other experts, they could locate no unpublished negative results.

Based on data from the trials, the researchers calculated an overall "effect size" for the two compounds: the figure 0.2 is considered a small effect; 0.5, moderate; and 0.8, large. The researchers calculated an effect size for glucosamine of 0.44 and for chondroitin sulfate of 0.78, but reported that these values "were diminished when only high-quality or large trials were considered."

"The results of this analysis performed by Boston University researchers underscore the critical public health need to test these agents in a rigorous way," said Dr. Stephen E. Straus, director of the NCCAM. "The NCCAM and NIAMS have jointly initiated the largest multicenter study to date of glucosamine and chondroitin sulfate in order to provide Americans with definitive answers about their effectiveness for osteoarthritis," Straus concluded. The University of Utah School of Medicine is coordinating a nine-center effort in over 1,000 patients, with recruitment to begin later this year.

In the meantime, says Dr. McAlindon, he would not discourage patients from trying these compounds, "but there is a possibility that they might not work," and that substances labeled as these compounds might not even contain them, due to a lack of regulation. Both the Arthritis Foundation and the American College of Rheumatology have issued statements[2] urging patients with osteoarthritis not to stop proven treatments and disease-management techniques and to let their physicians know if they are considering use of these compounds.

The mission of the NIAMS is to support research into the causes, treatment, and prevention of arthritis and musculoskeletal and skin diseases, the training of basic and clinical scientists to carry out this research, and the dissemination of information on the progress of research in these diseases. More information on NIAMS is available at www.nih.gov/niams/. The NIH multicenter study is described at http://www.niams.nih.gov/ne/press/1999/09_15.htm.

Notes

1. McAlindon TM, LaValley MP, Gulin JP, Felson DM. Glucosamine and Chondroitin Sulfate for Treatment of Osteoarthritis: A Systematic Quality Assessment and Meta-analysis. *JAMA*. 2000;283:1469-1475. Accompanying editorial: Towheed TE, Tassos PA. Glucosamine and Chondroitin for Treating Symptoms of Osteoarthritis: Evidence is Widely Touted but Incomplete. *JAMA*. 2000;283:1483-4.

2. These statements are available at: http://www.arthritis.org/resource/statements/glucosamine.asp and http://www.rheumatology.org/patients/hotline/970127.html, respectively.

Chapter 79

Genetic Engineering Studies May Lead to Development of More Effective Pain Relievers

Morphine and related compounds, called opiates, are among the most effective pain-relieving medications currently available. If administered properly, they rarely produce addiction. However, patients who take these medications for more than several days develop a tolerance to them, meaning that they must take increasingly higher doses to achieve the same level of pain relief. Unfortunately, when patients take higher doses of opiates, they are more likely to experience side effects.

Differences in Degree

Although all opiates cause physiological tolerance with prolonged administration, the degree of tolerance produced can vary considerably from drug to drug, even under similar conditions. Researchers have noted many factors that may contribute to these differences in "tolerogenicity."

Dr. Mark von Zastrow and his colleagues at the University of California, San Francisco and Los Angeles campuses, have been exploring one of these factors—how various opiate drugs affect the regulation of opioid receptors, proteins on the surface of some nerve cells in the brain and spinal cord. Understanding how opiates differ in their effects on these receptors may help explain the biological underpinnings

"Genetic Engineering Studies May Lead to Development of More Effective Pain Relievers," by Steven Stocker, *NIDA Notes*, National Institute on Drug Abuse (NIDA), Volume 15, Number 3, 2000.

of opiate tolerance and may be useful in developing improved opiate analgesics, Dr. von Zastrow believes.

Morphine and many other opiates produce analgesia by activating a type of opioid receptor called the mu opioid receptor. When this receptor is activated, it may or may not undergo endocytosis—movement from the surface of the cell to the cell's interior. Research has demonstrated that some opiate drugs cause mu receptor endocytosis, while others do not. Dr. von Zastrow and his colleagues believe that differences in this process of endocytosis may be a determining factor in whether or not a drug will produce tolerance.

A Case of Biochemical Compensation

The researchers have examined the effects on the mu opioid receptor of morphine; DAMGO, a derivative of one of the body's native opioids; etorphine, an opiate used in veterinary medicine; and methadone, an opiate medication used to treat heroin addiction.

Their studies have found that when DAMGO, etorphine, and methadone activate opioid receptors, the receptors are rapidly internalized. Morphine, on the other hand, activates the receptors, but does so with no detectable endocytosis.

Understanding how opiates differ in their effects on these receptors may help explain the biological underpinnings of opiate tolerance and may be useful in developing improved opiate analgesics.

"Morphine may change the shape of the opioid receptor so that it is not internalized," Dr. von Zastrow says. Thus, he explains, the receptor continues to be exposed to activation by the morphine. "My colleagues and I believe that endocytosis of the opioid receptor is essential for normal homeostasis in the nervous system. We hypothesize that, as morphine continues to activate the immobilized receptor, biochemical events inside the cell compensate for this abnormally prolonged activation. In other words, by immobilizing the receptor and continuing to activate it, morphine forces a pathological change in the signaling circuitry that underlies drug tolerance and, perhaps, dependence."

"If this theory is correct, it means that scientists might be able to develop new opioid analgesics that would not produce tolerance," says Dr. Jonathan Pollock of NIDA's (National Institute on Drug Abuse) Division of Neuroscience and Behavioral Research. "These compounds would both activate the mu opioid receptor and allow its internalization."

To test their theory, Dr. von Zastrow and his colleagues are using genetic engineering techniques in a project to develop mice that, instead of mu opioid receptors, have a different type of opioid receptor that can internalize when morphine attaches to it. "If our theory of opioid tolerance is correct, morphine should produce less tolerance in the mice containing these genetically engineered receptors," he says.

Sources

Keith, D.E.; Murray, S.R.; Zaki, P.A.; Chu, P.C.; Lissin, D.V.; Kang, L.; Evans, C.J.; and von Zastrow, M. Morphine activates opioid receptors without causing their rapid internalization. *Journal of Biological Chemistry*, 271(32): 19021-4, 1996.

Whistler, J.L.; Chuang, H.; Chu, L.Y.; and von Zastrow, M. Functional dissociation of mu opioid receptor signaling and endocytosis: Implications for the biology of opiate tolerance and addiction. *Neuron*, 23:737-746, 1999.

Whistler, J.L., and von Zastrow, M. Regulated internalization of opioid receptors: Implications for the biology of opiate tolerance. *The Neuroscientist*, in press.

— by Steven Stocker, NIDA NOTES *Contributing Writer*

Chapter 80

Analgesia Alternatives

NIDA's (National Institute on Drug Abuse) commitment to basic neuroscience research continues to result in important advances in the understanding of pain and how it might be controlled more effectively. NIDA-supported studies of the pain-relieving, or analgesic, properties of addictive drugs and how they work have broadened the horizon for analgesia research, as scientists discover that pain relief can be effected through a variety of processes.

"There are multiple pain-relieving mechanisms and many pieces to the puzzle of how they work," says Dr. Lindsay Hough, a NIDA-funded researcher at the Albany Medical College in New York. By putting these pieces together, NIDA-supported researchers hope to develop new pain-relief strategies and improve existing analgesia medications.

A main focus of NIDA-supported analgesia research is to develop medications that relieve pain without producing unwanted side effects. Opiate analgesics such as morphine are among the most effective medications currently available for treating long-term pain. Nonetheless, because many opiates have addictive side effects, physicians often under-prescribe them because they or their patients fear that the use of these medications could lead to opiate addiction. These perceptions linger even though studies have found that the fear of becoming addicted to opiates used clinically to treat pain is unfounded.

"NIDA Research Expands Horizon for Analgesia Alternatives," by John A. Bowersox, *NIDA Notes*, National Institute on Drug Abuse (NIDA), Volume 11, Number 2, March/April 1996.

Still, these fears and debilitating side effects, such as nausea, sedation, confusion, and constipation, that opiate medications can produce limit their effectiveness and contribute to the need for alternative analgesics.

NIDA-supported researchers are addressing this need through a number of experimental approaches. These include:

- developing opioid compounds, synthetic derivatives of opiates, that promote pain relief without producing the euphoria, or "high," that can lead to addiction;

- developing "promoter compounds" that enhance the pain-relieving effects of opioids so that smaller doses can be used; and

- developing nonopioid analgesics that function through a different pain-relief process and presumably will not produce the negative side effects of opioids.

Research conducted by Dr. Hough and his colleagues holds promise for the development of clinically useful nonopioid analgesics. For years, says Dr. Hough, scientists have known that the brain activates a number of pain-relieving systems in response to stress. Several of these systems appear to require histamine, a natural substance released by the body during stress. Histamine produces a variety of effects associated with the stress response, including the stimulation of gastric secretion, the constriction of muscles of the respiratory system, and the dilation of blood vessels.

Dr. Hough added to the number of known effects of histamine by showing that, in rats, morphine does not produce optimal analgesia unless histamine is released from a brainstem structure called the dorsal raphe nucleus or its surrounding tissue, known as the periaqueductal grey. He also found that histamine itself can produce analgesia when injected into this same part of the brain. Histamine-induced analgesia can be inhibited by simultaneously injecting morphine antagonists, compounds that interfere with the interactions between morphine and brain cells, into the same brain region. These findings, he says, suggest that histamine works with morphine or other opioid compounds to relieve pain through a shared brain pathway.

In recent studies, Dr. Hough and his colleagues showed that certain compounds derived from histamine can induce powerful analgesia in rats. Most importantly, says Dr. Hough, the histamine derivatives, unlike histamine, are not blocked by opiate antagonists. This finding implies the existence of a pain relief pathway in the brain that functions independently of the pathway used by morphine and other opiates.

"We think the histaminergic system is central to analgesia," says Dr. Hough, referring to the nerve cells and brain regions that use histamine as their neurotransmitter, or chemical messenger. Although still at an early stage, Dr. Hough's research into histamine-derived analgesics could lead to a new class of nonopioid pain relief medications.

While NIDA-supported researchers such as Dr. Hough are trying to develop novel pain-relief strategies that are not mediated by opioid compounds, others are trying to improve existing opioid medications by finding ways to enhance their analgesic properties.

Researchers have long known that amphetamines and other central nervous system stimulants increase the analgesia induced by opioid medications. Anecdotal evidence suggests that medications that activate brain regions that use the neurotransmitters serotonin and norepinephrine can produce similar effects. NIDA-funded researchers hope to exploit these effects through the development of a pain-relief strategy known as enhancement or promoter therapy.

The principal aim of enhancement therapy research is to identify nonanalgesic drugs that can selectively enhance the pain-relieving effects of morphine and other opiates, says NIDA researcher Dr. Danny Shen. This approach ultimately could allow physicians to prescribe smaller doses of opioids while achieving the same or greater degrees of pain relief. Smaller doses of opioids also could make the detrimental side effects of these medications less of a consideration in treatment decisions.

Dr. Shen and Dr. Barbara Coda, his colleague at the Fred Hutchinson Cancer Research Center in Seattle, are investigating whether compounds that either promote or prolong the activity of serotonin, a neurotransmitter that some neurons use to communicate with each other, can enhance analgesia.

In a NIDA-supported study, these investigators confirmed the long-held belief that activation of the brain's serotonergic pathways can enhance opiate-induced analgesia in people. In this study, subjects who were given fenfluramine, an appetite suppressant that promotes the release of serotonin from neurons, required 25 to 50 percent less morphine to relieve their pain than did those who received a placebo.

Dr. Shen is continuing this research to test a class of antidepressant medications known as selective serotonin re-uptake inhibitors (SSRIs). As their name suggests, SSRIs inhibit serotonin-releasing neurons from taking the neurotransmitter back up after it has been released. Thus, serotonin remains in the spaces between neurons, free to repeatedly activate those that have serotonin receptors.

A consortium of NIDA-supported investigators that includes Dr. Shen, Dr. Christopher Bernards of the University of Washington, and Dr. Tony L. Yaksh of the University of California at San Diego is trying to determine the best way to deliver opiate analgesics directly to the spinal cord. Dr. Yaksh was the first to demonstrate that opiates with an action limited to the spinal cord could produce a powerful analgesia. This work has led to the characterization of other spinal receptor systems that also can produce analgesia.

Spinal drug delivery reduces the discomfort that morphine can cause. However, some morphine is still able to seep into the bloodstream and thus be carried into the brain and other organs, where opiates' side effects originate. Researchers suspect that improving the spinal administration of opioids could present yet another opportunity to exploit the analgesic properties of opiates while bypassing their harmful or unpleasant side effects.

Sources

Coda, B.A.; Hill, H.F.; Schaffer, R.L.; Luger, T.J.; Jacobson, R.C.; and Chapman, C.R. Enhancement of morphine analgesia by fenfluramine in subjects receiving tailored opioid infusions. *Pain* 52:85-91, 1993.

Thoburn, K.K.; Hough, L.B.; Nalwalk, J.W.; and Mischler, S.A. Histamine-induced modulation of nociceptive responses. *Pain* 58:29-37, 1994.

Yaksh, T.L., and Rudy, T.A. Analgesia mediated by a direct spinal action of narcotics. *Science* 192:1357-1358, 1976.

—by John A. Bowersox, NIDA Notes Contributing Writer

Chapter 81

Research Eases Concerns about Use of Opioids

Many physicians limit their use of powerful opioid pain medications because they think that patients may become addicted to them. Now, accumulating evidence from a series of National Institute on Drug Abuse (NIDA)-funded studies indicates that the abuse potential of opioid medications is generally low in healthy, non-drug-abusing volunteers. The findings from this research could help to improve the use of opioid medications to treat a variety of pain conditions.

The term "opioids" describes morphine and other natural and synthetic chemicals that are structurally similar to morphine. Opioids include codeine and meperidine and other medications that are used to treat pain, as well as heroin, an abused drug. Research has provided much information about the addictive mechanisms and mood-altering and behavioral effects of opioids in opioid abusers. However, little is known about whether non-opioid-abusers being treated for postoperative pain experience similar effects.

"There is a prevailing notion that patients can readily become addicted to opioid medications, but it is not based on scientific evidence," says Dr. James Zacny of the University of Chicago. This belief in a high risk of addiction often leads to underuse of opioid medications for pain relief and causes unnecessary suffering in patients, he says. While research shows that several opioid medications commonly used for post-operative pain relief are likely to be abused by opioid abusers,

"Research Eases Concerns about Use of Opioids to Relieve Pain," by Robert Mathias, *NIDA Notes*, National Institute on Drug Abuse (NIDA), Volume 15, Number 1, 2000.

few studies have examined their abuse potential and subjective effects in people who don't abuse drugs.

For the last 7 years, Dr. Zacny has conducted a series of studies aimed at filling this critical gap in clinical knowledge. His research has examined the subjective and behavioral effects of powerful opioid medications, such as morphine and fentanyl, in non-drug-abusers. Dr. Zacny's research was recently recognized with a NIDA MERIT Award that will enable him to continue and expand his work.

"Most of what is known today about the mood-altering, psychomotor, and reinforcing aspects of opiates among people who don't abuse opioid drugs has come from Dr. Zacny's research," says Dr. Cora Lee Wetherington of NIDA's Division of Neuroscience and Behavioral Research. Generally, he has found that non-drug-abusing volunteers who are given these drugs do not report feeling the euphoria that opioid abusers do, she says. They also experience more drowsiness and impairment of psychomotor functions such as reaction time and eye-hand coordination from opioids than do opioid abusers, she adds.

Dr. Zacny's research also has shown that pain may modulate some of the subjective and behavioral effects produced by opioids in non-drug-abusers. In one study, non-opioid-abusing volunteers immersed their forearms either in ice-cold water, inducing constant pain, or lukewarm water, inducing no pain. When volunteers were given intravenous morphine while experiencing pain from the ice water, they reported feeling less euphoric, lightheaded, and sleepy than they felt following morphine administration when their arm was immersed in lukewarm water. However, regardless of whether or not they were experiencing pain, study participants did not feel the same amount of euphoria from morphine that drug abusers report, Dr. Zacny says.

"In our studies, we find the majority of healthy non-drug-abusing volunteers do not report euphoria after being administered opioids in the lab either with or without pain," Dr. Zacny stresses. "Since euphoria appears to be a factor in opioid abuse, it seems that the abuse potential of these opioid medications is generally low in such people," he says. Further clinical studies now are needed to assess the range of effects experienced by patients who receive opioid medications in hospitals, as opposed to laboratory settings, Dr. Zacny says. "Such studies could tell us if patients who have been given an opioid following an operation experience absolutely no euphoria or if some patients do experience such an effect."

Currently, Dr. Zacny is studying other opioids with different mechanisms of action that are commonly given for pain relief following operations. This research is examining the extent to which different doses of meperidine, butorphanol, and nalbuphine administered in the presence of a painful stimulus produce such subjective effects as sedation, he says. "Our findings should give clinicians a better sense of how patients are feeling from these drugs."

Dr. Zacny also is studying the behavioral effects of oral opioids, such as oxycodone (Percodan) and hydrocodone (found in Vicodin), and propoxyphene (Darvon), that sometimes are given to people with pain that is expected to last for a few days to a week. None of these medications, which typically are given following such procedures as outpatient surgery or extraction of wisdom teeth, have been carefully scrutinized for their behavioral effects, he says. Characterizing these effects in people in pain without a history of drug dependence could aid in assessing these medications' abuse liability in this population and determining if they significantly impair performance, Dr. Zacny says.

In the future, Dr. Zacny would like to examine how opioid medications affect non-drug-abusing patients who receive them on a long-term basis for chronic pain. This research could have clinical implications for people suffering from such conditions as cancer, osteoarthritis, or even chronic lower back pain, he says. For example, research into long-term use of these medications could help determine if repeated use leads to euphoria in these patients, could provide information about possible cognitive and psychomotor impairments, and could establish whether and how tolerance to their effects develops over time.

Studies of the effects of opioids in chronic pain patients will be complex and will have to consider many other factors affecting chronic pain patients' reactions to these drugs. These factors include different disease states, coexisting conditions, such as depression, and other medications, Dr. Zacny says. "The MERIT Award will enable me to enter this realm of research where the potential for gaining important new information is very great," he says.

Source

Conley, K.M.; Toledano, A.Y.; Apfelbaum, J.L.; and Zacny, J.P. The modulating effects of a cold water stimulus on opioid effects in volunteers. *Psychopharmacology*, 131:313-320, 1997.

— by Robert Mathias, NIDA NOTES Staff Writer

Chapter 82

Genes and Drugs Influence Codeine's Effectiveness

To cleanse itself of toxic substances or drugs, the body often mobilizes enzymes that help convert harmful compounds to less toxic ones or transform drugs into inactive products. But one such enzyme has a different effect on the common pain-relieving drug codeine: instead of dismantling the drug into inert components, the liver enzyme known as CYP2D6 converts codeine into its active therapeutic form, morphine. In fact, codeine's beneficial effects depend on the activity of CYP2D6.

Unfortunately, for about 20 million people in the United States — including about 8 percent of Caucasians, 6 percent of African Americans, and 1 percent of Asians — codeine offers little or no pain relief because they lack CYP2D6. In other individuals, codeine's effects are readily altered by medications that alter CYP2D6 activity. In a series of studies conducted at the National Center for Research Resources (NCRR)-supported General Clinical Research Center at Vanderbilt University in Nashville, Tennessee, Dr. Alastair J. J. Wood and his colleagues are working to define how drug interactions and individual variations in CYP2D6 activity affect codeine's analgesic properties. Their findings should alert physicians to the possibility that codeine might be ineffective in some patients, and that concurrent use of CYP2D6-inhibiting medications should be avoided or carefully monitored in all individuals.

National Center for Research Resources (NCRR), *NCRR Reporter*, April 1998.

"Codeine is unusual in that it does not exert its effects directly on the body like most drugs, but by its conversion to morphine," explains Dr. Wood, professor of medicine and pharmacology at Vanderbilt University. Morphine then binds to opiate receptors in the central nervous system and sets off a cascade of reactions that reduce the sensation of pain, inhibit respiration and cognitive ability, and constrict pupils.

A clinical study of 10 people with normal CYP2D6 and six without active enzyme helped the Vanderbilt researchers to firmly establish the mechanism of codeine action. The investigators administered in random, double-blind fashion codeine or codeine plus quinidine, a drug that inhibits CYP2D6—in addition to proper controls that included placebo administrations—to the study participants and then tested their blood for morphine and morphine metabolites and assessed their respiration, cognitive ability, and pupil size.

People with normal CYP2D6, but not those who lacked active enzyme, had morphine in their blood after codeine administration and showed the typical respiratory, cognitive, and pupillary effects. When the participants received both codeine and quinidine, morphine levels decreased almost tenfold in people with normal CYP2D6 and the respiratory, cognitive, and pupillary effects were also significantly reduced. In people without CYP2D6, codeine produced no measurable effects, thus showing that this enzyme was needed to activate the drug.

Like most drugs, the amount of codeine required for effective pain relief varies from individual to individual and typically increases over time because a person's sensitivity to the drug diminishes with prolonged use. But people who lack CYP2D6 activity get no pain relief from codeine—at any dose. In most cases, says Dr. Wood, "If a patient doesn't get the effect, the physician gives more of the drug. But here we have a situation where a proportion of the population gets absolutely no effect from the drug. It's actually predictable."

CYP2D6 also processes many other drugs, including some antidepressants and drugs involved in controlling blood pressure and heart arrhythmias. But in contrast to codeine, these drugs act directly. They are broken down to inactive metabolites by CYP2D6 and cleared from the body. "A lack of the enzyme in these cases would result in a prolonged activity of the drug and potential toxicity due to accumulation," Dr. Wood explains.

The Vanderbilt researchers also discovered a link between race and codeine sensitivity that went beyond the simple correlation with the presence or absence of CYP2D6. In a study of ten white men and eight

Chinese men—all of whom produced normal levels of the enzyme—Dr. Wood and his colleagues found that both codeine and morphine were consistently less effective in the Asians than in the Caucasians.

"Even with CYP2D6, the Chinese men produced less morphine from codeine. And both codeine and morphine were cleared from the bodies of the Chinese men much more quickly than in the Caucasians, thus reducing the overall effects of opiate," says Dr. Wood. This increased metabolism of codeine and morphine takes place via the action of enzymes other than CYP2D6, he adds.

Paradoxically, the Chinese men who had decreased codeine/morphine sensitivity (unrelated to CYP2D6 activity) were more likely to develop the nauseating side effects of codeine, Dr. Wood says. Although the exact pharmacologic mechanisms for this effect are poorly understood, the researchers speculate that they are caused by the activation of different receptors by morphine and other codeine metabolites.

In addition to exploring the genetic and ethnic aspects of codeine effectiveness, the researchers also examined how other drugs might alter the effects of codeine. In their most recent study, the scientists found that the antituberculosis drug rifampin blocked codeine-induced analgesia. Although this effect might seem similar to that of quinidine, which inhibits CYP2D6, the underlying mechanisms are in fact quite distinct. "Our experiments indicate that rifampin does not block CYP2D6 activity but instead increases the rate of other pathways of codeine metabolism in the body," says Dr. Wood. "This reduces the levels of morphine in the bloodstream, which in turn results in a decreased pain-killing effect."

These codeine effectiveness studies have important implications for physicians deciding which medications to prescribe. For example, prescribing codeine to alleviate pain in patients being treated with quinidine—an antiarrhythmia heart drug—would have little pain-relieving effect, which may prompt physicians or patients to administer higher than recommended doses, which are still likely to produce little pain relief.

Patients are often reluctant to ask for additional pain killers, afraid they may be considered potential drug abusers or weaklings; therefore, they may stoically endure unnecessary pain. In addition to considering potential drug interactions, "physicians need to be aware that this CYP2D6-lacking population exists and to adopt alternate strategies for pain management in these cases," emphasizes Dr. Wood. "Most of the people who complain that their pain persists despite medication are not wimps. They are quite simply not capable of responding to codeine."

Additional Reading

Caraco, Y., Sheller, J., and Wood, A. J. J., Pharmacogenetic determinants of codeine induction by rifampin: The impact on codeine's respiratory, psychomotor and miotic effects. *Journal of Pharmacology and Experimental Therapeutics* 281:330-336, 1997.

Caraco, Y., Sheller, J., and Wood, A. J. J., Pharmacogenetic determination of the effects of codeine and prediction of drug interactions. *Journal of Pharmacology and Experimental Therapeutics* 278:1165-1174, 1996.

— by Neeraja Sankaran

These studies were supported by the Clinical Research area of the National Center for Research Resources and by the National Institute of General Medical Sciences.

For more information about NCRR's Clinical Research area, see http://www.ncrr.nih.gov/clinical.htm

Chapter 83

Gene Therapy for Pain

National Institutes of Health (NIH) scientists are attacking chronic pain with a novel form of gene therapy that targets the spinal cord. Though still in the animal testing stage, this approach has overcome one of the major obstacles to gene therapy as a way to manipulate spinal cord function. Rather than injecting genes directly into a localized area of the spinal cord, the pain-relieving gene is introduced into the sheath of tissue that surrounds the cord. From that strategic location, the gene can pump out its product and bathe many nerves, thus extending the range of its pain-numbing effect. The investigators hope that this simplified approach can be used to generate a variety of products in the tissue surrounding nerves, including factors that could stimulate new nerve growth.

The study, carried out by scientists from the National Institute of Dental and Craniofacial Research (NIDCR) and the University of Pennsylvania, was reported in the May 1, 1999 issue of *Human Gene Therapy*.

"We are totally pumped up that this approach is working in an animal model," said Dr. Mike Iadarola, chief of NIDCR's Neuronal Gene Expression Unit. "The animal studies have shown us that genes are readily taken up by the connective tissue cells that surround the central nervous system. So, given the right gene, our approach has application to a broad range of conditions, from pain control to spinal

National Institute of Dental and Craniofacial Research (NIDCR), *NIDCR Research Digest* July 1999.

cord injury and disorders like multiple sclerosis and Parkinson's disease."

Release of Beta-endorphin

In the study, investigators used an adenovirus—similar to a cold virus—to deliver the beta-endorphin gene to the rat spinal cord. The virus particles were injected into the spinal fluid, where they were readily taken up by the protective sheath of connective tissue, called the pia mater, which surrounds the cord. Within 24 hours the sheath cells began secreting beta-endorphin, one of the body's natural sedatives for alleviating pain.

"The incredible simplicity and relative noninvasiveness of this approach provides a new frame of reference for gene therapy of the nervous system," said co-author, Dr. Alan Finegold, previously with NIDCR's Pain and Neurosensory Mechanisms Branch and now in the private sector.

The spinal cord was selected as the target for the beta-endorphin gene, not only because of its ease of access, but also because it is the first processing point for relaying pain signals to the brain, and pain can be effectively controlled at this location. The idea was to have beta-endorphin block pain signals before they reached the brain, where pain perception occurs.

The researchers observed that beta-endorphin levels in the spinal fluid increased nearly ten-fold following a single injection of virus. Cellular analysis confirmed that sheath cells, not spinal cord neurons, were the source of beta-endorphin.

Effectiveness Demonstrated in Rats

To determine if the method had a therapeutic effect, the investigators used the rat "hindpaw" model for evaluating pain response. It is based on the time that elapses before a rat voluntarily pulls its paw away from a heat lamp. The system allows a rat to be tested for the normal pain response in one paw and the so-called "hyperalgesic" response in the other paw, which has been inflamed by injection of an irritant. This latter type of super-sensitive pain results in rapid paw withdrawal and is used as a model for the chronic pain of cancer or arthritis.

The rats responded to beta-endorphin by exhibiting a delayed response in pulling the inflamed paw away from the heat source, a sign that the hyperalgesic pain sensation was reduced. An added bonus was the observation that the non-inflamed paw had a normal withdrawal response. This points not only to a lack of toxicity from the treatment procedure but also to a selective therapeutic effect for beta-endorphin. The results are similar to a person getting relief from chronic cancer pain, yet not losing the normal sense of feeling to react to painful stimuli. The reason for this distinction is not completely understood, but scientists feel that inflammation may help activate receptors on the affected nerves, making them more responsive to the blocking effect of beta-endorphin.

Determining the Site of Injection

Development of this novel method evolved from some preliminary trial and error testing. Initial attempts were aimed at injecting virus directly into neural tissues. "We discovered early-on that brain and spinal cord were not a hospitable environment for direct injection of virus," said Dr. Iadarola. "There are physical barriers that prevent the virus from infiltrating the space between the neurons, keeping any beneficial effects very localized. We shifted our approach to the spinal fluid, which we thought would be an excellent medium to expose a wide swath of neurons to the therapeutic virus."

What they observed however, was the protective sheath of connective tissues that coats the spinal cord acted like a sponge, soaking up the virus and preventing direct contact with nerve tissue. What initially appeared as an obstacle turned out to be the makings of a new approach for gene therapy to the nervous system. Although the nerve cells could not be made to effectively take up the gene, they wound up being exposed to beta-endorphin that was produced by neighboring sheath cells.

As with other studies that have used adenoviruses to deliver genes, the effects of beta-endorphin were not permanent. Production peaked after 3–7 days and tailed off dramatically by day 15. However, the investigators are optimistic that improvements in vector design will result in a single injection that provides long-term gene expression, not only of beta-endorphin, but genes to treat a variety of spinal cord and brain disorders.

Working with Drs. Iadarola and Finegold was Dr. Andrew Mannes from the University of Pennsylvania, Department of Anesthesiology.

—by Wayne Little

Chapter 84

Brain Chemistry and Pain Relief

A unique study that looked at chemical activity in the brains of human volunteers while they experienced sustained pain and reported how they felt is providing new insights into the importance of the body's natural painkiller system—and the reasons why each of us experiences pain differently.

The results confirm long-suspected connections between pain-dampening changes in brain chemistry and the senses and emotions experienced by people in pain. The findings may help researchers better understand prolonged pain and find more effective ways to relieve it.

Results from the brain imaging study were published in the July 13, 2001 issue of *Science* by NIDCR-supported researchers from the University of Michigan Health System and School of Dentistry. It is the first study to combine sustained, induced pain with simultaneous brain scan monitoring of a key neurochemical system and the self-reported pain ratings of human participants.

The research cements the critical role of the mu opioid system, in which naturally produced chemicals called endogenous opioids, or endorphins, match up with receptors on the surface of brain cells and reduce or block the spread of pain messages from the body through the brain. The mu opioid receptor in particular has been found to be a major target for both the body's own painkillers, as well as for drugs

"Study Gives Glimpse of Human Brain's Natural Painkiller System in Action," *NIDCR Research Digest*, National Institute of Dental and Craniofacial Research (NIDCR), August 1, 2001.

such as heroin, morphine, methadone, synthetic pain medications and anesthetics, which also numb pain.

The study found that the onset and slow release of jaw muscle pain over 20 minutes caused a surge in the release of the chemicals. It also found that the flood of those chemicals coincided with a reduction in the amount of pain and pain-related emotions the volunteers said they felt. Specific brain regions, especially those already known to play a role in affective, or emotional, responses, and those known to help process signals from the body's sensory systems, had the biggest increase in the level of opioids when pain was introduced. The research also revealed major variation among volunteers in the baseline and pain-induced levels of opioids.

"This result gives us new appreciation for the power of our brain's own anti-pain system, and shows how brain chemistry regulates sensory and emotional experiences," said lead author Jon-Kar Zubieta, M.D., Ph.D., assistant professor of psychiatry and radiology at the University of Michigan Medical School and assistant research scientist in the Mental Health Research Institute.

Zubieta and his colleagues used positron emission tomography, or PET, a technique that allowed them to have a unique window into the chemical activity of the volunteers' brains. To narrow their view to the mu opioid receptor system, they attached short-lived radioactive carbon atoms to minute quantities of a molecule known to bind only to mu opioid receptors. This gave them a tracer whose radioactive decay signals, followed over time, allowed them to measure the release of endogenous opioids and the activation of the mu opioid receptors.

With their view onto the brain's pain mechanism ready, the researchers looked at prolonged jaw pain, mimicking the chronic condition of temporomandibular joint disorder (TMJ). To stimulate TMJ's symptoms, they devised a way to inject high-concentration salt water directly into each volunteer's jaw muscle, which caused a painful sensation that continued only as long as water was injected. A placebo solution that does not cause pain also was used for comparison. Rather than limiting the pain to a few seconds as in prior studies examining pain, they administered the solutions for 20 minutes. This allowed them to achieve the brain conditions and emotions much more closely related to those seen in chronic pain conditions like TMJ.

While the volunteers were scanned during the two injections, they were asked to rate how much pain they were feeling, giving a rating via a computerized system every 15 seconds. The same computer system then controlled the intensity of the pain stimulus so that each volunteer's own rating would be about the same throughout the 20 minutes. This allowed the researchers to compare the response of the brain's anti-pain system across individual subjects. Afterward, the volunteers completed a questionnaire about how the experience made them feel.

The results, said Zubieta, showed a brain chemistry response that was strongest in the brain regions where sensation and emotion are rooted—a response tied directly to the ratings of the pain experience that the volunteers gave. "We saw an intense activation of the mu opioid system in areas such as the amygdala, the thalamus, the hypothalamus, the frontal cortex, and the nucleus accumbens, as much as a 12 percent change over baseline conditions," he added. "And the higher the level of activation, the lower the scores the volunteers gave for pain-related sensations and emotions like feelings of the unpleasantness of pain."

The results also showed wide individual variations in the intensity of the brain anti-pain response, which correlated with the individual's sensory and affective responses to the pain experience— even though the computer system had ensured that all participants had experienced similar pain intensity. The activation of the anti-pain response was dramatic in some volunteers when the placebo and pain-inducing conditions were compared, while in others the response was much less pronounced. And those who had the biggest change tended to rate the experience of pain, both in its sensory and emotional aspects, the lowest.

"This may help explain why some people are more sensitive or less sensitive than others when it comes to painful sensations," Zubieta explained. "We show that people vary both in the number of receptors that they have for these anti-pain brain chemicals, and in their ability to release the anti-pain chemicals themselves. Both of these factors appear to determine the emotional and sensory aspects of a painful experience. Such variability in the pain response system may help explain why some people react to pain and pain medications differently. It may also be quite relevant to why some people, but not others, develop chronic pain conditions."

In addition to Dr. Zubieta, the research team included Yolanda Smith of the Department of Obstetrics and Gynecology; Joshua Bueller and Yanjun Xu of the Department of Psychiatry and Mental Health Research Institute; Michael Kilbourn, Douglas Jewett, Charles Meyer, and Robert Koeppe from the Department of Radiology; and Christian Stohler from the School of Dentistry.

Chapter 85

A New Way to Inhibit Nerve Pain

Scientists funded by the National Institute of Neurological Disorders and Stroke (NINDS) may soon be able to reduce sensitivity to stimuli that are associated with chronic neuropathic and inflammatory pain by disabling certain nerve cells that send pain signals to the brain.

Research reported in the November 19, 1999, issue of *Science* shows that, in an animal model, combining substance P with the ribosome-inactivating protein saporin (SAP) will inhibit the pain associated with nerve injury when administered before or after the development of neuropathic pain and will significantly reduce sensitivity to stimuli associated with inflammatory pain. Previous data have suggested that in the peripheral nervous system, neuropathic and inflammatory pain arise from different mechanisms and are conveyed to the spinal cord by distinct groups of primary afferent neurons. Study findings suggest that these different types of pain conditions, which can arise via different mechanisms, may be conveyed to the spinal cord by the same substance P receptor-expressing neurons. Further, the study found that, following substance P-SAP treatment, opiates such as morphine remain a viable therapy for breakthrough pain. This discovery could lead to new treatments for chronic pain and the development of more targeted pain-relieving drug therapy.

"New Target Identified for Chronic Pain Therapy," National Institute of Neurological Disorders and Stroke (NINDS), November 18, 1999; reviewed July 1, 2001.

Researchers at the University of Minnesota injected a combination of substance P (a neurotransmitter known to stimulate pain receptors) and SAP into the dorsal horn of the spinal cord in rats. Receptors for substance P—large molecules found on the surface of spinal cord nerve cells—served as portals for the compound's entry. Within days, the targeted neurons, located in the outer layer of the spinal cord along its entire length, absorbed the compound and were neutralized. Results indicate the substance P-SAP treatment reduced the number of spinal cord neurons that express substance P receptor as well as lessened the pain response to thermal and mechanically induced pain following nerve injury, inflammation, and the long-term effects of pain produced by capsaicin injection. The results appear to be long-lasting and do not affect other nerve cells.

Scientists already know that spinal cord neurons that express substance P receptors play a role in pain, but their specific role in signaling—relaying or conveying pain signals—is not entirely understood.

Investigators believe that these results suggest that this small group of neurons that express substance P play a critical role in communicating chronic pain information from the spinal cord to the thalamus, the brain's pain center.

The concept of using specific receptors to introduce therapeutic compounds may pave the way for a new pain therapy. Such compounds might be first introduced through a lumbar puncture, a technique commonly used for collecting spinal fluid. The compounds would then serve to relay information through the spinal cord to the thalamus, thus blocking pain signals.

"These findings are extremely important to the study of peripheral and neuropathic pain and our treatment of persons with persistent pain," says Patrick Mantyh, Ph.D., of the University of Minnesota and the Veterans Affairs Medical Center in Minneapolis, who led the study. "We were able to administer a potential treatment and specifically channel it to certain cells, disabling them. We can now focus on the biology of these cells and look at new ways of silencing these cells in other types of persistent pain."

"This discovery is critically important to our understanding of the pain process," says Cheryl Kitt, Ph.D., program director for pain at the NINDS. "Understanding pain pathway changes at the cellular level offers great potential for more effective treatment for pain."

Scientists now need to perform toxicology studies in large animals to demonstrate the safety and efficacy of this treatment in another species. If these studies are successful, approval would be sought to treat terminally ill patients who have severe chronic pain (cancer pain) to determine the extent of the relief of chronic pain in humans.

The NINDS, part of the National Institutes of Health located in Bethesda, Maryland, is the nation's leading supporter of research on the brain and nervous system and a lead agency in the Congressionally designated Decade of the Brain. The NINDS celebrated its 50th anniversary in the year 2000.

—Originally prepared by Paul Girolami,
NINDS Office of Communications and Public Liaison.

Chapter 86

Natural Compound May Offer New Treatment for Chronic Pain

National Institute on Drug Abuse (NIDA)-supported researchers Drs. George Wilcox and Carolyn Fairbanks at the University of Minnesota in Minneapolis and Dr. Robert Yezierski at the University of Miami have demonstrated that a recently discovered compound appears to alleviate chronic pain. The investigators, led by Dr. Wilcox, are studying agmatine, an amino-acid-like substance produced in the brain. They have found that in laboratory mice and rats, agmatine appears to relieve chronic pain caused by nerve damage and inflammation. (See "Acute vs. Chronic Pain," below.)

The research team injected either agmatine or saline solution into the spines of rodents that had pain associated with nerve damage due to chemically induced inflammation or surgically induced spinal cord injury. The researchers found that the animals treated with agmatine showed reduced sensitivity to this pain.

"Agmatine seems to interrupt the cascade of changes that occur in the nervous system after nerve damage," says Dr. Wilcox. Agmatine, thought to be a neurotransmitter like dopamine or serotonin—substances that act as chemical messengers between nerve cells—counters the effect of another brain chemical, glutamate. Glutamate, which is released in large quantities following injuries, promotes pain by damaging and destroying nerve cells.

"Natural Compound May Offer New Treatment for Chronic Pain," by Susan Gonzales, *NIDA Notes*, National Institute on Drug Abuse (NIDA), Volume 16, Number 3, 2001.

"Agmatine is not a typical pain reliever," says Dr. Fairbanks. "It appears to selectively reduce the chronic pain resulting from nerve damage or inflammation, but not the acute pain caused by normal injury."

In the study with rodents, Dr. Wilcox notes, "the relief provided by agmatine appeared to be permanent, unlike the temporary relief provided by medications like morphine." Moreover, agmatine seemed to produce none of the serious side effects seen with morphine and related drugs, such as sedation, respiratory depression, and loss of coordination.

Agmatine still has to go through many stages of testing before scientists will know if it can be a safe and effective treatment for people. Meanwhile, these early findings with the compound are hopeful for chronic pain sufferers.

Acute vs. Chronic Pain

Physical pain comes in two varieties: acute and chronic. Acute pain can occur during transient illnesses or after an injury or surgery and goes away once the condition clears up or wound heals. In acute pain, pain-specific nerves respond to noxious stimulation or injury by releasing chemicals that transmit pain signals to the spinal column and brain. This type of pain can be treated effectively with short-term use of opioids or other pain-relievers, which generally pose a minuscule risk of addiction.

In contrast, chronic pain may be caused by nerve damage, chronic diseases such as cancer and arthritis, and degenerative conditions such as spinal cord injury. While chronic pain is complex and not well understood, research suggests that prolonged disease states or tissue injury may sensitize certain nerves in pain-signaling pathways. As a result, these nerves may continue sending pain signals to the brain even when the pain-causing condition has been resolved.

Chronic pain is a difficult-to-treat, persistent condition that often requires long-term use of medications. With prolonged use of opioids, some patients require increasing doses to control their pain and patients may develop withdrawal symptoms if the drug is stopped. NIDA-funded researchers have been spearheading the exploration for new painkillers that are effective in treating chronic pain but do not produce withdrawal symptoms and are not addicting.

NIDA's Dr. David Thomas says, "In addition to our interest in how opioids work and in developing better opioids for the treatment of pain, we are searching for alternatives to opioids because of their abuse potential and because they are not effective for reducing some types of pain, such as pain caused by nerve damage and inflammation."

Source

Fairbanks, C.A.; Schreiber, K.L.; Brewer, K.L.; Yu, C-G.; Stone, L.S.; Kitto, K.F.; Nguyen, H.O.; Grocholski, B.M.; Shoeman, D.W.; Kehl, L.J.; Regunathan, S.; Reis. D.J.; Yezierski, R.P.; and Wilcox, G.L. Agmatine reverses pain induced by inflammation, neuropathy, and spinal cord injury. *Proceedings of the National Academy of Sciences* 97(19):10584-10589, 2000.

— *by Susan Gonzales,* NIDA NOTES *Contributing Writer*

Chapter 87

Pain in Newborns Alters Nerve Circuitry

Newborns who experience tissue injury and pain during critical periods of development may undergo a permanent rewiring of their nervous system that increases their sensitivity to pain later in life.

Working with an animal model, scientists at the National Institute of Dental and Craniofacial Research (NIDCR) have provided the first physical evidence that pain and inflammation in newborns alters the development of pain pathway circuitry, causing a stronger response to pain in adulthood. The study, which appears in the July 28, 2000 issue of *Science*, calls attention to the need to assess the long-term effects of pain and tissue injury on human newborns.

"Although we have yet to directly link animal research findings to what happens in human infants, one is tempted to speculate that similar changes as those identified in the animals may occur in newborn humans exposed to pain and inflammation," said Dr. M. A. Ruda, principal investigator on the study and chief of NIDCR's Cellular Neuroscience Section.

Each year, more than 400,000 babies in the U.S. are born either prematurely or at a low birth weight. Of these, 25,000 are considered to be extremely premature—born at 27 weeks of gestation or less. While 10 or 15 years ago most of these micropreemies did not live, it is no longer unusual for them to survive, thanks to advances in medical technology. Yet these tiny babies face a host of problems. Not only

National Institute of Dental and Craniofacial Research (NIDCR), "Animal Model Shows Pain and Tissue Injury in Newborns Alters Nerve Circuitry and Reaction to Pain Later in Life", July 27, 2000.

are they confronted with the trauma of living in the outside world too soon, but available medical procedures used to keep them alive and monitor their progress may cause pain and tissue injury. Heel sticks to draw blood, the insertion of IV lines and nasogastric tubes, and the use of ventilators are some of the modern technologies and procedures that are both miraculous and difficult.

"A premature infant can be thought of as still in the fetal time of their life when the basic elements of brain development are occurring," explained Dr. Ruda. "Abnormal stimulation during these critical developmental time points can abnormally wire the brain."

There has been considerable debate over the existence of pain in newborns and its management. As late as the mid-1980's, surgery was performed on infants without benefit of anesthesia, the belief being that even if babies did experience pain, they would forget about it. Since then, studies of the biological response to pain and the facial expressions of newborns during traumatic procedures document that they do indeed respond to pain. Today, pain from traumatic surgeries in newborns is carefully managed with anesthesia and analgesics.

Scientists have learned that by 24 weeks gestation, very immature pain transmission pathways are already in place. The development of these pathways continues postnatally. What newborns lack are fully developed and functional pain inhibitory systems. These typically develop several weeks after a full-term baby is born.

"Unlike other sensory modalities such as vision and hearing that require the input of sight and sound for their appropriate development, pain pathways normally develop in the absence of, or with little exposure to, painful stimulation. However, medical procedures shortly after birth can expose the nervous system to pain, the developmental effects of which we are just learning," said Dr. Ruda.

In their study, Dr. Ruda and her colleagues used newborn rat pups to explore the effect of tissue injury and pain on the development of pain pathways. An irritant was injected into the left hind paw of the pups to induce swelling. One group received the injection when they were one day old, an age equivalent to 24 weeks gestation in humans. A second group received the injection 14 days after birth, equivalent to adolescence in humans. Swelling and redness occurred shortly after the injection and persisted for 5–7 days in both groups.

When the animals were examined as adults, it was found that rats who received the left hind paw injection on day one had an increase in the density of nerve fibers on the left side of the dorsal horn, the layered structure in the spinal cord that propels pain signals up to the brain. Even at the level of individual nerve cells, the response to pain was increased. Spinal cord segments also exhibited an increase in pain input on the left neonatal treated side, including areas that normally would not be expected to display this. The picture was very different for the rats that received the injection on postnatal day 14. The patterns of nerve fibers in this group looked like those of normal rats. The researchers surmise that the critical time point responsible for a change in input had passed by day 14, so that neuronal circuits were not altered by the tissue injury and pain.

Adult rats that experienced left hind paw tissue injury and swelling on day one also reacted more strongly to pain as adults. When an irritant was injected into their left hind paw and the paw was exposed to heat, they were much quicker to withdraw it than normal rats. The changes that occurred because of tissue injury and pain are likely not limited to the spinal cord but could also involve higher centers of the brain that are part of pain pathways, suggest the researchers.

"Our study adds pain to the emerging list of early birth stimuli that we are discovering have a lifelong impact and suggests that further study is warranted to develop approaches to limit or prevent those effects," added Dr. Ruda.

Collaborating with Dr. Ruda on the study were Drs. Qing-Dong Ling, Andrea G. Hohmann, Yuan Bo Peng, and Toshiya Tachibana from the Cellular Neuroscience Section, Pain and Neurosensory Mechanisms Branch, NIDCR. The National Institute of Dental and Craniofacial Research is one of the federal National Institutes of Health, located in Bethesda, MD.

Part Six

Additional Help
and Information

Chapter 88

Pain Terms You Should Know

Acroparesthesia: 1) Paresthesia of one or more of the extremities. 2) Nocturnal paresthesia involving the hands, most often of middle-aged women; formerly attributed to a lesion in the thoracic outlet, but now known to be a classic symptom of carpal tunnel syndrome.

Acupuncture: Puncture with long, fine needles: 1) An ancient Asian system of therapy. 2) More recently, acupuncture anesthesia or analgesia.

Analgesia: A neurologic or pharmacologic state in which painful stimuli are so moderated that, though still perceived, they are no longer painful.

Anesthesia: Loss of sensation resulting from pharmacologic depression of nerve function or from neurologic dysfunction.

Anesthesiology: The medical specialty concerned with the pharmacological, physiological, and clinical basis of anesthesia and related fields, including resuscitation, intensive respiratory care, and acute and chronic pain.

Angina pectoris: Severe constricting pain in the chest, often radiating from the precordium to a shoulder (usually left) and down the arm, due to ischemia of the heart muscle usually caused by coronary disease.

Arthralgia: Pain in a joint, especially one not inflammatory in character.

Biofeedback: A training technique that enables an individual to gain some element of voluntary control over autonomic body functions; based on the learning principle that a desired response is learned when received information such as a recorded increase in skin temperature (feedback) indicates that a specific thought complex or action has produced the desired physiological response.

Cardiodynia: Pain in the heart. (Synonym: Cardialgia.)

Carpal tunnel syndrome: The most common nerve entrapment syndrome, characterized by nocturnal hand paresthesia and pain, and sometimes sensory loss and wasting in the median hand distribution; affects women more than men and is often bilateral; caused by chronic entrapment of the median nerve at the wrist, within the carpal tunnel.

Cauda equina: The bundle of spinal nerve roots arising from the lumbosacral enlargement and medullary cone and running through the lumbar cistern (subarachnoid space) within the vertebral canal below the first lumbar vertebra; it comprises the roots of all the spinal nerves below the first lumbar.

Cauda equina syndrome: Involvement, often asymmetric, of multiple roots making up the cauda equina (i.e., L2–S3 roots), manifested by pain, paresthesia, and weakness; often bladder and bowel sphincter function is unaffected because of sacral sparing (lack of compromise of the S2, S3, and S4 roots).

Causalgia: Persistent severe burning pain, usually following injury of a peripheral nerve (especially median and tibial) or the brachial plexus, accompanied by trophic changes.

Cervical disk syndrome: Pain, paresthesias, and sometimes weakness in the area of the distribution of one or more cervical roots, due to pressure of a protruded cervical intervertebral disk. (Synonym: Cervical compression syndrome.)

Dysmenorrhea: Difficult and painful menstruation.

Dyspareunia: Occurrence of pain during sexual intercourse.

Dyspepsia: Impaired gastric function or "upset stomach" due to some disorder of the stomach; characterized by epigastric pain, sometimes burning, nausea, and gaseous eructation. (Synonym: Gastric indigestion.)

Eburnation: A change in exposed subchondral bone in degenerative joint disease in which it is converted into a dense substance with a smooth surface like ivory. (Synonym: bone sclerosis.)

Esophageal reflux; gastroesophageal reflux: Regurgitation of the contents of the stomach into the esophagus, possibly into the pharynx where they can be aspirated between the vocal cords and down into the trachea; symptoms of burning pain and acid taste result; pulmonary complications of aspiration are dependent upon the amount, content, and acidity of the aspirate.

Fascia (plural: fasciae, fascias): A sheet of fibrous tissue that envelops the body beneath the skin; it also encloses muscles and groups of muscles, and separates their several layers or groups.

Fibromyalgia: A syndrome of chronic pain of musculoskeletal origin but uncertain cause. The American College of Rheumatology has established diagnostic criteria that include pain on both sides of the body, both above and below the waist, as well as in an axial distribution (cervical, thoracic, or lumbar spine or anterior chest); additionally there must be point tenderness in at least 11 of 18 specified sites.

Flashing pain syndrome: Sudden, intermittent, and severe brief episodes of pain, without apparent cause, in the distribution of a spinal dermatome; resembles in character the pain of tic douloureux.

General anesthesia: Loss of ability to perceive pain associated with loss of consciousness produced by intravenous or inhalation anesthetic agents.

General anesthetics: Drugs used either by the intravenous route or by inhalation that render the subject unconscious and incapable of perceiving pain as might otherwise occur in surgery.

Gout: A disorder of purine metabolism, occurring especially in men, characterized by a raised but variable blood uric acid level and severe recurrent acute arthritis of sudden onset resulting from deposition of crystals of sodium urate in connective tissues and articular cartilage; most cases are inherited, resulting from a variety of abnormalities of purine metabolism. The familial aggregation is for the most part galtonian with a threshold of expression determined by the solubility of uric acid. However, gout is also a feature of the Lesch-Nyhan syndrome, an X-linked disorder.

Herpes zoster: An infection caused by a herpesvirus (varicella-zoster virus), characterized by an eruption of groups of vesicles on one side of the body following the course of a nerve due to inflammation of ganglia and dorsal nerve roots resulting from activation of the virus, which in many instances has remained latent for years following a primary chickenpox infection; the condition is self-limited but may be accompanied by or followed by severe postherpetic pain.

Hypnosis: An artificially induced trancelike state, resembling somnambulism, in which the subject is highly susceptible to suggestion, oblivious to all else, and responds readily to the commands of the hypnotist; its scientific validity has been accepted and rejected through several cycles during the past two centuries.

Idiopathic neuralgia: Nerve pain not due to any apparent cause.

Iliotibial band syndrome: A syndrome of knee pain that may result from inflammation due to mechanical friction of the iliotibial band and the lateral femoral epicondyle.

Intermittent claudication: A condition caused by ischemia of the muscles; characterized by attacks of lameness and pain brought on by walking, chiefly in the calf muscles; however, the condition may occur in other muscle groups. (Synonyms: myasthenia angiosclerotica, Charcot syndrome.)

Interstitial cystitis: A chronic inflammatory condition of unknown etiology involving the epithelium and muscularis of the bladder, resulting in reduced bladder capacity, pain relieved by voiding, and severe bladder irritative symptoms.

Intractable pain: Pain resistant or refractory to ordinary analgesic agents.

Ischemia: Local anemia due to mechanical obstruction (mainly arterial narrowing or disruption) of the blood supply.

Local anesthetics: Drugs used for the interruption of the nerve transmission of pain sensations. They act at the site of application to prevent perception of pain; examples include procaine and lidocaine.

Migraine: A symptom complex occurring periodically and characterized by pain in the head (usually unilateral), vertigo, nausea and vomiting, photophobia, and scintillating appearances of light. Classified as classic migraine, common migraine, cluster headache, hemiplegic migraine, ophthalmoplegic migraine, and ophthalmic migraine. (Synonyms: bilious headache, blind headache, sick headache, vascular headache, hemicrania.)

Myalgia: Muscular pain. (Synonym: myodynia.)

Myofascial syndrome: Irritation of the muscles and fascia of the back and neck causing acute and chronic pain not associated with any neurologic or bony evidence of disease; presumed to arise primarily from poorly understood changes in the muscle and fascia themselves.

Neuralgia: Pain of a severe, throbbing, or stabbing character in the course or distribution of a nerve. (Synonym: neurodynia.)

Neuropathy: A disease involving the cranial nerves or the peripheral or autonomic nervous system. (Synonyms: neuritis, neuropathia.)

Nociceptive: Capable of appreciation or transmission of pain.

Opiate receptors: Regions of the brain that have the capacity to bind morphine; some, along the aqueduct of Sylvius and in the center median, are in areas related to pain, but others, as in the striatum, are not related.

Osteoarthritis: Arthritis characterized by erosion of articular cartilage, either primary or secondary to trauma or other conditions, which becomes soft, frayed, and thinned with eburnation of subchondral bone and outgrowths of marginal osteophytes; pain and loss of function result; mainly affects weight-bearing joints, is more common in older persons. (Synonyms: degenerative arthritis, arthrosis, degenerative joint disease, osteoarthrosis.)

Paresthesia: An abnormal sensation, such as of burning, pricking, tickling, or tingling.

Patient-controlled analgesia (PCA): A method for control of pain based upon a pump for the constant intravenous or, less frequently, epidural infusion of a dilute narcotic solution that includes a mechanism for the self-administration at predetermined intervals of a predetermined amount of the narcotic solution should the infusion fail to relieve pain. (Synonyms: outpatient anesthesia, patient-controlled anesthesia.)

Phantom limb pain: The sensation that an amputated limb is still present, often associated with painful paresthesia. (Synonyms: stump hallucination, phantom limb, pseudesthesia, pseudoesthesia.)

Polymyalgia: Pain in several muscle groups.

Polyneuropathy: 1) A disease process involving a number of peripheral nerves (literal sense). 2) A nontraumatic generalized disorder of peripheral nerves, affecting the distal fibers most severely, with proximal shading (for example, the feet are affected sooner or more severely than the hands), and typically symmetrically; most often affects motor and sensory fibers almost equally, but can involve either one solely or very disproportionately; classified as axon degenerating (axonal), or demyelinating; many causes, particularly metabolic and toxic; familial or sporadic in nature.

Posttraumatic neck syndrome: A clinical complex of pain, tenderness, tight neck musculature, vasomotor instability, and ill-defined symptoms such as dizziness and blurred vision as the result of trauma to the neck. Also variously termed occipital or suboccipital neuralgia or neuritis; cervical tension syndrome; cervical myospasm, myositis, or fibrositis. (Synonyms: cervical fibrositis, cervical tension syndrome.)

Psychogenic pain disorder: A disorder in which the principal complaint is pain that is out of proportion to objective findings and that is related to psychological factors.

Psychophysiology: The science of the relation between psychologic and physiologic processes; for example, elements of autonomic nervous system activity activated by emotion.

Radial tunnel syndrome: Pain in the lateral aspect of the elbow and forearm without motor or sensory deficits, resulting from compression of the radial nerve, at any of various sites along its course, as it passes the elbow and the proximal forearm.

Referred pain: Pain from deep structures perceived as arising from a surface area remote from its actual origin; the area where the pain is appreciated is innervated by the same spinal segment(s) as the deep structure. (Synonym: telalgia.)

Reflex sympathetic dystrophy (RSD): Diffuse persistent pain usually in an extremity often associated with vasomotor disturbances, trophic changes, and limitation or immobility of joints; frequently follows some local injury. (See Also: Causalgia.) (Synonyms: sympathetic reflex dystrophy, shoulder-hand syndrome.)

Runner's knee: An overuse syndrome of anterior knee pain associated with excessive lateral motion of the patella during activity. (Synonym: patellofemoral stress syndrome.)

Sciatica: Pain in the lower back and hip radiating down the back of the thigh into the leg, initially attributed to sciatic nerve dysfunction (hence the term), but now known to usually be due to herniated lumbar disk compromising a nerve root, most commonly the L5 or S1 root. (Synonyms: sciatic neuralgia, sciatic neuritis.)

Shin-splints: Tenderness and pain with induration and swelling of pretibial muscles, following athletic overexertion by the untrained; it may be a mild form of anterior tibial compartment syndrome.

Subchondral: Beneath or below the cartilages of the ribs.

Substance P: A peptide neurotransmitter composed of 11 amino acid residues (with the carboxyl group amidated), normally present in minute quantities in the nervous system and intestines of humans and various animals and found in inflamed tissue, that is primarily involved in pain transmission and is one of the most potent compounds affecting smooth muscle (dilation of blood vessels and contraction of intestine) and thus presumed to play a role in inflammation.

Trigeminal neuralgia: Severe, paroxysmal bursts of pain in one or more branches of the trigeminal nerve; often induced by touching trigger points in or about the mouth. (Synonyms: Fothergill disease, epileptiform neuralgia, facial neuralgia, Fothergill neuralgia, trifacial neuralgia, tic douloureux.)

Trigeminal: Relating to the fifth cranial or trigeminus nerve.

Chapter 89

How to Find Pain-Related Medical Information

You May Want More Information

Searching for medical information can be confusing, especially for first-timers. However, if you are patient and stick to it, you can find a wealth of information. Today's computer technology is making it easier than ever for people to track down medical and health information. There are also many other sources of medical information available in textbooks, journal articles, and reference books and from healthcare organizations. This chapter explains how to locate these important sources of information.

Where to Find Medical Information

- Community library
- Federal Government clearinghouses
- Associations and voluntary organizations
- Medical, hospital, or university libraries
- Personal physician
- Nurse, pharmacist, dietitian, or other health professional
- Telephone or fax services
- Computer databases
- The internet

Start with Your Community Library

Most people have a library in or near their community, and it's a good place to start to look for medical information. Before going to the library, you may find it helpful to make a list of topics you want information about and questions you have. Also, if you've received a National Institute of Arthritis and Musculoskeletal and Skin Diseases (NIAMS) or National Arthritis and Musculoskeletal and Skin Diseases Information Clearinghouse (NAMSIC), information package, you'll notice the list of additional references at the end of most articles. You may want to get a copy of some of these articles. Your topic list and the information package will make it easier for the librarian to direct you to the best resources.

Basic Medical References

Many community libraries have a collection of basic medical references. These references may include medical dictionaries or encyclopedias, drug information handbooks, basic medical and nursing textbooks, and directories of physicians and medical specialists (listings of doctors). You may also wish to find magazine articles on a certain topic. Look in the *Reader's Guide to Periodical Literature* for articles on health and medicine that were published in consumer magazines.

Other Resources

Infotrac, a CD-ROM computer database you're most likely to find at a public library, indexes hundreds of popular magazines and newspapers, as well as some medical journals such as the *Journal of the American Medical Association* and *New England Journal of Medicine*. Your library may also carry MEDLINE®, *Index Medicus, Abridged Index Medicus*, or the *Cumulative Index to Nursing and Allied Health Literature* in print format or on a computer database. The *Consumer Health and Nutrition Index* may be available in print form as well. These resources will help you find journal articles written for health professionals. Many of the indexes have abstracts that provide a summary of each journal article. Articles published in medical journals can be technical, but they may be the most current source of information on medical topics.

Interlibrary Loans

Although most community libraries don't have a large collection of medical and nursing journals, your librarian may be able to get copies of the articles you want. Interlibrary loans allow your librarian to request a copy of an article from a library that carries that particular medical journal. Your library may charge a fee for this service.

Medical and Health Directories

You may find many useful medical and health information directories at your library. Ask your librarian about the following resources: (Names of resources and organizations included in this text are provided as examples only, and their inclusion does not mean that they are endorsed by the National Institutes of Health or any other Government agency. Also, if a particular resource or organization is not mentioned, this does not mean or imply that it is unsatisfactory.)

- White, B.J., & Madone, E., editors. *The Self-Help Sourcebook: The Comprehensive Reference of Self-Help Group Resources*. 6th edition. Denville, NJ: Northwest Covenant Medical Center, 1997—lists over 700 organizations that offer support groups.

- Rees, A., editor. *The Consumer Health Information Sourcebook*. 5th edition. Phoenix, AZ: Oryx Press, 1997—lists information clearinghouses, books, and other resources.

- *Medical and Health Information Directory*. 9th edition. Detroit, MI: Gale Research, 1997—includes publications, organizations, libraries, and health services (three volumes).

- *Directory of Physicians in the United States*. Chicago, IL: American Medical Association (AMA) updated yearly—provides information such as address, medical school attended, year of license, specialty, and certifications for physicians who are members of the AMA.

- *The Official ABMS Directory of Board Certified Medical Specialists*. New Providence, NJ: Marquis Who's Who, updated yearly—provides information on physicians certified in various specialties by the American Board of Medical Specialists.

- *Health Hotlines*—a booklet of toll-free numbers of health information hotlines available from the National Library of Medicine (NLM) or on the internet at http://sis.nlm.nih.gov/hotlines/.

If you find a particularly useful book at the library, you can buy a copy at your local bookstore. If the book isn't in stock, your bookstore can probably order a copy for you.

Some medical references have been converted from book form to a CD-ROM or floppy disk for use on a personal computer. If you have a computer with a CD-ROM drive, color monitor, and sound card, you can use compact disks to locate medical information. Check with your local bookstore or computer store for software programs that contain health information.

Some Popular References for the Home Library

American Medical Association Complete Guide to Women's Health. 1996; and *American Medical Association Family Medical Guide.* 3rd edition. 1994. New York, NY: Random House (available in book and CD-ROM format).

Everything You Need To Know About Medical Tests. Springhouse, PA: Springhouse Corporation, 1996.

Johns Hopkins Symptoms and Remedies: The Complete Home Medical Reference. New York, NY: Medletter Associates, Inc., 1995.

Mayo Clinic Family Health. 3rd edition. New York, NY: William Morrow, Inc., 1997 (available as a book, CD-ROM, or computer disk).

Professional Guide to Disease. 6th edition. Springhouse, PA: Springhouse Corporation, 1998.

The Columbia University College of Physicians and Surgeons Complete Home Medical Guide. 3rd edition. New York, NY: Crown Publishers, 1995.

The Merck Manual of Medical Information (Home Edition). Rahway, NJ: The Merck Publishing Group, 1997.

Take Advantage of Services Provided by the Federal Government and Other Organizations

Federal Government

The Federal Government operates a number of clearinghouses and information centers— National Arthritis and Musculoskeletal and Skin Diseases Information Clearinghouse (NAMSIC) is one of them. Services vary but may include publications, referrals, and answers to consumer inquiries. To obtain a free list of Federal information clearinghouses, visit the National Health Information Center's home page (http://NHIC-nt.health.org/), write to P.O. Box 1133, Washington, DC 20013–1133, or call (800) 336–4797.

Associations and Voluntary Organizations

Many associations and voluntary organizations are excellent sources of information. Some are devoted to specific diseases or conditions, such as the Scleroderma Foundation, National Alopecia Areata Foundation, National Psoriasis Foundation, and numerous others. Other organizations, such as the American Association of Retired Persons, serve a particular population group and provide a variety of information, including health-related topics. Your librarian or a NAMSIC information specialist can help you locate appropriate organizations and support networks. Many of these organizations offer referrals, publications, newsletters, educational programs, and local support groups. Your doctor may be able to tell you about support groups in your community as well.

Examples of Health-Related Associations and Organizations

- American Academy of Dermatology
- American College of Rheumatology
- American Academy of Orthopaedic Surgeons
- Arthritis Foundation
- American Skin Association
- Lupus Foundation of America

There are many more organizations; call NAMSIC for additional information.

Look for a Medical Library

Medical libraries can usually be found at medical, nursing, and dental schools; large medical centers; and community hospitals. Not all hospital or academic libraries are open to the public, but a librarian at your community library may be able to give you information about the closest medical library open to the public. Medical libraries may also be listed in your telephone book under "hospitals," "schools," or "universities." In addition, you can call the National Network of Libraries of Medicine of the National Library of Medicine

(NLM), National Institutes of Health, at (800) 338–7657 to find the location of the nearest regional medical library.

A medical library has a large collection of resources, including many medical and nursing textbooks and a comprehensive collection of medical and health-related journals. Although you may not be allowed to check out materials, most libraries have photocopiers you can use to copy material you want to take home.

Library Resources

- Medical dictionaries
- Medical encyclopedias
- Directories of board-certified medical specialists
- Medical and health information directories
- Medical, nursing, and allied health textbooks
- Medical and diagnostic laboratory testing manuals
- Drug reference books
- Computer databases

Investigate Other Options for Finding Information

People who are unable to get to a community or medical library have several options for finding additional medical information. Some community libraries provide access to online databases that can be searched from a home computer via a modem. In addition, your doctor, nurse, pharmacist, or dietitian, or the patient education department at your local hospital may be able to provide you with pamphlets, brochures, and journal articles or direct you to classes, seminars, and health screenings.

Use Telephone and Fax Services

Some communities have a telephone medical service that allows callers to listen to audiotapes on certain disease topics. Also, your health insurance company or health maintenance organization may have a nurse available to answer health-related questions over the telephone.

If you have access to a fax machine, you can get health information from some organizations in just a few minutes. If a faxback system is available, use the telephone on your fax machine to call the faxback number of the organization and listen to the instructions. In most cases, you can request a list or menu of information to be sent to you first. To get information quickly by fax from NAMSIC, dial (301) 881–2731 from a fax machine telephone to access *NIAMS Fast Facts*. Request document number 5 to receive a list of topics. You can get fact sheets on many different topics from *NIAMS Fast Facts*.

Other organizations also have information available by fax; for example, the Centers for Disease Control and Prevention at (404) 332–4565. Your librarian can help you locate other fax services.

Explore Computer Databases

The computer has become an important tool for helping people locate medical and health information quickly and easily. Most software and information services are user friendly and allow people with no formal training in computer searching to use databases to obtain information. Using a computer at home or in the library, you can find health information by searching CD-ROM databases, searching online on the internet, or using a health-related software program.

As mentioned earlier, many public libraries have Infotrac, a database that includes consumer health information. It indexes popular magazines and newspapers and 2 to 4 years' worth of medical publications. Medical libraries have more extensive medical databases. Start with the following list and ask your librarian to help you find the most appropriate CD-ROM or online (internet) databases for your needs:

- MEDLARS (Medical Literature Analysis and Retrieval Systems). For more technical information, you can search one of the MEDLARS databases. MEDLARS is a collection of over 40 databases created by or available from the National Library of Medicine (see below for more information on the NLM). Some of these databases are available only in CD-ROM format, while others are online.

- MEDLINE®. The largest and best known of the MEDLARS databases, MEDLINE® contains citations and often abstracts for over 9 million articles in 3,900 biomedical journals on all aspects of biomedicine and allied health fields from 1966 to the present. MEDLINE® is available at medical and university libraries, at some community libraries, and through a variety of fee-based and free internet sites, including the NLM website at http://www.nlm.nih.gov/.

587

- DIRLINE®. This database, a part of MEDLARS, contains location and description information about a wide variety of resources, including organizations, research resources, projects, databases, and electronic bulletin boards concerned with health and biomedicine. The database is available online through the NLM at no fee.

- CHID (Combined Health Information Database). Developed and managed by health-related agencies of the Federal Government, this database can help people find information and educational resources such as brochures, books, and audiovisuals on selected topics. CHID contains 18 subfiles, including the Arthritis and Musculoskeletal and Skin Diseases subfile. It is available on the internet at no fee at http://chid.nih.gov/.

Search the Internet

The internet is a worldwide network of computers that can exchange information almost instantaneously. The world wide web (abbreviated www in computer addresses), or more simply, the web, is a system of electronic documents, linked together and available on the internet for anyone with a computer, a modem, and an internet provider account. While the terms "internet" and "world wide web" are often used interchangeably, the web is actually the part of the internet that supports the use of graphics, pictures, sound, and even video.

If you have access to the web, you can find information on everything from the latest medical research to facts on particular conditions. You may have access at home or at work to internet databases through a commercial service such as America Online or through a local internet provider. Many public libraries have computer stations that provide internet access.

You'll find extensive health and medical information on the internet. America Online and other internet providers and sites offer MEDLINE®; some sites may charge a search fee. The internet also offers other resources such as bulletin boards, online publications, forums for discussion of current medical issues, and online support groups. For example, the American Self-Help Clearinghouse offers an online version of its *Self-Help Sourcebook* at http://www.cmhc.com/selfhelp/welcome.htm/ that provides information on support groups and networks available in your community and throughout the world. The site also provides a link to the Self-Help Resource Room that contains information about online support groups and other health resources.

Help with Searching on the Internet

Searching for health information on the internet can be confusing and difficult. The sheer volume of information can be overwhelming, and people often find it difficult to narrow down search topics or find specific websites. Although an internet search engine such as YA-HOO!® or Infoseek is meant to help you find information, search results on specific topics often reveal thousands of websites, many of which may be unrelated to the information you want. You may want to get a copy of a reference book that provides tips on how to find health information on the internet. *Health Online*, by Tom Ferguson, M.D. (Addison-Wesley Publishing Company, 1996), is an example of one reference that can help you use the internet to find health information and support groups.

National Library of Medicine

You can search the NLM's MEDLINE® database, free of charge, on the web. The link to this database can be found on the NLM home page at http://www.nlm.nih.gov/. You can conduct a search in one of two web-based products, PubMed or Internet Grateful Med. Both provide you with free access to MEDLINE® and, for a fee, allow you to use Loansome Doc Delivery Service to order copies of articles. PubMed links you to publishers' sites for approximately 100 full-text journals; some are by subscription only. Internet Grateful Med also gives you access to other databases, including AIDSLINE, HealthSTAR, AIDSDRUGS, and AIDSTRIALS.

healthfinder®

To help people find health information on the internet, the Federal Government's Department of Health and Human Services has developed a website—healthfinder® (http://www.healthfinder.gov/). This site serves as a gateway or point of entry to the broad range of consumer health information resources produced by the Federal Government and many of its partners. healthfinder® includes a searchable index and locator aids for news, publications, online journals, support and self-help groups, online discussions, and toll-free numbers.

Some Health Resources to Check Out on the WWW

National Institute of Arthritis and Musculoskeletal and Skin Diseases
http://www.nih.gov/niams/

National Institutes of Health
http://www.nih.gov/

CHID
http://chid.nih.gov/

healthfinder®
http://www.healthfinder.gov/

National Library of Medicine
http://www.nlm.nih.gov/

Agency for Health Care Policy and Research
http://www.ahcpr.gov/

Arthritis Foundation
http://www.arthritis.org/

American Academy of Dermatology
http://www.aad.org/

Don't Believe Everything You Read

As you make purchases for your home library or search the internet, keep in mind that not all information is written by qualified medical experts. Your doctor or a health organization may be able to recommend some good books or helpful internet sites. When looking for health information on the internet, don't believe everything you see. Articles published in peer-reviewed medical journals are checked for accuracy, but anyone can put information on the internet, so there's no guarantee that the information you find is accurate or up-to-date. In addition, many companies set up websites primarily to sell their products. It may be helpful to ask a health professional about the information you find on the internet, particularly before you buy any products. If you search and shop with care, you can add some medically sound reference materials to your home library and find accurate information on the internet.

Use Information Wisely

It can be hard to judge the accuracy and credibility of medical information you read in books or magazines, see on television, or find on the internet. Even people with medical backgrounds sometimes find this task challenging. Following are some important tips to help you decide what information is believable and accurate.

Books, Articles, and Television Reports

- Compare several different resources on the same topic. Check two or three other articles or books to see whether the information or advice is similar.

- Check the author's credentials by looking up his or her affiliations, such as university and medical school attended, associations, and lists of other publications. For doctors, this information can be found in one of the physician directories at your library or on the AMA's website at http://www.ama-assn.org/ (click on AMA Physician Select). You can also call the American Board of Medical Specialists at (800) 776–2378 to see whether a physician is board certified in his or her specialty. Your librarian can help you find other resources to check the credentials of nonphysicians.

- Ask yourself if the information or advice "rings true." That is, is it feasible, plausible, and common sense, or is it wishful thinking or sensationalism?

- Look for a list of references at the end of the article or book. Information that is backed up by other medical professionals and researchers is more likely to be accurate.

- Check out your information source. Was the article published in a peer-reviewed journal? Look for a list of editorial or review board members at the beginning of a journal. In a peer-reviewed journal, articles are reviewed by other qualified members of the profession for accuracy and reliability.

- Look very carefully at information published in newspapers and magazines or reported on television. Most reporters are journalists rather than medical experts. In addition, newspapers and television reporters may use sensationalism to attract more readers or viewers. Medical facts and statistics can be misrepresented or incomplete. Check to see whether the newspaper or magazine cites a source for its information and includes the credentials of the persons cited.

- Examine a magazine's list of editors. Do medical experts serve as editors and review articles? Be especially wary of personal testimonials of miracle cures. There's often no way of judging whether the story is true. Furthermore, don't trust medical

591

product advertisements claiming miracle cures or spectacular results.

The Internet

- Compare the information you find on the internet with other resources. Check two or three articles in the medical literature or medical textbooks to see whether the information or advice is similar.

- Check the author's or organization's credentials. They should be clearly displayed on the website. If the credentials are missing, consider this a red flag. Unfortunately, there are many phony doctors and other health professionals making false claims on the internet.

- Find out if the website is maintained by a reputable health organization. Remember that no one regulates information on the internet. Anyone can set up a home page and claim anything. Some reliable websites providing health information include Government agencies, health foundations and associations, and medical colleges.

- Be wary of websites advertising and selling products that claim to improve your health. More important, be very careful about giving out credit-card information on the internet. Further, even if nothing is being sold on a website, ask yourself if the site host has an interest in promoting a particular product or service.

- Ask yourself whether the information or advice seems to contradict what you've learned from your doctor. If so, talk to your doctor to clarify the differences in the information.

- Be cautious when using information found on bulletin boards or during "chat" sessions with others. Testimonials and personal stories are based on one person's experience rather than on objective facts or proven medical research.

To Make Informed Decisions about Your Health Care, You Need to Understand Your Health Problem

Medical information, especially material written for health care providers, can be hard to understand, confusing, and sometimes frightening. As you read through your materials, write down any words or information you don't understand or find confusing. Make a list of your questions and concerns. During your next office visit, ask your doctor, nurse, or other health professional to review the information with you so that you understand clearly how it might be helpful to you.

If the medical information you gathered is for a personal health problem, you may want to share what you found with your spouse, other family members, or a close friend. Family members and friends who understand your health problem are better able to provide needed support and care. Finally, you might want to consider joining a support group in your community.

Chapter 90

Pain Treatment Facility Classification

Facilities for the treatment of patients with chronic pain have developed rapidly in the past fifteen years. There have been few, if any, governmental or professional standards or controls for such patient care facilities, even in the developed nations of the world. In the United States of America, pain treatment facilities that exist within hospitals are theoretically evaluated under the aegis of the Joint Committee on the Accreditation of Hospitals, but the accreditation process does not specifically assess the pain treatment facility. Freestanding pain treatment programs and those within hospitals may also obtain voluntary certification from the Commission on Accreditation of Rehabilitation Facilities through a program instituted with assistance from the American Pain Society in 1983. In other countries, both governmental agencies and the national chapters of the International Association for the Study of Pain (IASP®) have developed some standards. Governmental health care systems in some countries regulate all aspects of the provision of health care, and the freedom to establish new types of health care delivery is limited.

The International Association for the Study of Pain believes that patients throughout the world would benefit from the establishment of a set of desirable characteristics for pain treatment facilities. Although

Excerpted from "Desirable Characteristics for Pain Treatment Facilities," Task Force on Guidelines for Desirable Characteristics for Pain Treatment Facilities, International Association for the Study of Pain®. © 1990, reviewed for currency in 2001; reprinted with permission. Full text is available online at www.iasp-pain.org/desirabl.html.

IASP itself does not plan to offer certification or accreditation, the standards set forth in this chapter can serve as a guideline for both practitioners and those governmental or professional organizations involved in the establishment of standards for this type of health care delivery. The field of pain management has been viewed with skepticism by many physicians and health policy and funding administrators; reasonable guidelines should be established and adhered to by reputable treatment facilities.

It is important to recognize that not every patient referred to a pain treatment facility requires the services of a large number of health care professionals. Nonetheless, many pain patients do require the services of multiple disciplines and resources must be available to effectively manage the patient. It is on the basis of the types of resources available that the following classification scheme has been proposed.

Pain treatment facility: A generic term used to describe all forms of pain treatment facilities without regard to personnel involved or types of patients served. Pain unit is a synonym for pain treatment facility.

Multidisciplinary pain center: An organization of health care professionals and basic scientists which includes research, teaching and patient care related to acute and chronic pain. This is the largest and most complex of the pain treatment facilities and ideally would exist as a component of a medical school or teaching hospital. Clinical programs must be supervised by an appropriately trained and licensed clinical director; a wide array of health care specialists is required, such as physicians, psychologists, nurses, physical therapists, occupational therapists, vocational counselors, social workers and other specialized health care providers.

The disciplines of health care providers required is a function of the varieties of patients seen and the health care resources of the community. The members of the treatment team must communicate with each other on a regular basis, both about specific patients and about overall development. Health care services in a multidisciplinary pain clinic must be integrated and based upon multidisciplinary assessment and management of the patient. Inpatient and outpatient programs are offered in such a facility.

Multidisciplinary pain clinic: A health care delivery facility staffed by physicians of different specialties and other non-physician health care providers who specialize in the diagnosis and management of patients with chronic pain. This type of facility differs from a Multidisciplinary Pain Center only because it does not include research and teaching activities in its regular programs. A Multidisciplinary pain clinic may have diagnostic and treatment facilities which are outpatient, inpatient or both.

Pain clinic: A health care delivery facility focusing upon the diagnosis and management of patients with chronic pain. A pain clinic may specialize in specific diagnoses or in pains related to a specific region of the body. A pain clinic may be large or small but it should never be a label for an isolated solo practitioner. A single physician functioning within a complex health care institution which offers appropriate consultative and therapeutic services could qualify as a pain clinic, if chronic pain patients were suitably assessed and managed. The absence of interdisciplinary assessment and management distinguishes this type of facility from a multidisciplinary pain center or clinic. Pain clinics can, and should be encouraged to, carry out research, but it is not a required characteristic of this type of facility.

Modality-oriented clinic: This is a health care facility which offers a specific type of treatment and does not provide comprehensive assessment or management. Examples include nerve block clinic, transcutaneous nerve stimulation clinic, acupuncture clinic, biofeedback clinic, etc. Such a facility may have one or more health care providers with different professional training; because of its limited treatment options and the lack of an integrated, comprehensive approach, it does not qualify for the term, multidisciplinary.

Chapter 91

Information Resources for Pain Patients

Administration on Aging
Department of Health and Human Services (DHHS)
330 Independence Avenue, SW
Washington, DC 20201
Toll Free: 800-677-1116
(Eldercare Locator)
Phone: 202-619-7501
TTY: 800-877-8339
Fax: 202-260-1012
Website: http://www.aoa.gov
E-Mail: AoAInfo@aoa.gov

Agency for Healthcare Research and Quality
Publications Clearinghouse
P.O. Box 8547
Silver Spring, MD 20907-8547
Toll Free: 800-358-9295
Phone: 410-381-3150
TDD: 888-586-6340
Website: http://www.ahrq.gov
E-Mail: ahrqpubs@ahrq.gov

American Academy of Family Physicians (AAFP)
11400 Tomahawk Creek Parkway
Leawood, KS 66211-2672
Toll Free: 800-274-2237
Phone: 913-906-6000
Fax: 913-906-6094
Website: http://familydoctor.org
E-Mail: email@familydoctor.org

American Academy of Neurology (AAN)
1080 Montreal Avenue
St. Paul, MN 55116
Phone: 651-695-1940
Fax: 651-695-2791
Website: http://www.aan.com
E-Mail: web@aan.com

Resources in this chapter were compiled from several sources deemed reliable; all contact information was verified and updated in February 2002.

American Academy of Orthopaedic Surgeons (AAOS)
6300 North River Road
Rosemont, IL 60018-4262
Toll Free: 800-346-AAOS
Phone: 847-823-7186
Fax: 847-823-8125
Website: http://www.aaos.org
E-Mail: custserv@aaos.org

American Academy of Pain Management
13947 Mono Way, #A
Sonora, CA 95370
Phone: 209-533-9744
Website: http://
www.aapainmanage.org
E-Mail:
aapm@aapainmanage.org

American Academy of Physical Medicine and Rehabilitation (AAPMR)
One IBM Plaza, Suite 2500
Chicago, IL 60611-3604
Phone: 312-464-9700
Fax: 312-464-0227
Website: http://www.aapmr.org
E-Mail: info@aapmr.org

American Association of Endodontists
211 East Chicago Ave.
Suite 1100
Chicago, IL 60611-2691
Toll Free: 800-872-3636
Phone: 312-266-7255
Fax: 312-266-9867
Website: http://www.aae.org
E-Mail: info@aae.org

American Association of Neurological Surgeons/ Congress of Neurological Surgeons
5550 Meadowbrook Drive
Rolling Meadows, IL 60025
Toll Free: 888-566-2267
Phone: 847-378-0500
Fax: 847-378-0600
Website: http://
www.neurosurgery.org
E-Mail: info@aans.org

American Cancer Society (ACS)
1599 Clifton Road, NE
Atlanta, GA 30329
Toll Free: 800-ACS-2345 (227-2345)
Phone: 404-320-3333
Fax: 404-329-5787
Website: http://www.cancer.org

American Chiropractic Association (ACA)
1701 Clarendon Boulevard
Arlington, VA 22209
Toll Free: 800-986-4636
Phone: 703-276-8800
Fax: 703-243-2593
Website: http://
www.amerchiro.org
E-Mail:
memberinfo@amerchiro.org

American Chronic Pain Association
P.O. Box 850
Rocklin, CA 95677-0850
Phone: 916-632-0922
Website: http://www.theacpa.org

American College of Sports Medicine (ACSM)
401 W. Michigan St.
Indianapolis, IN 46206-3233
Phone: 317-637-9200
Fax: 317-634-7817
Website: http://www.acsm.org

American College of Surgeons (ACS)
633 North St. Clair Street
Chicago, IL 60611-3211
Phone: 312-202-5000
Fax: 312-202-5001
Website: http://www.facs.org
E-Mail: postmaster@facs.org

American Council for Headache Education
19 Mantua Road
Mt. Royal, NJ 08061
Phone: 856-423-0258
Fax: 856-423-0082
Website: http://www.achenet.org
E-Mail: achehq@talley.com

American Dental Association (ADA)
211 East Chicago Avenue
Chicago, IL 60611
Phone: 312-440-2500
Fax: 312-440-2800
Website: http://www.ada.org

American Diabetes Association (ADA)
1701 North Beauregard Street
Arlington, VA 22311
Toll Free: 800-DIABETES
Phone: 703-549-1500
Website: http://www.diabetes.org

American Heart Association (AHA)
7272 Greenville Avenue
Dallas, TX 75231
Toll Free: Phone: 800-AHA-USA1
(242-8721)
Fax: 214-706-2139
Website: http://www.americanheart.org

American Medical Association (AMA)
515 North State Street
Chicago, IL 60610
Toll Free: 800-621-8335
Phone: 312-464-5000
Fax: 312-464-5600
Website: http://www.ama-assn.org

American Occupational Therapy Association, Inc. (AOTA)
4720 Montgomery Lane
P.O. Box 31220
Bethesda, MD 20824-1220
Phone: 301-652-2682
Fax: 301-652-7711
TDD: 800-377-8555
Website: http://www.aota.org
E-Mail: praota@aota.org

American Osteopathic Association
142 East Ontario Street
Chicago, IL 60611
Toll Free: 800-621-1773
Phone: 312-202-8000
Fax: 312-202-8200
Website: http://www.aoa-net.org
E-Mail: info@aoa-net.org

601

American Pain Foundation
201 N. Charles Street, Suite 710
Baltimore, MD 21202
Toll Free: 888-615-7246
Phone: 410-385-5276
Website: http://
www.painfoundation.org
E-Mail: info@painfoundation.org

American Pain Society
4700 W. Lake Avenue
Glenview, IL 60025
Phone: 847-375-4715
Fax: 877-734-8758
Website: http://
www.ampainsoc.org
E-Mail: info@ampainsoc.org

American Pharmaceutical Association (APhA)
2215 Constitution Avenue, NW
Washington, DC 20037-2985
Toll Free: 800-237-2742
Phone: 202-628-4410
Fax: 202-783-2351
Website: http://
www.pharmacyandyou.org
E-Mail:
webmaster@mail.aphanet.org

American Physical Therapy Association (APTA)
1111 North Fairfax Street
Alexandria, VA 22314
Toll Free: 800-999-2782, ext. 3395
Phone: 703-684-2782
Fax: 703-684-7343
TDD: 703-683-6748
Website: http://www.apta.org

American Society of Anesthesiologists
520 N. Northwest Hwy.
Park Ridge, IL 60068-2573
Phone: 847-825-5586
Fax: 847-825-1692
Website: http://www.asahq.org
E-Mail: mail@asahq.org

Arthritis Foundation (AF)
National Office
1330 West Peachtree Street
Atlanta, GA 30309
Toll Free: 800-283-7800
Phone: 404-965-7537
Fax: 404-872-0457
Website: http://
www.arthritis.org
E-Mail: help@arthritis.org

Association for the Care of Children's Health
Dalhouise University
Halifax, Nova Scotia B3H 4J1
Canada
Phone: 902-494-3581
Fax: 902-464-6585
Website: http://www.pediatric-pain.ca

Cancer Care
275 7th Avenue, 22nd Floor
New York, NY 10001
Toll Free: 800-813-4673
Phone: 212-712-8400
Website: http://
www.cancercare.org
E-Mail: info@cancercare.org

*Centers for Disease Control
and Prevention (CDC)*
1600 Clifton Road
Atlanta, GA 30333
Toll Free: 800-311-3435
Phone: 404-639-3311
TTY: 800-255-0135
Fax: 404-639-7392
Website: http://www.cdc.gov
E-Mail: netinfo@cdc.gov

*Dannemiller Memorial
Education Foundation*
12500 Network Blvd., Suite 101
San Antonio, TX 78249-3302
Toll Free: 800-328-2308
Phone: 210-641-8329
Website: http://www.pain.com
E-Mail: dannemiller@pain.com

*Department of Veterans
Affairs (VA)*
Office of Public Affairs
810 Vermont Avenue, NW
Washington, DC 20420
Toll Free: 800-827-1000
Website: http://www.va.gov

*Disabled American
Veterans (DAV)*
3725 Alexandria Pike
Cold Spring, KY 41076
Phone: 859-441-7300
Website: http://www.dav.org

Fibromyalgia Network
P.O. Box 31750
Tuscon, AZ 85751-1750
Toll Free: 800-853-2929
Phone: 520-290-5508
Website: http://
www.fmnetnews.com

*Food and Drug
Administration (FDA)*
HFE88
5600 Fishers Lane
Rockville, MD 20857
Toll Free: 888-INFO-FDA
Website: http://www.fda.gov

*The International Pelvic
Pain Society*
Women's Medical Plaza, Ste. 402
2006 Brookwood Medical Ctr. Dr.
Birmingham, AL 35209
Toll Free: 800-624-9676
Phone: 205-877-2950
Website: http://
www.pelvicpain.org

National Cancer Institute
Public Inquiries Office
Building 31, Room 10A03
31 Center Drive MSC 2580
Bethesda, MD 20892-2580
Toll Free: 800-4-CANCER
Phone: 301-435-3848
TTY: 800-332-8615
Website: http://www.nci.nih.gov
E-Mail: webmaster@cancer.gov

*National Center for
Complementary and
Alternative Medicine
(NCCAM) Clearinghouse*
P.O. Box 7923
Silver Spring, MD 20898
Toll Free: 888-644-6226
TTY: 866-464-3615
Fax: 866-464-3616
Website: http://
www.nccam.nih.gov
E-Mail: info@nccam.nih.gov

National Chronic Pain Outreach Association
P.O. Box 274
Millboro, VA 25560
Phone: 540-862-9437
Fax: 540-862-9485

National Council on Patient Information and Education (NCPIE)
4915 Saint Elmo Avenue
Suite 505
Bethesda, MD 20814-6082
Phone: 301-656-8565
Fax: 301-656-4464
Website: http://
www.talkaboutrx.org
E-Mail: ncpie@erols.com

National Chronic Pain Outreach
P.O. Box 274
Millboro, VA 24460
Phone: 540-862-9437
Fax: 540-862-9485
E-Mail: ncpoa@cfw.com

National Diabetes Information Clearinghouse (NDIC)
National Institute of Diabetes and Digestive and Kidney Diseases (NIDDK)
1 Information Way
Bethesda, MD 20892-3560
Toll Free: 800-860-8747
Phone: 301-654-3327
Fax: 301-907-8906
Website: http://
www.niddk.nih.gov
E-Mail: ndic@info.niddk.nih.gov

National Family Caregivers Association (NFCA)
10400 Connecticut Avenue, #500
Kensington, MD 20895-3944
Toll Free: 800-896-3650
Fax: 301-942-2302
Website: http://
www.nfcacares.org
E-Mail: info@nfcacares.org

National Headache Foundation
428 West St. James Place
Second Floor
Chicago, IL 60614-2750
Toll Free: 888-643-5552
Phone: 773-388-6399
Fax: 773-525-7357
Website: http://
www.headaches.org
E-Mail: info@headaches.org

National Heart, Lung, and Blood Institute (NHLBI) Information Center
P.O. Box 30105
Bethesda, MD 20824-0105
Toll Free: 800-575-WELL (9355)
(recorded information)
Phone: 301-592-8573
Fax: 301-592-8563
Website: http://
www.nhlbi.nih.gov
E-Mail:
NHLBIinfo@rover.nhlbi.nih.gov

National Hospice and Palliative Care Organization (NHPCO)
1700 Diagonal Road, Suite 300
Alexandria, VA 22314
Toll Free: 800-658-8898 (Hospice Helpline and Locator)
Phone: 703-837-1500
Fax: 703-837-1233
Website: http://www.nhpco.org
E-Mail: info@nhpco.org

National Hospice Foundation (NHF)
1700 Diagonal Road, Suite 300
Alexandria, VA 22314
Toll Free: 800-338-8619
Phone: 703-516-4928
Fax: 703-837-1233
Website: http://www.hospiceinfo.org
E-Mail: info@nhpco.org

National Institute of Arthritis and Musculoskeletal and Skin Diseases (NIAMS)
1 AMS Circle
Bethesda, MD 20892-3675
Toll Free: 877-22-NIAMS (226-4267)
Phone: 301-495-4484
TTY: 301-565-2966
Fax: 301-718-6366
Website: http://www.niams.nih.gov
E-Mail: NIAMSInfo@mail.nih.gov

National Institute of Dental and Craniofacial Research
Bethesda, MD 20892-2290
Phone: 301-496-4261
Phone: 301-402-7364 (National Oral Health Information Clearinghouse—NOHIC)
Fax: 301-907-8830
TTY: 301-656-7581
Website: http://www.nidcr.nih.gov
Website: http://www.nohic.nidcr.nih.gov
E-Mail: nidcrinfo@mail.nih.gov
E-Mail: nohic@nidcr.nih.gov

National Institute of Diabetes and Digestive and Kidney Diseases (NIDDK)
3 Information Way
Bethesda, MD 20892-3580
Toll Free: 800-891-5390
Phone: 301-654-4415
Fax: 301-907-8906
Website: http://www.niddk.nih.gov
E-Mail: nkudic@info.niddk.nih.gov

National Institute of Neurological Disorders and Stroke (NINDS)
Office of Communications and Public Liaison
Bethesda, MD 20892-2540
Toll Free: 800-352-9424
Phone: 301-496-5751
Fax: 301-402-2186
Website: http://www.ninds.nih.gov
E-Mail: info@ninds.nih.gov

National Library of Medicine (NLM)
National Institutes of Health
Bethesda, MD 20894
Toll Free: 888-FIND-NLM (346-3656)
Phone: 301-594-5983
Fax: 301-496-4450
Website: http://www.nlm.nih.gov (MEDLINE)
Website: http://medlineplus.gov (MEDLINEplus)
Website: www.clinicaltrials.gov (Clinical Trials database)
E-Mail: custserv@nlm.nih.gov

National Rehabilitation Information Center (NARIC)
4200 Forbes Boulevard
Suite 202
Lanham, MD 20706
Toll Free: 800-346-2742
Phone: 301-459-5900
Fax: 301-562-2401
Website: http://www.naric.com
E-Mail:
naricinfo@heitechservices.com

National Vulvodynia Association
P.O. Box 4491
Silver Spring, MD
20914-4491
Phone: 301-299-0775
Fax: 301-299-3999
Website: http://www.nva.org
E-Mail: mate@nva.org

The Neuropathy Association
60 E. 42nd Street, Suite 942
New York, NY 10165
Toll Free: 800-247-6968
Phone: 212-692-0662
Website: http://www.neuropathy.org
E-Mail: info@neuropathy.org

North American Chronic Pain Association of Canada
60 Lorne Avenue
Dartmouth, Nova Scotia B2Y 3E7
Canada
Toll Free: 866-470-7246
Phone: 902-463-5587
Website: http://www.chronicpaincanada.org
E-Mail:
nacpac@chronicpaincanada.org

Reflex Sympathetic Dystrophy
P.O.Box 502
Milford, CT 06460
Phone: 203-877-3790
Website: http://www.rsds.org

Resource Center for Pain Medicine and Palliative Care
Beth Israel Medical Center
First Avenue at 16th Street
New York, NY, 10003
Toll Free: 877-620-9999
Phone: 212-844-1411
Fax: 212-844-1465
Website: http://www.stoppain.org
E-Mail:
mayday@bethisraelny.org

TMJ Association, Ltd.
P.O. Box 26770
Milwaukee, WI 53226
Phone 414-259-3223
Website: http://www.tmj.org
E-Mail: info@tmj.org

**Trigeminal Neuralgia
Association**
2801 SW Archer Rd., Suite C
Gainsville, FL 32608
Phone: 352-376-9955
Fax: 352-376-8688
Website: http://www.tna-
support.org
E-Mail: tnanational@tna-
support.org

U. C. Davis Pain Center
2315 Stockton Blvd.
Sacramento, CA 95817
Phone: 916-734-2011
Website: http://
www.pain.ucdavis.edu
E-Mail:
publicaffairs@ucdavis.edu

Vulvar Pain Foundation
203½ North Main Street
Suite 203
Graham, NC 27253
Phone: 336-226-0704
Fax: 336-226-8518
Website: http://
www.vulvarpainfoundation.org

**Well Spouse Foundation
(WSF)**
P.O. Box 30093
Elkins Park, PA 19027
Toll Free: 800-838-0879
Phone: 212-685-8815
Fax: 212-685-8676
Website: http://
www.wellspouse.org
E-Mail: info@wellspouse.org

Chapter 92

Additional Reading about Pain

Books

Catalano, Ellen M.; Hardin, Kimeron N. Tupper, Shelby P. *The Chronic Pain Control Workbook: A Step-by-Step Guide for Coping with and Overcoming Pain*. Oakland, CA: Hew Harbinger Publications, 1996. ISBN 1572240504.

Catalano, Ellen M.; Hardin, Kimeron N.; Beattie, Melody. *Chronic Pain Control Workbook*. New York, NY: Fine Communications, 1997. ISBN 1567312101.

Caudill, Margaret A. *Managing Pain before It Manages You, Revised Edition*. New York: Guilford, 2002. ISBN 1572307188.

Chaitow, Leon. *Conquer Pain the Natural Way: A Practical Guide*. San Francisco, CA: Chronicle Books, 2002. ISBN 0811835804.

Chevelen, Eric M.; Smith, Wesley J. *Power Over Pain: How to Get the Pain Control You Need*. Steubenville, OH: International Task Force, 2002. ISBN 0971094608.

Egoscue, Pete; Gittines, Roger. *Pain Free: A Revolutionary Method for Stopping Chronic Pain*. New York, NY: Bantam Doubleday Dell Publishers, 2000. ISBN 0553379887.

Resources listed in this chapter were compiled from several sources. Inclusion does not constitute endorsement. This list is not considered complete; it is merely intended to serve as a starting point for readers interested in pursuing additional information. Websites were all verified and accessed in February 2002.

Egoscue, Pete; Gittines, Roger. *Pain Free for Women*. New York, NY: Bantam Books, 2002. ISBN 0553801058.

Fransen, Jenny; Russel, I. John. *The Fibromyalgia Help Book: Practical Guide to Living Better with Fibromyalgia*. Saint Paul, MN: Smith House, 1997. ISBN 0961522143.

Grady, K.M.; Severn, A.M.; Eldridge, P. *Key Topics in Chronic Pain, Second Edition*. Oxford: BIOS Scientific, 2002. ISBN 1859960383.

Hardy, Paul Aj. *Chronic Pain Management: The Essentials*. London: Greenwich Medical Media, 1997. ISBN 1900151855.

Kazanowski, Mary K.; Laccetti, Margaret Saul. *Pain*. Thorofare, NJ: Slack, 2002. ISBN 1556425228.

Klein, Arthur C. *Chronic Pain: The Complete Guide to Relief*. New York, NY: Carroll and Graf, 2001. ISBN 0786708344.

Marcus, Norman J.; Arbeiter, Jean S. *Freedom from Pain: The Breakthrough Method of Pain Relief Based on the New York Pain Treatment Program at Lenox Hill Hospital*. New York, NY: Simon and Schuster, 1995. ISBN 067151653.

Starlanyl, Devin J.; Copeland, Mary Ellen. *Fibromyalgia and Chronic Myofascial Pain: A Survival Manual, Second Edition*. Oakland, CA: New Harbinger Publications, 2001. ISBN 1572242388.

Swanson, David W. (ed). *Mayo Clinic on Chronic Pain*. New York, NY: Kensington Publishing Corp., 1999. ISBN 189300502X.

Magazine/Journal Articles

Adams, Nancy J.; Plane, Mary Beth; Fleming, Michael F.; Mundt, Marlon P.; Saunders, Laura A.; Stauffacher, Ellyn A. "Opioids and the Treatment of Chronic Pain in a Primary Care Sample," *Journal of Pain and Symptom Management*, vol. 22, no. 3, pp. 791(6), September 2001.

Aeschbach, Armin; Mekhail, Nagy A. "Common Nerve Blocks in Chronic Pain Management," *Anesthesiology Clinics of North America*, vol. 18, no. 2, pp. 429(32), 2000.

Ashburn, Michael A.; Staats, Peter S. "Pain: Management of Chronic Pain. *The Lancet*, vol. 353, no. 9167, p. 1865, May 29, 1999.

Ashby, J. S.; Scott Lenhart, R. "Prayer as a Coping Strategy for Chronic Pain Patients," *Rehabilitation Psychology*, vol. 39, no. 3, p. 205, 1994.

Assendelft, W. J.; Koes, B. W.; van der Heijden, G. J.; Bouter, L. M. "The Efficacy of Chiropractic Manipulation for Back Pain: Blinded Review of Relevant Randomized Clinical Trials," *Journal of Manipulative and Physiological Therapeutics*, vol. 15, no. 8, pp. 487-94, October 1992.

Barkin, Robert L.; Barkin, Diana. "Pain Management—Pharmacologic Management of Acute and Chronic Pain: Focus on Drug Interactions and Patient-Specific Pharmacotherapeutic Selection," *Southern Medical Journal*, vol. 94, no. 8, pp. 756(15), August 2001.

Berman, B.M.; Singh, B.B.; Hartnoll, S.M., Singh, B.K.; Reilly, D. "Primary Care Physicians and Complementary-Alternative Medicine: Training, Attitudes, and Practice Patterns," *Journal of the American Board of Family Practice*, vol. 11, no. 4, pp. 272-281, 1998.

Bonelli, Raphael M.; Reisecker, Franz Koltringer, Peter. "Prevention of Chronic Pain in Whiplash Injury," *Journal of Pain and Symptom Management*, vol. 21, no. 2, p. 92, February 2001.

Bush, Ellen Greene; Rye, Mark S.; Brant, Curtis R.; Emery, Erin; Pargament, Kenneth I.; Riessinger, Camala A. "Religious Coping with Chronic Pain," *Applied Psychophysiology and Biofeedback*, vol. 24, no. 4, pp. 249-260, 2000.

Cassuto, J.; Liss, S.; Bennett, A. "The Use of Modulated Energy Carried on a High Frequency Wave for the Relief of Intractable Pain," *International Journal of Clinical Pharmacological Research*, vol. 13, no. 4, pp. 239-41, 1993.

"Chronic Pain Management—The Patient's Perspective," *Nursing Standard*, vol. 15, no. 52, pp. 33(6), 2001.

Clark, J. David. "Chronic Pain Prevalence and Analgesic Prescribing in a General Medical Population," *Journal of Pain and Symptom Management*, vol. 23, no. 2, pp. 131(7), February 2002.

Cohen, I.; Rainville, J. "Aggressive Exercise as Treatment for Chronic Low Back Pain," *Sports Medicine*, vol. 32, no. 1, pp. 75-82, 2002.

Cole, Barbara H.; Brunk, Quincealea. "Holistic Interventions for Acute Pain Episodes: An Integrative Review," *Journal of Holistic Nursing*, vol. 17, no. 4, pp. 385-397, December 1999.

Cote, P.; Mior, S. A.; Vernon, H. "The Short-Term Effect of a Spinal Manipulation on Pain/Pressure Threshold in Patients with Chronic Mechanical Low Back Pain," *Journal of Manipulative and Physiological Therapeutics*, vol. 17, no. 6, pp. 364-8, 1994.

Crasilneck, H.B. "The Use of the Crasilneck Bombardment Technique in Problems of Intractable Organic Pain," *American Journal of Clinical Hypnosis*, vol. 37, no. 4, pp. 255-66, 1995.

Diamond, Jamie. "Pain Relief. New Research and Better Treatments Can Help You Cope with Chronic Pain." *Parents*. vol. 73, no. 4, p. 45, April 1, 1998.

Diamond, M. P.; Bieber, E. "Pelvic Adhesions and Pelvic Pain: Opinions on Cause and Effect Relationship and When to Surgically Intervene," *Gynaecological Endoscopy,* vol. 10, no. 4, pp. 211-216, August 2001.

Dijkstra, Arie; Vlaeyen, Johan W. S.; Rijnen, Heidi; Nielson, Warren. "Readiness to Adopt the Self-Management Approach to Cope with Chronic Pain in Fibromyalgic Patients," *Pain*, vol. 90, no. 1, pp. 37(10), 2001.

Fahy, C.; Jones, N.S. "Nasal Polyposis and Facial Pain," *Clinical Otolaryngology,* vol. 26, no. 6, pp. 510-513, December 2001.

Fineberg, John. "A World of Pain Treatment Options—Multidisciplinary Pain Management Centers Offer a Range of Treatment Options for Patients Living with Chronic Pain," *Minnesota Medicine*, vol. 84, no. 7, pp. 18(2), July 2001.

"Forum: What Is the Role of Psychiatry in the Management of Chronic Pain?" *Harvard Medical School Mental Health Letter*. vol.16, no.3, p.8, September 1999.

Goloff, Marc S. "Insight into the Chronic Pain Patient," *Journal of Pain and Symptom Management*, vol. 21, no. 1, p. 85, January 2001.

Herr, Keela. "Chronic Pain in the Older Patient: Management Strategies," *Journal of Gerontological Nursing*, vol. 28, no. 2, 2002.

Kerns, R.D.; Rosenberg, R. "Predicting Responses to Self-Management Treatments for Chronic Pain: Application of the Pain Stages of Change Model," *Pain*, vol. 84, no. 1, pp. 49(8), 2000.

Labbe, E.E. "Treatment of Childhood Migraine with Autogenic Training and Skin Temperature Biofeedback: A Component Analysis," *Headache*, vol. 35, no. 1, pp. 10-3, January 1995.

McCracken, Lance M.; Gross, Richard T. "Does Anxiety Affect Coping with Chronic Pain?" *The Clinical Journal of Pain*, vol. 9, no. 4, pp. 253-259, December 1993.

Marcus, Dawn A. "Treatment of Nonmalignant Chronic Pain," *American Family Physician*. vol. 61, no. 5, pp. 1331(14), March 2000.

Meyers, John C. "The Pharmacist's Role in Palliative Care and Chronic Pain Management," *Drug Topics*, vol. 141, no. 1, p. 98(8), January 6, 1997.

Mounce, K. "Back Pain," *Rheumatology*, vol. 41, no. 1, pp. 1(5), 2002.

Rosendahl, Iris. "Painful Truth: Consumers Seek Options in Chronic Pain Management," *Drug Topics*, vol. 138, no. 22, p. 39, November 21,1994.

Scannel, Kate A. "Internal Medicine: The Voice of Pain," *Healthline*, vol. 16 no. 1, p.6-7, January 1997.

Schanberg, L.E.; Lefebvre, J.C.; Keefe, F.J.; Kredich, D.W.; Gil, K.M. "Pain Coping and the Pain Experience in Children with Juvenile Chronic Arthritis," *Pain*, vol. 73, no. 2, pp. 181(10), 1998.

Schenker, M.; Kay, S. "Mechanical Neuropathy at the Thoracic Outlet and Associated Pain Syndrome," *Current Orthopaedics*, vol. 15, no. 4, pp. 264-274, 2001.

Sloman, R. "Relaxation and the Relief of Cancer Pain," *Nursing Clinics of North America*, vol. 30, no. 4, pp. 697-709, 1995.

Snow-Turek, A.L.; Norris, M.P.; Tan, G. "Active and Passive Coping Strategies in Chronic Pain Patients," *Pain*, vol. 64, no. 3, 455(8), 1996.

Syrjala, K. L.; Donaldson, G. W.; Davis, M. W.; Kippes, M. E.; Carr, J. E. "Relaxation and Imagery and Cognitive-Behavioral Training Reduce Pain during Cancer Treatment: A Controlled Clinical Trial," *Pain*, vol. 63, no. 2, pp. 189-98, 1995.

Tan, Gabriel; Jensen, Mark P.; Robinson-Whelen, Susan; Thornby, John I.; Monga, Trilok N. "Coping with Chronic Pain: A Comparison of Two Measures," *Pain*, vol. 90, no. 1, pp. 127(8), 2001.

Treadwell, Marsha J.; Franck, Linda S.; Vichinsky, Elliott. "Using Quality Improvement Strategies to Enhance Pediatric Pain Assessment," *International Journal for Quality in Health Care*, vol. 14, no. 1, pp. 39(9), February 2002.

Turner, Judith A. "Chronic Pain Problems at Specific Stages of Life," *Journal of Pain and Symptom Management*, vol 19, no. 6, p. 479, June 2000.

Twomey, L.; Taylor, J. "Exercise and Spinal Manipulation in the Treatment of Low Back Pain," *Spine*, vol. 20, no. 5, pp. 615-9, 1995.

Winfield, John B. "Pain in Fibromyalgia," *Rheumatic Diseases Clinics of North America*. vol. 25, no. 1, pp. 55(26), 1999.

Wittink, Harriet. "Chronic Pain Management: A Qualitative Study of Elderly People's Preferred Coping Strategies and Barriers to Management." *Physical Therapy*, vol. 80, no. 10, p. 1049, October 2000.

Young, Melinda G. "Chronic Pain Management in the Elderly," *Patient Care*, vol. 34, no. 18, p. 31, September 30, 2000.

Web Pages

American Academy of Pain Management
http://www.aapainmanage.org

American Academy of Pain Medicine
http://www.painmed.org

American Chronic Pain Association
http://www.theacpa.org

American Pain Foundation
http://www.painfoundation.org

Central Pain Syndrome Alliance
http://www.centralpain.org

City of Hope: Pain Resource Center
http://prc.coh.org

healthfinder®
http://www.healthfinder.gov

International Association for the Study of Pain
http://www.iasp-pain.org

International Center for the Control of Pain in Children and Adults
http://www.nursing.uiowa.edu/AdultPain/index1.htm
http://www.nursing.uiowa.edu/PedsPain/index1.htm

M.A.G.N.U.M. Migraine Awareness Group
http://www.migraines.org

Mayday Pain Project
www.painandhealth.org

MGH Neurosurgical Service
http://neurosurgery.mgh.harvard.edu

Medical Information Network: Chronic Pain
http://www2.rpa.net/~lrandall

National Foundation for the Treatment of Pain
http://www.paincare.org

National Pain Foundation
http://www.painconnection.org

NeurologyChannel
http://www.neurologychannel.com

Oregon's Pain Management Program
http://www.hr.state.or.us/pain/welcome.html

Pain.com
http://www.pain.com

Pain Medicine and Palliative Care
http://www.stoppain.org

Rest Ministries, Inc.
http://www.restministries.org

University of California, Davis Pain Center
http://pain.ucdavis.edu

Index

Index

Page numbers followed by 'n' indicate a footnote. Page numbers in *italics* indicate a table or illustration.

children
  gastroesophageal reflux disease 188
  headache 185
  otitis media 142–43
  pain 53–56
"Children and Pain" (NIH) 53n
chlorpromazine 458, 476
chondrocalcinosis *see* gout
chondroitin 527–34
chronic disease, defined 157
chronic nonmalignant pain 27–30, 59
chronic pain
  versus acute pain 21–23, 564–65
  agmatine 563–65
  anesthesia 13
  defined 245
  depression 479–82
  described 3, 78, 88
  gender factor 46
  sexual expression 495–97
  sleep disorders 499–503
  statistics 57
  survey 65–66
  treatment 67–72, 439–41
"Chronic Pain - Hope Through Research" (NINDS) 3n
"Chronic Pain in America: Roadblocks to Relief" (Roper Starch) 65n
chronic pelvic pain
  defined 245–46
  described 235–39
  diagnosis 239–41
  treatment 242–45
  see also interstitial cystitis
chronic pelvic pain syndrome, defined 246
chronic reproductive organ pain 43–44
chronic testicular pain 44
Cilcoat, Howard 367
cimetidine 190, 458
cingulotomy, described 12–13
Cipro (quinolone) 475
circumcision pain 49–50
Citroma 476
City of Hope: Pain Resource Center, Web site address 614
"Classification and Treatment of Vulvodynia" (Marinoff) 319n

clindamycin 475
clinical psychophysiology, described 425–28
clinical trials
  arthritis 527–34
  defined 408–9
  randomized controlled, defined 410
clonazepam 353
clonidine hydrochloride 250, 353, 354, 476
cluster headache 178, 179–80
Coda, Barbara 541
codeine
  alcohol interaction 459
  cancer pain 95
  genetic factor 547–50
  kidney disorders 466
  pain management 366
  shingles 285
cognitive-behavioral therapy
  arthritis 83
  pain treatment 58
cognitive therapy
  pain management 345–47
  phantom pain 250
  stump pain 251
colchicine
  defined 167, 476
  gout 165
cold treatment
  arthritis 80
  pain management 344, 397–98
collagen, defined 158
Collins, Kathy 433n
collision dyspareunia, defined 278
Combined Health Information Database (CHID)
  contact information 414–15
  Web site address 590
comfort measures, pain management 50–51
complementary treatment
  pain management 348–49, 356, 397–400
  pain research 523–26
"Complex Regional Pain Syndrome" (Beth Israel Medical Center) 135n

tipped uterus *see* retroverted uterus
Titralac 190
tizanidine 250, 353
TMJ Association, Ltd., contact information 607
TMJ syndrome *see* temporomandibular joint dysfunction
tobacco use
  gastroesophageal reflux disease 189
  interstitial cystitis 201
tolbutamide 457
Tolectin (tometin) 477
tolerance, pain medications 361–64
tometin 477
tooth pain 311–13
  see also dental pain
"Tooth Pain Guide" (American Association of Endodontists) 311n
Topamax (topiramate) 353
tophus
  defined 168
  gout 164–65
topiramate 353
traction, neck pain 227
traction headache 183
traditional Chinese medicine, defined 410
  see also acupuncture
transcription, described 34
transcutaneous electrical nerve stimulation (TENS)
  arthritis 15, 80
  complex regional pain syndrome 139
  defined 247
  described 6
  interstitial cystitis 200–201
  low back pain 14
  pain management 331, 344, 355
  pain treatment 24
  post-herpetic neuralgia 286
  reflex sympathetic dystrophy syndrome 268
  stump pain 251
transient ischemic attack (TIA), headache 183
tricyclic antidepressants
  alcohol interactions 457
  pain management 352

tricyclic antidepressants, continued
  vulvar pain 322–23
  see also antidepressants
trifacial neuralgia, defined 579
trigeminal, defined 579
trigeminal nerves, described 19
trigeminal neuralgia
  chronic pain 23
  defined 579
  described 315–17
  headache 184
  pain 4
  treatment 9, 15
Trigeminal Neuralgia Association, contact information 607
trigger points, defined 247
Trileptal 323
trochlear nerves, described 19
trophic changes, described 137–38
tuberculosis, treatment 476
tumor necrosis factor 391
Tums 190, 475
Turk, Dennis 46–47
Tylenol (acetaminophen)
  alcohol interaction 459
  arthritis 80
  cancer pain 94
  described 475
  pain management 330, 351
Tylox 95
tyramine 457

U

ultrasound
  dyspareunia 276
  shoulder pain 295
The United States Pharmacopeial Convention, Inc., contact information 478
University of California, Davis Pain Center
  contact information 607
  Web site address 615
University of Iowa College of Nursing, publications
  anxiety 487n
  hypnosis 433n

Health Reference Series
COMPLETE CATALOG

Adolescent Health Sourcebook

Basic Consumer Health Information about Common Medical, Mental, and Emotional Concerns in Adolescents, Including Facts about Acne, Body Piercing, Mononucleosis, Nutrition, Eating Disorders, Stress, Depression, Behavior Problems, Peer Pressure, Violence, Gangs, Drug Use, Puberty, Sexuality, Pregnancy, Learning Disabilities, and More

Along with a Glossary of Terms and Other Resources for Further Help and Information

Edited by Chad T. Kimball. 658 pages. 2002. 0-7808-0248-9. $78.

■

AIDS Sourcebook, 1st Edition

Basic Information about AIDS and HIV Infection, Featuring Historical and Statistical Data, Current Research, Prevention, and Other Special Topics of Interest for Persons Living with AIDS

Along with Source Listings for Further Assistance

Edited by Karen Bellenir and Peter D. Dresser. 831 pages. 1995. 0-7808-0031-1. $78.

"One strength of this book is its practical emphasis. The intended audience is the lay reader . . . useful as an educational tool for health care providers who work with AIDS patients. Recommended for public libraries as well as hospital or academic libraries that collect consumer materials."
— *Bulletin of the Medical Library Association, Jan '96*

"This is the most comprehensive volume of its kind on an important medical topic. Highly recommended for all libraries."   — *Reference Book Review, '96*

"Very useful reference for all libraries."
— *Choice, Association of College and Research Libraries, Oct '95*

"There is a wealth of information here that can provide much educational assistance. It is a must book for all libraries and should be on the desk of each and every congressional leader. Highly recommended."
— *AIDS Book Review Journal, Aug '95*

"Recommended for most collections."
— *Library Journal, Jul '95*

■

AIDS Sourcebook, 2nd Edition

Basic Consumer Health Information about Acquired Immune Deficiency Syndrome (AIDS) and Human Immunodeficiency Virus (HIV) Infection, Featuring Updated Statistical Data, Reports on Recent Research and Prevention Initiatives, and Other Special Topics of Interest for Persons Living with AIDS, Including New Antiretroviral Treatment Options, Strategies for Combating Opportunistic Infections, Information about Clinical Trials, and More

Along with a Glossary of Important Terms and Resource Listings for Further Help and Information

Edited by Karen Bellenir. 751 pages. 1999. 0-7808-0225-X. $78.

"Highly recommended."
— *American Reference Books Annual, 2000*

"Excellent sourcebook. This continues to be a highly recommended book. There is no other book that provides as much information as this book provides."
— *AIDS Book Review Journal, Dec-Jan 2000*

"Recommended reference source."
— *Booklist, American Library Association, Dec '99*

"A solid text for college-level health libraries."
— *The Bookwatch, Aug '99*

Cited in *Reference Sources for Small and Medium-Sized Libraries, American Library Association, 1999*

■

Alcoholism Sourcebook

Basic Consumer Health Information about the Physical and Mental Consequences of Alcohol Abuse, Including Liver Disease, Pancreatitis, Wernicke-Korsakoff Syndrome (Alcoholic Dementia), Fetal Alcohol Syndrome, Heart Disease, Kidney Disorders, Gastrointestinal Problems, and Immune System Compromise and Featuring Facts about Addiction, Detoxification, Alcohol Withdrawal, Recovery, and the Maintenance of Sobriety

Along with a Glossary and Directories of Resources for Further Help and Information

Edited by Karen Bellenir. 613 pages. 2000. 0-7808-0325-6. $78.

"This title is one of the few reference works on alcoholism for general readers. For some readers this will be a welcome complement to the many self-help books on the market. Recommended for collections serving general readers and consumer health collections."
— *E-Streams, Mar '01*

"This book is an excellent choice for public and academic libraries."
— *American Reference Books Annual, 2001*

"Recommended reference source."
— *Booklist, American Library Association, Dec '00*

"Presents a wealth of information on alcohol use and abuse and its effects on the body and mind, treatment, and prevention." — *SciTech Book News, Dec '00*

"Important new health guide which packs in the latest consumer information about the problems of alcoholism." — *Reviewer's Bookwatch, Nov '00*

SEE ALSO *Drug Abuse Sourcebook, Substance Abuse Sourcebook*

Allergies Sourcebook, 1st Edition

Basic Information about Major Forms and Mechanisms of Common Allergic Reactions, Sensitivities, and Intolerances, Including Anaphylaxis, Asthma, Hives and Other Dermatologic Symptoms, Rhinitis, and Sinusitis

Along with Their Usual Triggers Like Animal Fur, Chemicals, Drugs, Dust, Foods, Insects, Latex, Pollen, and Poison Ivy, Oak, and Sumac; Plus Information on Prevention, Identification, and Treatment

Edited by Allan R. Cook. 611 pages. 1997. 0-7808-0036-2. $78.

■

Allergies Sourcebook, 2nd Edition

Basic Consumer Health Information about Allergic Disorders, Triggers, Reactions, and Related Symptoms, Including Anaphylaxis, Rhinitis, Sinusitis, Asthma, Dermatitis, Conjunctivitis, and Multiple Chemical Sensitivity

Along with Tips on Diagnosis, Prevention, and Treatment, Statistical Data, a Glossary, and a Directory of Sources for Further Help and Information

Edited by Annemarie S. Muth. 598 pages. 2002. 0-7808-0376-0. $78.

■

Alternative Medicine Sourcebook, First Edition

Basic Consumer Health Information about Alternatives to Conventional Medicine, Including Acupressure, Acupuncture, Aromatherapy, Ayurveda, Bioelectromagnetics, Environmental Medicine, Essence Therapy, Food and Nutrition Therapy, Herbal Therapy, Homeopathy, Imaging, Massage, Naturopathy, Reflexology, Relaxation and Meditation, Sound Therapy, Vitamin and Mineral Therapy, and Yoga, and More

Edited by Allan R. Cook. 737 pages. 1999. 0-7808-0200-4. $78.

"Recommended reference source."
  —Booklist, American Library Association, Feb '00

"A great addition to the reference collection of every type of library." —American Reference Books Annual, 2000

■

Alternative Medicine Sourcebook, Second Edition

Basic Consumer Health Information about Alternative and Complementary Medical Practices, Including Acupuncture, Chiropractic, Herbal Medicine, Homeopathy, Naturopathic Medicine, Mind-Body Interventions, Ayurveda, and Other Non-Western Medical Traditions

Along with Facts about such Specific Therapies as Massage Therapy, Aromatherapy, Qigong, Hypnosis, Prayer, Dance, and Art Therapies, a Glossary, and Resources for Further Information

Edited by Dawn D. Matthews. 650 pages. 2002. 0-7808-0605-0. $78.

Alzheimer's, Stroke & 29 Other Neurological Disorders Sourcebook, 1st Edition

Basic Information for the Layperson on 31 Diseases or Disorders Affecting the Brain and Nervous System, First Describing the Illness, Then Listing Symptoms, Diagnostic Methods, and Treatment Options, and Including Statistics on Incidences and Causes

Edited by Frank E. Bair. 579 pages. 1993. 1-55888-748-2. $78.

"Nontechnical reference book that provides reader-friendly information."
  —Family Caregiver Alliance Update, Winter '96

"Should be included in any library's patient education section." —American Reference Books Annual, 1994

"Written in an approachable and accessible style. Recommended for patient education and consumer health collections in health science center and public libraries." —Academic Library Book Review, Dec '93

"It is very handy to have information on more than thirty neurological disorders under one cover, and there is no recent source like it." —Reference Quarterly, American Library Association, Fall '93

SEE ALSO Brain Disorders Sourcebook

■

Alzheimer's Disease Sourcebook, 2nd Edition

Basic Consumer Health Information about Alzheimer's Disease, Related Disorders, and Other Dementias, Including Multi-Infarct Dementia, AIDS-Related Dementia, Alcoholic Dementia, Huntington's Disease, Delirium, and Confusional States

Along with Reports Detailing Current Research Efforts in Prevention and Treatment, Long-Term Care Issues, and Listings of Sources for Additional Help and Information

Edited by Karen Bellenir. 524 pages. 1999. 0-7808-0223-3. $78.

"Provides a wealth of useful information not otherwise available in one place. This resource is recommended for all types of libraries."
  —American Reference Books Annual, 2000

"Recommended reference source."
  —Booklist, American Library Association, Oct '99

■

Arthritis Sourcebook

Basic Consumer Health Information about Specific Forms of Arthritis and Related Disorders, Including Rheumatoid Arthritis, Osteoarthritis, Gout, Polymyalgia Rheumatica, Psoriatic Arthritis, Spondyloarthropathies, Juvenile Rheumatoid Arthritis, and Juvenile Ankylosing Spondylitis

Along with Information about Medical, Surgical, and Alternative Treatment Options, and Including Strategies for Coping with Pain, Fatigue, and Stress

Edited by Allan R. Cook. 550 pages. 1998. 0-7808-0201-2. $78.

"... accessible to the layperson."
—*Reference and Research Book News, Feb '99*

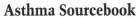

Asthma Sourcebook

Basic Consumer Health Information about Asthma, Including Symptoms, Traditional and Nontraditional Remedies, Treatment Advances, Quality-of-Life Aids, Medical Research Updates, and the Role of Allergies, Exercise, Age, the Environment, and Genetics in the Development of Asthma

Along with Statistical Data, a Glossary, and Directories of Support Groups, and Other Resources for Further Information

Edited by Annemarie S. Muth. 628 pages. 2000. 0-7808-0381-7. $78.

"A worthwhile reference acquisition for public libraries and academic medical libraries whose readers desire a quick introduction to the wide range of asthma information." — *Choice, Association of College & Research Libraries, Jun '01*

"Recommended reference source."
— *Booklist, American Library Association, Feb '01*

"Highly recommended." — *The Bookwatch, Jan '01*

"There is much good information for patients and their families who deal with asthma daily."
— *American Medical Writers Association Journal, Winter '01*

"This informative text is recommended for consumer health collections in public, secondary school, and community college libraries and the libraries of universities with a large undergraduate population."
— *American Reference Books Annual, 2001*

Attention Deficit Disorder Sourcebook, First Edition

Basic Consumer Health Information about Attention Deficit/Hyperactivity Disorder in Children and Adults, Including Facts about Causes, Symptoms, Diagnostic Criteria, and Treatment Options Such as Medications, Behavior Therapy, Coaching, and Homeopathy

Along with Reports on Current Research Initiatives, Legal Issues, and Government Regulations, and Featuring a Glossary of Related Terms, Internet Resources, and a List of Additional Reading Material

Edited by Dawn D. Matthews. 450 pages. 2002. 0-7808-0624-7. $78.

Back & Neck Disorders Sourcebook

Basic Information about Disorders and Injuries of the Spinal Cord and Vertebrae, Including Facts on Chiropractic Treatment, Surgical Interventions, Paralysis, and Rehabilitation

Along with Advice for Preventing Back Trouble

Edited by Karen Bellenir. 548 pages. 1997. 0-7808-0202-0. $78.

"The strength of this work is its basic, easy-to-read format. Recommended."
— *Reference and User Services Quarterly, American Library Association, Winter '97*

Blood & Circulatory Disorders Sourcebook

Basic Information about Blood and Its Components, Anemias, Leukemias, Bleeding Disorders, and Circulatory Disorders, Including Aplastic Anemia, Thalassemia, Sickle-Cell Disease, Hemochromatosis, Hemophilia, Von Willebrand Disease, and Vascular Diseases

Along with a Special Section on Blood Transfusions and Blood Supply Safety, a Glossary, and Source Listings for Further Help and Information

Edited by Karen Bellenir and Linda M. Shin. 554 pages. 1998. 0-7808-0203-9. $78.

"Recommended reference source."
— *Booklist, American Library Association, Feb '99*

"An important reference sourcebook written in simple language for everyday, non-technical users. "
— *Reviewer's Bookwatch, Jan '99*

Brain Disorders Sourcebook

Basic Consumer Health Information about Strokes, Epilepsy, Amyotrophic Lateral Sclerosis (ALS/Lou Gehrig's Disease), Parkinson's Disease, Brain Tumors, Cerebral Palsy, Headache, Tourette Syndrome, and More

Along with Statistical Data, Treatment and Rehabilitation Options, Coping Strategies, Reports on Current Research Initiatives, a Glossary, and Resource Listings for Additional Help and Information

Edited by Karen Bellenir. 481 pages. 1999. 0-7808-0229-2. $78.

"Belongs on the shelves of any library with a consumer health collection." — *E-Streams, Mar '00*

"Recommended reference source."
— *Booklist, American Library Association, Oct '99*

SEE ALSO *Alzheimer's, Stroke & 29 Other Neurological Disorders Sourcebook, 1st Edition*

Breast Cancer Sourcebook

Basic Consumer Health Information about Breast Cancer, Including Diagnostic Methods, Treatment Options, Alternative Therapies, Self-Help Information, Related Health Concerns, Statistical and Demographic Data, and Facts for Men with Breast Cancer

Along with Reports on Current Research Initiatives, a Glossary of Related Medical Terms, and a Directory of Sources for Further Help and Information

Edited by Edward J. Prucha and Karen Bellenir. 580 pages. 2001. 0-7808-0244-6. $78.

"Recommended reference source."
—*Booklist, American Library Association, Jan '02*

"This reference source is highly recommended. It is quite informative, comprehensive and detailed in nature, and yet it offers practical advice in easy-to-read language. It could be thought of as the 'bible' of breast cancer for the consumer." —*E-Streams, Jan '02*

"The broad range of topics covered in lay language make the *Breast Cancer Sourcebook* an excellent addition to public and consumer health library collections."
—*American Reference Books Annual 2002*

"From the pros and cons of different screening methods and results to treatment options, *Breast Cancer Sourcebook* provides the latest information on the subject."
—*Library Bookwatch, Dec '01*

"This thoroughgoing, very readable reference covers all aspects of breast health and cancer. . . . Readers will find much to consider here. Recommended for all public and patient health collections."
—*Library Journal, Sep '01*

SEE ALSO Cancer Sourcebook for Women, 1st and 2nd Editions, Women's Health Concerns Sourcebook

■

Breastfeeding Sourcebook

Basic Consumer Health Information about the Benefits of Breastmilk, Preparing to Breastfeed, Breastfeeding as a Baby Grows, Nutrition, and More, Including Information on Special Situations and Concerns Such as Mastitis, Illness, Medications, Allergies, Multiple Births, Prematurity, Special Needs, and Adoption

Along with a Glossary and Resources for Additional Help and Information

Edited by Jenni Lynn Colson. 388 pages. 2002. 0-7808-0332-9. $78.

SEE ALSO Pregnancy & Birth Sourcebook

■

Burns Sourcebook

Basic Consumer Health Information about Various Types of Burns and Scalds, Including Flame, Heat, Cold, Electrical, Chemical, and Sun Burns

Along with Information on Short-Term and Long-Term Treatments, Tissue Reconstruction, Plastic Surgery, Prevention Suggestions, and First Aid

Edited by Allan R. Cook. 604 pages. 1999. 0-7808-0204-7. $78.

"This is an exceptional addition to the series and is highly recommended for all consumer health collections, hospital libraries, and academic medical centers."
—*E-Streams, Mar '00*

"This key reference guide is an invaluable addition to all health care and public libraries in confronting this ongoing health issue."
—*American Reference Books Annual, 2000*

"Recommended reference source."
—*Booklist, American Library Association, Dec '99*

SEE ALSO Skin Disorders Sourcebook

■

Cancer Sourcebook, 1st Edition

Basic Information on Cancer Types, Symptoms, Diagnostic Methods, and Treatments, Including Statistics on Cancer Occurrences Worldwide and the Risks Associated with Known Carcinogens and Activities

Edited by Frank E. Bair. 932 pages. 1990. 1-55888-888-8. $78.

Cited in *Reference Sources for Small and Medium-Sized Libraries, American Library Association, 1999*

"Written in nontechnical language. Useful for patients, their families, medical professionals, and librarians."
—*Guide to Reference Books, 1996*

"Designed with the non-medical professional in mind. Libraries and medical facilities interested in patient education should certainly consider adding the *Cancer Sourcebook* to their holdings. This compact collection of reliable information . . . is an invaluable tool for helping patients and patients' families and friends to take the first steps in coping with the many difficulties of cancer."
—*Medical Reference Services Quarterly, Winter '91*

"Specifically created for the nontechnical reader . . . an important resource for the general reader trying to understand the complexities of cancer."
—*American Reference Books Annual, 1991*

"This publication's nontechnical nature and very comprehensive format make it useful for both the general public and undergraduate students."
—*Choice, Association of College and Research Libraries, Oct '90*

■

New Cancer Sourcebook, 2nd Edition

Basic Information about Major Forms and Stages of Cancer, Featuring Facts about Primary and Secondary Tumors of the Respiratory, Nervous, Lymphatic, Circulatory, Skeletal, and Gastrointestinal Systems, and Specific Organs; Statistical and Demographic Data; Treatment Options; and Strategies for Coping

Edited by Allan R. Cook. 1,313 pages. 1996. 0-7808-0041-9. $78.

"An excellent resource for patients with newly diagnosed cancer and their families. The dialogue is simple, direct, and comprehensive. Highly recommended for

patients and families to aid in their understanding of cancer and its treatment."
— *Booklist Health Sciences Supplement, American Library Association, Oct '97*

"The amount of factual and useful information is extensive. The writing is very clear, geared to general readers. Recommended for all levels." — *Choice, Association of College & Research Libraries, Jan '97*

■

Cancer Sourcebook, 3rd Edition

Basic Consumer Health Information about Major Forms and Stages of Cancer, Featuring Facts about Primary and Secondary Tumors of the Respiratory, Nervous, Lymphatic, Circulatory, Skeletal, and Gastrointestinal Systems, and Specific Organs

Along with Statistical and Demographic Data, Treatment Options, Strategies for Coping, a Glossary, and a Directory of Sources for Additional Help and Information

Edited by Edward J. Prucha. 1,069 pages. 2000. 0-7808-0227-6. $78.

"This title is recommended for health sciences and public libraries with consumer health collections."
— *E-Streams, Feb '01*

". . . can be effectively used by cancer patients and their families who are looking for answers in a language they can understand. Public and hospital libraries should have it on their shelves."
— *American Reference Books Annual, 2001*

"Recommended reference source."
— *Booklist, American Library Association, Dec '00*

■

Cancer Sourcebook for Women, 1st Edition

Basic Information about Specific Forms of Cancer That Affect Women, Featuring Facts about Breast Cancer, Cervical Cancer, Ovarian Cancer, Cancer of the Uterus and Uterine Sarcoma, Cancer of the Vagina, and Cancer of the Vulva; Statistical and Demographic Data; Treatments, Self-Help Management Suggestions, and Current Research Initiatives

Edited by Allan R. Cook and Peter D. Dresser. 524 pages. 1996. 0-7808-0076-1. $78.

". . . written in easily understandable, non-technical language. Recommended for public libraries or hospital and academic libraries that collect patient education or consumer health materials."
— *Medical Reference Services Quarterly, Spring '97*

"Would be of value in a consumer health library. . . . written with the health care consumer in mind. Medical jargon is at a minimum, and medical terms are explained in clear, understandable sentences."
— *Bulletin of the Medical Library Association, Oct '96*

"The availability under one cover of all these pertinent publications, grouped under cohesive headings, makes this certainly a most useful sourcebook." — *Choice, Association of College & Research Libraries, Jun '96*

"Presents a comprehensive knowledge base for general readers. Men and women both benefit from the gold mine of information nestled between the two covers of this book. Recommended."
— *Academic Library Book Review, Summer '96*

"This timely book is highly recommended for consumer health and patient education collections in all libraries." — *Library Journal, Apr '96*

SEE ALSO *Breast Cancer Sourcebook, Women's Health Concerns Sourcebook*

■

Cancer Sourcebook for Women, 2nd Edition

Basic Consumer Health Information about Gynecologic Cancers and Related Concerns, Including Cervical Cancer, Endometrial Cancer, Gestational Trophoblastic Tumor, Ovarian Cancer, Uterine Cancer, Vaginal Cancer, Vulvar Cancer, Breast Cancer, and Common Non-Cancerous Uterine Conditions, with Facts about Cancer Risk Factors, Screening and Prevention, Treatment Options, and Reports on Current Research Initiatives

Along with a Glossary of Cancer Terms and a Directory of Resources for Additional Help and Information

Edited by Karen Bellenir. 604 pages. 2002. 0-7808-0226-8. $78.

SEE ALSO *Breast Cancer Sourcebook, Women's Health Concerns Sourcebook*

■

Cardiovascular Diseases & Disorders Sourcebook, 1st Edition

Basic Information about Cardiovascular Diseases and Disorders, Featuring Facts about the Cardiovascular System, Demographic and Statistical Data, Descriptions of Pharmacological and Surgical Interventions, Lifestyle Modifications, and a Special Section Focusing on Heart Disorders in Children

Edited by Karen Bellenir and Peter D. Dresser. 683 pages. 1995. 0-7808-0032-X. $78.

". . . comprehensive format provides an extensive overview on this subject." — *Choice, Association of College & Research Libraries, Jun '96*

". . . an easily understood, complete, up-to-date resource. This well executed public health tool will make valuable information available to those that need it most, patients and their families. The typeface, sturdy non-reflective paper, and library binding add a feel of quality found wanting in other publications. Highly recommended for academic and general libraries. "
— *Academic Library Book Review, Summer '96*

SEE ALSO *Healthy Heart Sourcebook for Women, Heart Diseases & Disorders Sourcebook, 2nd Edition*

653

Caregiving Sourcebook

Basic Consumer Health Information for Caregivers, Including a Profile of Caregivers, Caregiving Responsibilities and Concerns, Tips for Specific Conditions, Care Environments, and the Effects of Caregiving

Along with Facts about Legal Issues, Financial Information, and Future Planning, a Glossary, and a Listing of Additional Resources

Edited by Joyce Brennfleck Shannon. 600 pages. 2001. 0-7808-0331-0. $78.

"An ideal addition to the reference collection of any public library. Health sciences information professionals may also want to acquire the *Caregiving Sourcebook* for their hospital or academic library for use as a ready reference tool by health care workers interested in aging and caregiving." —*E-Streams, Jan '02*

"Essential for most collections."
—*Library Journal, Apr 1, 2002*

"Recommended reference source."
—*Booklist, American Library Association, Oct '01*

■

Colds, Flu & Other Common Ailments Sourcebook

Basic Consumer Health Information about Common Ailments and Injuries, Including Colds, Coughs, the Flu, Sinus Problems, Headaches, Fever, Nausea and Vomiting, Menstrual Cramps, Diarrhea, Constipation, Hemorrhoids, Back Pain, Dandruff, Dry and Itchy Skin, Cuts, Scrapes, Sprains, Bruises, and More

Along with Information about Prevention, Self-Care, Choosing a Doctor, Over-the-Counter Medications, Folk Remedies, and Alternative Therapies, and Including a Glossary of Important Terms and a Directory of Resources for Further Help and Information

Edited by Chad T. Kimball. 638 pages. 2001. 0-7808-0435-X. $78.

"A good starting point for research on common illnesses. It will be a useful addition to public and consumer health library collections."
—*American Reference Books Annual 2002*

"Will prove valuable to any library seeking to maintain a current, comprehensive reference collection of health resources. . . . Excellent reference."
—*The Bookwatch, Aug '01*

"Recommended reference source."
—*Booklist, American Library Association, July '01*

■

Communication Disorders Sourcebook

Basic Information about Deafness and Hearing Loss, Speech and Language Disorders, Voice Disorders, Balance and Vestibular Disorders, and Disorders of Smell, Taste, and Touch

Edited by Linda M. Ross. 533 pages. 1996. 0-7808-0077-X. $78.

"This is skillfully edited and is a welcome resource for the layperson. It should be found in every public and medical library." —*Booklist Health Sciences Supplement, American Library Association, Oct '97*

■

Congenital Disorders Sourcebook

Basic Information about Disorders Acquired during Gestation, Including Spina Bifida, Hydrocephalus, Cerebral Palsy, Heart Defects, Craniofacial Abnormalities, Fetal Alcohol Syndrome, and More

Along with Current Treatment Options and Statistical Data

Edited by Karen Bellenir. 607 pages. 1997. 0-7808-0205-5. $78.

"Recommended reference source."
— *Booklist, American Library Association, Oct '97*

SEE ALSO Pregnancy & Birth Sourcebook

■

Consumer Issues in Health Care Sourcebook

Basic Information about Health Care Fundamentals and Related Consumer Issues, Including Exams and Screening Tests, Physician Specialties, Choosing a Doctor, Using Prescription and Over-the-Counter Medications Safely, Avoiding Health Scams, Managing Common Health Risks in the Home, Care Options for Chronically or Terminally Ill Patients, and a List of Resources for Obtaining Help and Further Information

Edited by Karen Bellenir. 618 pages. 1998. 0-7808-0221-7. $78.

"Both public and academic libraries will want to have a copy in their collection for readers who are interested in self-education on health issues."
—*American Reference Books Annual, 2000*

"The editor has researched the literature from government agencies and others, saving readers the time and effort of having to do the research themselves. Recommended for public libraries."
—*Reference and User Services Quarterly, American Library Association, Spring '99*

"Recommended reference source."
—*Booklist, American Library Association, Dec '98*

■

Contagious & Non-Contagious Infectious Diseases Sourcebook

Basic Information about Contagious Diseases like Measles, Polio, Hepatitis B, and Infectious Mononucleosis, and Non-Contagious Infectious Diseases like Tetanus and Toxic Shock Syndrome, and Diseases Occurring as Secondary Infections Such as Shingles and Reye Syndrome

Along with Vaccination, Prevention, and Treatment Information, and a Section Describing Emerging Infectious Disease Threats

Edited by Karen Bellenir and Peter D. Dresser. 566 pages. 1996. 0-7808-0075-3. $78.

Death & Dying Sourcebook

Basic Consumer Health Information for the Layperson about End-of-Life Care and Related Ethical and Legal Issues, Including Chief Causes of Death, Autopsies, Pain Management for the Terminally Ill, Life Support Systems, Insurance, Euthanasia, Assisted Suicide, Hospice Programs, Living Wills, Funeral Planning, Counseling, Mourning, Organ Donation, and Physician Training

Along with Statistical Data, a Glossary, and Listings of Sources for Further Help and Information

Edited by Annemarie S. Muth. 641 pages. 1999. 0-7808-0230-6. $78.

"Public libraries, medical libraries, and academic libraries will all find this sourcebook a useful addition to their collections."
— American Reference Books Annual, 2001

"An extremely useful resource for those concerned with death and dying in the United States."
— Respiratory Care, Nov '00

"Recommended reference source."
— Booklist, American Library Association, Aug '00

"This book is a definite must for all those involved in end-of-life care." — Doody's Review Service, 2000

■

Diabetes Sourcebook, 1st Edition

Basic Information about Insulin-Dependent and Non-insulin-Dependent Diabetes Mellitus, Gestational Diabetes, and Diabetic Complications, Symptoms, Treatment, and Research Results, Including Statistics on Prevalence, Morbidity, and Mortality

Along with Source Listings for Further Help and Information

Edited by Karen Bellenir and Peter D. Dresser. 827 pages. 1994. 1-55888-751-2. $78.

". . . very informative and understandable for the layperson without being simplistic. It provides a comprehensive overview for laypersons who want a general understanding of the disease or who want to focus on various aspects of the disease."
— Bulletin of the Medical Library Association, Jan '96

■

Diabetes Sourcebook, 2nd Edition

Basic Consumer Health Information about Type 1 Diabetes (Insulin-Dependent or Juvenile-Onset Diabetes), Type 2 (Noninsulin-Dependent or Adult-Onset Diabetes), Gestational Diabetes, and Related Disorders, Including Diabetes Prevalence Data, Management Issues, the Role of Diet and Exercise in Controlling Diabetes, Insulin and Other Diabetes Medicines, and Complications of Diabetes Such as Eye Diseases, Periodontal Disease, Amputation, and End-Stage Renal Disease

Along with Reports on Current Research Initiatives, a Glossary, and Resource Listings for Further Help and Information

Edited by Karen Bellenir. 688 pages. 1998. 0-7808-0224-1. $78.

"An invaluable reference." — Library Journal, May '00

Selected as one of the 250 "Best Health Sciences Books of 1999." — Doody's Rating Service, Mar-Apr 2000

"This comprehensive book is an excellent addition for high school, academic, medical, and public libraries. This volume is highly recommended."
— American Reference Books Annual, 2000

"Provides useful information for the general public."
— Healthlines, University of Michigan Health Management Research Center, Sep/Oct '99

". . . provides reliable mainstream medical information . . . belongs on the shelves of any library with a consumer health collection." — E-Streams, Sep '99

"Recommended reference source."
— Booklist, American Library Association, Feb '99

■

Diet & Nutrition Sourcebook, 1st Edition

Basic Information about Nutrition, Including the Dietary Guidelines for Americans, the Food Guide Pyramid, and Their Applications in Daily Diet, Nutritional Advice for Specific Age Groups, Current Nutritional Issues and Controversies, the New Food Label and How to Use It to Promote Healthy Eating, and Recent Developments in Nutritional Research

Edited by Dan R. Harris. 662 pages. 1996. 0-7808-0084-2. $78.

"Useful reference as a food and nutrition sourcebook for the general consumer." — Booklist Health Sciences Supplement, American Library Association, Oct '97

"Recommended for public libraries and medical libraries that receive general information requests on nutrition. It is readable and will appeal to those interested in learning more about healthy dietary practices."
— Medical Reference Services Quarterly, Fall '97

"An abundance of medical and social statistics is translated into readable information geared toward the general reader." — Bookwatch, Mar '97

"With dozens of questionable diet books on the market, it is so refreshing to find a reliable and factual reference book. Recommended to aspiring professionals, librarians, and others seeking and giving reliable dietary advice. An excellent compilation." — Choice, Association of College and Research Libraries, Feb '97

SEE ALSO Digestive Diseases & Disorders Sourcebook, Gastrointestinal Diseases & Disorders Sourcebook

■

Diet & Nutrition Sourcebook, 2nd Edition

Basic Consumer Health Information about Dietary Guidelines, Recommended Daily Intake Values, Vitamins, Minerals, Fiber, Fat, Weight Control, Dietary Supplements, and Food Additives

Along with Special Sections on Nutrition Needs throughout Life and Nutrition for People with Such Spe-

cific Medical Concerns as Allergies, High Blood Cho-
lesterol, Hypertension, Diabetes, Celiac Disease,
Seizure Disorders, Phenylketonuria (PKU), Cancer, and
Eating Disorders, and Including Reports on Current
Nutrition Research and Source Listings for Additional
Help and Information

Edited by Karen Bellenir. 650 pages. 1999. 0-7808-0228-
4. $78.

"This book is an excellent source of basic diet and
nutrition information."   — Booklist Health Sciences
    Supplement, American Library Association, Dec '00

"This reference document should be in any public
library, but it would be a very good guide for beginning
students in the health sciences. If the other books in
this publisher's series are as good as this, they should all
be in the health sciences collections."
    —American Reference Books Annual, 2000

"This book is an excellent general nutrition reference
for consumers who desire to take an active role in their
health care for prevention. Consumers of all ages who
select this book can feel confident they are receiving
current and accurate information."   — Journal of
    Nutrition for the Elderly, Vol. 19, No. 4, '00

"Recommended reference source."
    —Booklist, American Library Association, Dec '99

SEE ALSO Digestive Diseases & Disorders Sourcebook,
Gastrointestinal Diseases & Disorders Sourcebook

∎

Digestive Diseases
& Disorders Sourcebook

Basic Consumer Health Information about Diseases
and Disorders that Impact the Upper and Lower Digestive System, Including Celiac Disease, Constipation,
Crohn's Disease, Cyclic Vomiting Syndrome, Diarrhea,
Diverticulosis and Diverticulitis, Gallstones, Heartburn, Hemorrhoids, Hernias, Indigestion (Dyspepsia),
Irritable Bowel Syndrome, Lactose Intolerance, Ulcers,
and More

Along with Information about Medications and Other
Treatments, Tips for Maintaining a Healthy Digestive
Tract, a Glossary, and Directory of Digestive Diseases
Organizations

Edited by Karen Bellenir. 335 pages. 2000. 0-7808-0327-
2. $78.

"This title would be an excellent addition to all public
or patient-research libraries."
    —American Reference Books Annual, 2001

"This title is recommended for public, hospital, and
health sciences libraries with consumer health collections."   — E-Streams, Jul-Aug '00

"Recommended reference source."
    —Booklist, American Library Association, May '00

SEE ALSO Diet & Nutrition Sourcebook, 1st and 2nd
Editions, Gastrointestinal Diseases & Disorders
Sourcebook

Disabilities Sourcebook

Basic Consumer Health Information about Physical
and Psychiatric Disabilities, Including Descriptions of
Major Causes of Disability, Assistive and Adaptive
Aids, Workplace Issues, and Accessibility Concerns

Along with Information about the Americans with
Disabilities Act, a Glossary, and Resources for Additional Help and Information

Edited by Dawn D. Matthews. 616 pages. 2000. 0-7808-
0389-2. $78.

"It is a must for libraries with a consumer health section."   — American Reference Books Annual 2002

"A much needed addition to the Omnigraphics Health
Reference Series. A current reference work to provide
people with disabilities, their families, caregivers or
those who work with them, a broad range of information
in one volume, has not been available until now. . . . It
is recommended for all public and academic library reference collections."   — E-Streams, May '01

"An excellent source book in easy-to-read format covering many current topics; highly recommended for all
libraries."   — Choice, Association of College
                             and Research Libraries, Jan '01

"Recommended reference source."
    —Booklist, American Library Association, Jul '00

"An involving, invaluable handbook."
                         — The Bookwatch, May '00

∎

Domestic Violence &
Child Abuse Sourcebook

Basic Consumer Health Information about Spousal/
Partner, Child, Sibling, Parent, and Elder Abuse,
Covering Physical, Emotional, and Sexual Abuse, Teen
Dating Violence, and Stalking; Includes Information
about Hotlines, Safe Houses, Safety Plans, and Other
Resources for Support and Assistance, Community Ini-
tiatives, and Reports on Current Directions in Research
and Treatment

Along with a Glossary, Sources for Further Reading,
and Governmental and Non-Governmental Organizations Contact Information

Edited by Helene Henderson. 1,064 pages. 2001. 0-7808-
0235-7. $78.

"This is important information. The Web has many
resources but this sourcebook fills an important societal need. I am not aware of any other resources of this
type."   — Doody's Review Service, Sep '01

"Recommended for all libraries, scholars, and practitioners."   — Choice,
    Association of College & Research Libraries, Jul '01

"Recommended reference source."
    — Booklist, American Library Association, Apr '01

"Important pick for college-level health reference libraries."   — The Bookwatch, Mar '01

"Because this problem is so widespread and because
this book includes a lot of issues within one volume,
this work is recommended for all public libraries."
    —American Reference Books Annual, 2001

Drug Abuse Sourcebook

Basic Consumer Health Information about Illicit Substances of Abuse and the Diversion of Prescription Medications, Including Depressants, Hallucinogens, Inhalants, Marijuana, Narcotics, Stimulants, and Anabolic Steroids

Along with Facts about Related Health Risks, Treatment Issues, and Substance Abuse Prevention Programs, a Glossary of Terms, Statistical Data, and Directories of Hotline Services, Self-Help Groups, and Organizations Able to Provide Further Information

Edited by Karen Bellenir. 629 pages. 2000. 0-7808-0242-X. $78.

"Containing a wealth of information, this book will be useful to the college student just beginning to explore the topic of substance abuse. This resource belongs in libraries that serve a lower-division undergraduate or community college clientele as well as the general public." — Choice, Association of College and Research Libraries, Jun '01

"Recommended reference source." — Booklist, American Library Association, Feb '01

"Highly recommended." — The Bookwatch, Jan '01

"Even though there is a plethora of books on drug abuse, this volume is recommended for school, public, and college libraries." — American Reference Books Annual, 2001

SEE ALSO Alcoholism Sourcebook, Substance Abuse Sourcebook

■

Ear, Nose & Throat Disorders Sourcebook

Basic Information about Disorders of the Ears, Nose, Sinus Cavities, Pharynx, and Larynx, Including Ear Infections, Tinnitus, Vestibular Disorders, Allergic and Non-Allergic Rhinitis, Sore Throats, Tonsillitis, and Cancers That Affect the Ears, Nose, Sinuses, and Throat

Along with Reports on Current Research Initiatives, a Glossary of Related Medical Terms, and a Directory of Sources for Further Help and Information

Edited by Karen Bellenir and Linda M. Shin. 576 pages. 1998. 0-7808-0206-3. $78.

"Overall, this sourcebook is helpful for the consumer seeking information on ENT issues. It is recommended for public libraries." — American Reference Books Annual, 1999

"Recommended reference source." — Booklist, American Library Association, Dec '98

■

Eating Disorders Sourcebook

Basic Consumer Health Information about Eating Disorders, Including Information about Anorexia Nervosa, Bulimia Nervosa, Binge Eating, Body Dysmorphic Disorder, Pica, Laxative Abuse, and Night Eating Syndrome

Along with Information about Causes, Adverse Effects, and Treatment and Prevention Issues, and Featuring a Section on Concerns Specific to Children and Adolescents, a Glossary, and Resources for Further Help and Information

Edited by Dawn D. Matthews. 322 pages. 2001. 0-7808-0335-3. $78.

"Recommended for health science libraries that are open to the public, as well as hospital libraries. This book is a good resource for the consumer who is concerned about eating disorders." — E-Streams, Mar '02

"This volume is another convenient collection of excerpted articles. Recommended for school and public library patrons; lower-division undergraduates; and two-year technical program students." — Choice, Association of College & Research Libraries, Jan '02

"Recommended reference source." — Booklist, American Library Association, Oct '01

■

Endocrine & Metabolic Disorders Sourcebook

Basic Information for the Layperson about Pancreatic and Insulin-Related Disorders Such as Pancreatitis, Diabetes, and Hypoglycemia; Adrenal Gland Disorders Such as Cushing's Syndrome, Addison's Disease, and Congenital Adrenal Hyperplasia; Pituitary Gland Disorders Such as Growth Hormone Deficiency, Acromegaly, and Pituitary Tumors; Thyroid Disorders Such as Hypothyroidism, Graves' Disease, Hashimoto's Disease, and Goiter; Hyperparathyroidism; and Other Diseases and Syndromes of Hormone Imbalance or Metabolic Dysfunction

Along with Reports on Current Research Initiatives

Edited by Linda M. Shin. 574 pages. 1998. 0-7808-0207-1. $78.

"Omnigraphics has produced another needed resource for health information consumers." — American Reference Books Annual, 2000

"Recommended reference source." — Booklist, American Library Association, Dec '98

■

Environmentally Induced Disorders Sourcebook

Basic Information about Diseases and Syndromes Linked to Exposure to Pollutants and Other Substances in Outdoor and Indoor Environments Such as Lead, Asbestos, Formaldehyde, Mercury, Emissions, Noise, and More

Edited by Allan R. Cook. 620 pages. 1997. 0-7808-0083-4. $78.

"Recommended reference source." — Booklist, American Library Association, Sep '98

"This book will be a useful addition to anyone's library." — Choice Health Sciences Supplement, Association of College and Research Libraries, May '98

"... a good survey of numerous environmentally induced physical disorders ... a useful addition to anyone's library."
— *Doody's Health Sciences Book Reviews, Jan '98*

"... provide[s] introductory information from the best authorities around. Since this volume covers topics that potentially affect everyone, it will surely be one of the most frequently consulted volumes in the *Health Reference Series.*" — *Rettig on Reference, Nov '97*

■

Ethnic Diseases Sourcebook

Basic Consumer Health Information for Ethnic and Racial Minority Groups in the United States, Including General Health Indicators and Behaviors, Ethnic Diseases, Genetic Testing, the Impact of Chronic Diseases, Women's Health, Mental Health Issues, and Preventive Health Care Services

Along with a Glossary and a Listing of Additional Resources

Edited by Joyce Brennfleck Shannon. 664 pages. 2001. 0-7808-0336-1. $78.

"Recommended for health sciences libraries where public health programs are a priority."
— *E-Streams, Jan '02*

"Not many books have been written on this topic to date, and the *Ethnic Diseases Sourcebook* is a strong addition to the list. It will be an important introductory resource for health consumers, students, health care personnel, and social scientists. It is recommended for public, academic, and large hospital libraries."
— *American Reference Books Annual 2002*

"Recommended reference source."
— *Booklist, American Library Association, Oct '01*

"Will prove valuable to any library seeking to maintain a current, comprehensive reference collection of health resources.... An excellent source of health information about genetic disorders which affect particular ethnic and racial minorities in the U.S."
— *The Bookwatch, Aug '01*

■

Family Planning Sourcebook

Basic Consumer Health Information about Planning for Pregnancy and Contraception, Including Traditional Methods, Barrier Methods, Hormonal Methods, Permanent Methods, Future Methods, Emergency Contraception, and Birth Control Choices for Women at Each Stage of Life

Along with Statistics, a Glossary, and Sources of Additional Information

Edited by Amy Marcaccio Keyzer. 520 pages. 2001. 0-7808-0379-5. $78.

"Recommended for public, health, and undergraduate libraries as part of the circulating collection."
— *E-Streams, Mar '02*

"Information is presented in an unbiased, readable manner, and the sourcebook will certainly be a neces-

sary addition to those public and high school libraries where Internet access is restricted or otherwise problematic." — *American Reference Books Annual 2002*

"Recommended reference source."
— *Booklist, American Library Association, Oct '01*

"Will prove valuable to any library seeking to maintain a current, comprehensive reference collection of health resources.... Excellent reference."
— *The Bookwatch, Aug '01*

SEE ALSO Pregnancy & Birth Sourcebook

■

Fitness & Exercise Sourcebook, 1st Edition

Basic Information on Fitness and Exercise, Including Fitness Activities for Specific Age Groups, Exercise for People with Specific Medical Conditions, How to Begin a Fitness Program in Running, Walking, Swimming, Cycling, and Other Athletic Activities, and Recent Research in Fitness and Exercise

Edited by Dan R. Harris. 663 pages. 1996. 0-7808-0186-5. $78.

"A good resource for general readers." — *Choice, Association of College and Research Libraries, Nov '97*

"The perennial popularity of the topic ... make this an appealing selection for public libraries."
— *Rettig on Reference, Jun/Jul '97*

■

Fitness & Exercise Sourcebook, 2nd Edition

Basic Consumer Health Information about the Fundamentals of Fitness and Exercise, Including How to Begin and Maintain a Fitness Program, Fitness as a Lifestyle, the Link between Fitness and Diet, Advice for Specific Groups of People, Exercise as It Relates to Specific Medical Conditions, and Recent Research in Fitness and Exercise

Along with a Glossary of Important Terms and Resources for Additional Help and Information

Edited by Kristen M. Gledhill. 646 pages. 2001. 0-7808-0334-5. $78.

"This work is recommended for all general reference collections."
— *American Reference Books Annual 2002*

"Highly recommended for public, consumer, and school grades fourth through college."
— *E-Streams, Nov '01*

"Recommended reference source." — *Booklist, American Library Association, Oct '01*

"The information appears quite comprehensive and is considered reliable.... This second edition is a welcomed addition to the series."
— *Doody's Review Service, Sep '01*

"This reference is a valuable choice for those who desire a broad source of information on exercise, fitness, and chronic-disease prevention through a healthy lifestyle." —*American Medical Writers Association Journal, Fall '01*

"Will prove valuable to any library seeking to maintain a current, comprehensive reference collection of health resources. . . . Excellent reference." —*The Bookwatch, Aug '01*

■

Food & Animal Borne Diseases Sourcebook

Basic Information about Diseases That Can Be Spread to Humans through the Ingestion of Contaminated Food or Water or by Contact with Infected Animals and Insects, Such as Botulism, E. Coli, Hepatitis A, Trichinosis, Lyme Disease, and Rabies

Along with Information Regarding Prevention and Treatment Methods, and Including a Special Section for International Travelers Describing Diseases Such as Cholera, Malaria, Travelers' Diarrhea, and Yellow Fever, and Offering Recommendations for Avoiding Illness

Edited by Karen Bellenir and Peter D. Dresser. 535 pages. 1995. 0-7808-0033-8. $78.

"Targeting general readers and providing them with a single, comprehensive source of information on selected topics, this book continues, with the excellent caliber of its predecessors, to catalog topical information on health matters of general interest. Readable and thorough, this valuable resource is highly recommended for all libraries." —*Academic Library Book Review, Summer '96*

"A comprehensive collection of authoritative information." —*Emergency Medical Services, Oct '95*

■

Food Safety Sourcebook

Basic Consumer Health Information about the Safe Handling of Meat, Poultry, Seafood, Eggs, Fruit Juices, and Other Food Items, and Facts about Pesticides, Drinking Water, Food Safety Overseas, and the Onset, Duration, and Symptoms of Foodborne Illnesses, Including Types of Pathogenic Bacteria, Parasitic Protozoa, Worms, Viruses, and Natural Toxins

Along with the Role of the Consumer, the Food Handler, and the Government in Food Safety; a Glossary, and Resources for Additional Help and Information

Edited by Dawn D. Matthews. 339 pages. 1999. 0-7808-0326-4. $78.

"This book is recommended for public libraries and universities with home economic and food science programs." —*E-Streams, Nov '00*

"Recommended reference source." —*Booklist, American Library Association, May '00*

"This book takes the complex issues of food safety and foodborne pathogens and presents them in an easily understood manner. [It does] an excellent job of covering a large and often confusing topic." —*American Reference Books Annual, 2000*

Forensic Medicine Sourcebook

Basic Consumer Information for the Layperson about Forensic Medicine, Including Crime Scene Investigation, Evidence Collection and Analysis, Expert Testimony, Computer-Aided Criminal Identification, Digital Imaging in the Courtroom, DNA Profiling, Accident Reconstruction, Autopsies, Ballistics, Drugs and Explosives Detection, Latent Fingerprints, Product Tampering, and Questioned Document Examination

Along with Statistical Data, a Glossary of Forensics Terminology, and Listings of Sources for Further Help and Information

Edited by Annemarie S. Muth. 574 pages. 1999. 0-7808-0232-2. $78.

"Given the expected widespread interest in its content and its easy to read style, this book is recommended for most public and all college and university libraries." —*E-Streams, Feb '01*

"Recommended for public libraries." —*Reference & User Services Quarterly, American Library Association, Spring 2000*

"Recommended reference source." —*Booklist, American Library Association, Feb '00*

"A wealth of information, useful statistics, references are up-to-date and extremely complete. This wonderful collection of data will help students who are interested in a career in any type of forensic field. It is a great resource for attorneys who need information about types of expert witnesses needed in a particular case. It also offers useful information for fiction and nonfiction writers whose work involves a crime. A fascinating compilation. All levels." —*Choice, Association of College and Research Libraries, Jan 2000*

"There are several items that make this book attractive to consumers who are seeking certain forensic data. . . . This is a useful current source for those seeking general forensic medical answers." —*American Reference Books Annual, 2000*

■

Gastrointestinal Diseases & Disorders Sourcebook

Basic Information about Gastroesophageal Reflux Disease (Heartburn), Ulcers, Diverticulosis, Irritable Bowel Syndrome, Crohn's Disease, Ulcerative Colitis, Diarrhea, Constipation, Lactose Intolerance, Hemorrhoids, Hepatitis, Cirrhosis, and Other Digestive Problems, Featuring Statistics, Descriptions of Symptoms, and Current Treatment Methods of Interest for Persons Living with Upper and Lower Gastrointestinal Maladies

Edited by Linda M. Ross. 413 pages. 1996. 0-7808-0078-8. $78.

". . . very readable form. The successful editorial work that brought this material together into a useful and understandable reference makes accessible to all readers information that can help them more effectively understand and obtain help for digestive tract problems." —*Choice, Association of College & Research Libraries, Feb '97*

SEE ALSO *Diet & Nutrition Sourcebook, 1st and 2nd Editions, Digestive Diseases & Disorders*

Genetic Disorders Sourcebook, 1st Edition

Basic Information about Heritable Diseases and Disorders Such as Down Syndrome, PKU, Hemophilia, Von Willebrand Disease, Gaucher Disease, Tay-Sachs Disease, and Sickle-Cell Disease, Along with Information about Genetic Screening, Gene Therapy, Home Care, and Including Source Listings for Further Help and Information on More Than 300 Disorders

Edited by Karen Bellenir. 642 pages. 1996. 0-7808-0034-6. $78.

"Recommended for undergraduate libraries or libraries that serve the public."
— *Science & Technology Libraries, Vol. 18, No. 1, '99*

"Provides essential medical information to both the general public and those diagnosed with a serious or fatal genetic disease or disorder." — *Choice, Association of College and Research Libraries, Jan '97*

"Geared toward the lay public. It would be well placed in all public libraries and in those hospital and medical libraries in which access to genetic references is limited." — *Doody's Health Sciences Book Review, Oct '96*

Genetic Disorders Sourcebook, 2nd Edition

Basic Consumer Health Information about Hereditary Diseases and Disorders, Including Cystic Fibrosis, Down Syndrome, Hemophilia, Huntington's Disease, Sickle Cell Anemia, and More; Facts about Genes, Gene Research and Therapy, Genetic Screening, Ethics of Gene Testing, Genetic Counseling, and Advice on Coping and Caring

Along with a Glossary of Genetic Terminology and a Resource List for Help, Support, and Further Information

Edited by Kathy Massimini. 768 pages. 2001. 0-7808-0241-1. $78.

"Recommended for public libraries and medical and hospital libraries with consumer health collections."
— *E-Streams, May '01*

"Recommended reference source."
— *Booklist, American Library Association, Apr '01*

"Important pick for college-level health reference libraries." — *The Bookwatch, Mar '01*

Head Trauma Sourcebook

Basic Information for the Layperson about Open-Head and Closed-Head Injuries, Treatment Advances, Recovery, and Rehabilitation

Along with Reports on Current Research Initiatives

Edited by Karen Bellenir. 414 pages. 1997. 0-7808-0208-X. $78.

Headache Sourcebook

Basic Consumer Health Information about Migraine, Tension, Cluster, Rebound and Other Types of Headaches, with Facts about the Cause and Prevention of Headaches, the Effects of Stress and the Environment, Headaches during Pregnancy and Menopause, and Childhood Headaches

Along with a Glossary and Other Resources for Additional Help and Information

Edited by Dawn D. Matthews. 362 pages. 2002. 0-7808-0337-X. $78.

Health Insurance Sourcebook

Basic Information about Managed Care Organizations, Traditional Fee-for-Service Insurance, Insurance Portability and Pre-Existing Conditions Clauses, Medicare, Medicaid, Social Security, and Military Health Care

Along with Information about Insurance Fraud

Edited by Wendy Wilcox. 530 pages. 1997. 0-7808-0222-5. $78.

"Particularly useful because it brings much of this information together in one volume. This book will be a handy reference source in the health sciences library, hospital library, college and university library, and medium to large public library."
— *Medical Reference Services Quarterly, Fall '98*

Awarded "Books of the Year Award"
— *American Journal of Nursing, 1997*

"The layout of the book is particularly helpful as it provides easy access to reference material. A most useful addition to the vast amount of information about health insurance. The use of data from U.S. government agencies is most commendable. Useful in a library or learning center for healthcare professional students."
— *Doody's Health Sciences Book Reviews, Nov '97*

Health Reference Series Cumulative Index 1999

A Comprehensive Index to the Individual Volumes of the Health Reference Series, Including a Subject Index, Name Index, Organization Index, and Publication Index

Along with a Master List of Acronyms and Abbreviations

Edited by Edward J. Prucha, Anne Holmes, and Robert Rudnick. 990 pages. 2000. 0-7808-0382-5. $78.

"This volume will be most helpful in libraries that have a relatively complete collection of the Health Reference Series." — *American Reference Books Annual, 2001*

"Essential for collections that hold any of the numerous *Health Reference Series* titles."
— *Choice, Association of College and Research Libraries, Nov '00*

660

Healthy Aging Sourcebook

Basic Consumer Health Information about Maintaining Health through the Aging Process, Including Advice on Nutrition, Exercise, and Sleep, Help in Making Decisions about Midlife Issues and Retirement, and Guidance Concerning Practical and Informed Choices in Health Consumerism

Along with Data Concerning the Theories of Aging, Different Experiences in Aging by Minority Groups, and Facts about Aging Now and Aging in the Future; and Featuring a Glossary, a Guide to Consumer Help, Additional Suggested Reading, and Practical Resource Directory

Edited by Jenifer Swanson. 536 pages. 1999. 0-7808-0390-6. $78.

"Recommended reference source."
—Booklist, American Library Association, Feb '00

SEE ALSO Physical & Mental Issues in Aging Sourcebook

Healthy Heart Sourcebook for Women

Basic Consumer Health Information about Cardiac Issues Specific to Women, Including Facts about Major Risk Factors and Prevention, Treatment and Control Strategies, and Important Dietary Issues

Along with a Special Section Regarding the Pros and Cons of Hormone Replacement Therapy and Its Impact on Heart Health, and Additional Help, Including Recipes, a Glossary, and a Directory of Resources

Edited by Dawn D. Matthews. 336 pages. 2000. 0-7808-0329-9. $78.

"A good reference source and recommended for all public, academic, medical, and hospital libraries."
—Medical Reference Services Quarterly, Summer '01

"Because of the lack of information specific to women on this topic, this book is recommended for public libraries and consumer libraries."
—American Reference Books Annual, 2001

"Contains very important information about coronary artery disease that all women should know. The information is current and presented in an easy-to-read format. The book will make a good addition to any library." *—American Medical Writers Association Journal, Summer '00*

"Important, basic reference."
—Reviewer's Bookwatch, Jul '00

SEE ALSO Cardiovascular Diseases & Disorders Sourcebook, 1st Edition, Heart Diseases & Disorders Sourcebook, 2nd Edition, Women's Health Concerns Sourcebook

---

Heart Diseases & Disorders Sourcebook, 2nd Edition

Basic Consumer Health Information about Heart Attacks, Angina, Rhythm Disorders, Heart Failure, Valve Disease, Congenital Heart Disorders, and More, Including Descriptions of Surgical Procedures and Other Interventions, Medications, Cardiac Rehabilitation, Risk Identification, and Prevention Tips

Along with Statistical Data, Reports on Current Research Initiatives, a Glossary of Cardiovascular Terms, and Resource Directory

Edited by Karen Bellenir. 612 pages. 2000. 0-7808-0238-1. $78.

"This work stands out as an imminently accessible resource for the general public. It is recommended for the reference and circulating shelves of school, public, and academic libraries."
—American Reference Books Annual, 2001

"Recommended reference source."
—Booklist, American Library Association, Dec '00

"Provides comprehensive coverage of matters related to the heart. This title is recommended for health sciences and public libraries with consumer health collections."
—E-Streams, Oct '00

SEE ALSO Cardiovascular Diseases & Disorders Sourcebook, 1st Edition; Healthy Heart Sourcebook for Women

---

Household Safety Sourcebook

Basic Consumer Health Information about Household Safety, Including Information about Poisons, Chemicals, Fire, and Water Hazards in the Home

Along with Advice about the Safe Use of Home Maintenance Equipment, Choosing Toys and Nursery Furniture, Holiday and Recreation Safety, a Glossary, and Resources for Further Help and Information

Edited by Dawn D. Matthews. 606 pages. 2002. 0-7808-0338-8. $78.

Immune System Disorders Sourcebook

Basic Information about Lupus, Multiple Sclerosis, Guillain-Barré Syndrome, Chronic Granulomatous Disease, and More

Along with Statistical and Demographic Data and Reports on Current Research Initiatives

Edited by Allan R. Cook. 608 pages. 1997. 0-7808-0209-8. $78.

Infant & Toddler Health Sourcebook

Basic Consumer Health Information about the Physical and Mental Development of Newborns, Infants, and Toddlers, Including Neonatal Concerns, Nutrition Recommendations, Immunization Schedules, Common Pediatric Disorders, Assessments and Milestones, Safety Tips, and Advice for Parents and Other Caregivers

Along with a Glossary of Terms and Resource Listings for Additional Help

Edited by Jenifer Swanson. 585 pages. 2000. 0-7808-0246-2. $78.

"As a reference for the general public, this would be useful in any library."   —E-Streams, May '01

"Recommended reference source."
                —Booklist, American Library Association, Feb '01

"This is a good source for general use."
                —American Reference Books Annual, 2001

Injury & Trauma Sourcebook

Basic Consumer Health Information about the Impact of Injury, the Diagnosis and Treatment of Common and Traumatic Injuries, Emergency Care, and Specific Injuries Related to Home, Community, Workplace, Transportation, and Recreation

Along with Guidelines for Injury Prevention, a Glossary, and a Directory of Additional Resources

Edited by Joyce Brennfleck Shannon. 696 pages. 2002. 0-7808-0421-X. $78.

Kidney & Urinary Tract Diseases & Disorders Sourcebook

Basic Information about Kidney Stones, Urinary Incontinence, Bladder Disease, End Stage Renal Disease, Dialysis, and More

Along with Statistical and Demographic Data and Reports on Current Research Initiatives

Edited by Linda M. Ross. 602 pages. 1997. 0-7808-0079-6. $78.

Learning Disabilities Sourcebook

Basic Information about Disorders Such as Dyslexia, Visual and Auditory Processing Deficits, Attention Deficit/Hyperactivity Disorder, and Autism

Along with Statistical and Demographic Data, Reports on Current Research Initiatives, an Explanation of the Assessment Process, and a Special Section for Adults with Learning Disabilities

Edited by Linda M. Shin. 579 pages. 1998. 0-7808-0210-1. $78.

Named "Outstanding Reference Book of 1999."
                —New York Public Library, Feb 2000

"An excellent candidate for inclusion in a public library reference section. It's a great source of information. Teachers will also find the book useful. Definitely worth reading."
                —Journal of Adolescent & Adult Literacy, Feb 2000

"Readable . . . provides a solid base of information regarding successful techniques used with individuals who have learning disabilities, as well as practical suggestions for educators and family members. Clear language, concise descriptions, and pertinent information

for contacting multiple resources add to the strength of this book as a useful tool."   —Choice, Association of College and Research Libraries, Feb '99

"Recommended reference source."
                —Booklist, American Library Association, Sep '98

"A useful resource for libraries and for those who don't have the time to identify and locate the individual publications."   —Disability Resources Monthly, Sep '98

Liver Disorders Sourcebook

Basic Consumer Health Information about the Liver and How It Works; Liver Diseases, Including Cancer, Cirrhosis, Hepatitis, and Toxic and Drug Related Diseases; Tips for Maintaining a Healthy Liver; Laboratory Tests, Radiology Tests, and Facts about Liver Transplantation

Along with a Section on Support Groups, a Glossary, and Resource Listings

Edited by Joyce Brennfleck Shannon. 591 pages. 2000. 0-7808-0383-3. $78.

"A valuable resource."
                —American Reference Books Annual, 2001

"This title is recommended for health sciences and public libraries with consumer health collections."
                —E-Streams, Oct '00

"Recommended reference source."
                —Booklist, American Library Association, Jun '00

Lung Disorders Sourcebook

Basic Consumer Health Information about Emphysema, Pneumonia, Tuberculosis, Asthma, Cystic Fibrosis, and Other Lung Disorders, Including Facts about Diagnostic Procedures, Treatment Strategies, Disease Prevention Efforts, and Such Risk Factors as Smoking, Air Pollution, and Exposure to Asbestos, Radon, and Other Agents

Along with a Glossary and Resources for Additional Help and Information

Edited by Dawn D. Matthews. 678 pages. 2002. 0-7808-0339-6. $78.

Medical Tests Sourcebook

Basic Consumer Health Information about Medical Tests, Including Periodic Health Exams, General Screening Tests, Tests You Can Do at Home, Findings of the U.S. Preventive Services Task Force, X-ray and Radiology Tests, Electrical Tests, Tests of Blood and Other Body Fluids and Tissues, Scope Tests, Lung Tests, Genetic Tests, Pregnancy Tests, Newborn Screening Tests, Sexually Transmitted Disease Tests, and Computer Aided Diagnoses

Along with a Section on Paying for Medical Tests, a Glossary, and Resource Listings

Edited by Joyce Brennfleck Shannon. 691 pages. 1999. 0-7808-0243-8. $78.

"Recommended for hospital and health sciences libraries with consumer health collections."
—*E-Streams, Mar '00*

"This is an overall excellent reference with a wealth of general knowledge that may aid those who are reluctant to get vital tests performed."
—*Today's Librarian, Jan 2000*

"A valuable reference guide."
—*American Reference Books Annual, 2000*

■

Men's Health Concerns Sourcebook

Basic Information about Health Issues That Affect Men, Featuring Facts about the Top Causes of Death in Men, Including Heart Disease, Stroke, Cancers, Prostate Disorders, Chronic Obstructive Pulmonary Disease, Pneumonia and Influenza, Human Immunodeficiency Virus and Acquired Immune Deficiency Syndrome, Diabetes Mellitus, Stress, Suicide, Accidents and Homicides; and Facts about Common Concerns for Men, Including Impotence, Contraception, Circumcision, Sleep Disorders, Snoring, Hair Loss, Diet, Nutrition, Exercise, Kidney and Urological Disorders, and Backaches

Edited by Allan R. Cook. 738 pages. 1998. 0-7808-0212-8. $78.

"This comprehensive resource and the series are highly recommended."
—*American Reference Books Annual, 2000*

"Recommended reference source."
—*Booklist, American Library Association, Dec '98*

■

Mental Health Disorders Sourcebook, 1st Edition

Basic Information about Schizophrenia, Depression, Bipolar Disorder, Panic Disorder, Obsessive-Compulsive Disorder, Phobias and Other Anxiety Disorders, Paranoia and Other Personality Disorders, Eating Disorders, and Sleep Disorders

Along with Information about Treatment and Therapies

Edited by Karen Bellenir. 548 pages. 1995. 0-7808-0040-0. $78.

"This is an excellent new book . . . written in easy-to-understand language."
—*Booklist Health Sciences Supplement, American Library Association, Oct '97*

". . . useful for public and academic libraries and consumer health collections."
—*Medical Reference Services Quarterly, Spring '97*

"The great strengths of the book are its readability and its inclusion of places to find more information. Especially recommended."
—*Reference Quarterly, American Library Association, Winter '96*

". . . a good resource for a consumer health library."
—*Bulletin of the Medical Library Association, Oct '96*

"The information is data-based and couched in brief, concise language that avoids jargon. . . . a useful reference source."
—*Readings, Sep '96*

"The text is well organized and adequately written for its target audience."
—*Choice, Association of College and Research Libraries, Jun '96*

". . . provides information on a wide range of mental disorders, presented in nontechnical language."
—*Exceptional Child Education Resources, Spring '96*

"Recommended for public and academic libraries."
—*Reference Book Review, 1996*

■

Mental Health Disorders Sourcebook, 2nd Edition

Basic Consumer Health Information about Anxiety Disorders, Depression and Other Mood Disorders, Eating Disorders, Personality Disorders, Schizophrenia, and More, Including Disease Descriptions, Treatment Options, and Reports on Current Research Initiatives

Along with Statistical Data, Tips for Maintaining Mental Health, a Glossary, and Directory of Sources for Additional Help and Information

Edited by Karen Bellenir. 605 pages. 2000. 0-7808-0240-3. $78.

"Well organized and well written."
—*American Reference Books Annual, 2001*

"Recommended reference source."
—*Booklist, American Library Association, Jun '00*

■

Mental Retardation Sourcebook

Basic Consumer Health Information about Mental Retardation and Its Causes, Including Down Syndrome, Fetal Alcohol Syndrome, Fragile X Syndrome, Genetic Conditions, Injury, and Environmental Sources

Along with Preventive Strategies, Parenting Issues, Educational Implications, Health Care Needs, Employment and Economic Matters, Legal Issues, a Glossary, and a Resource Listing for Additional Help and Information

Edited by Joyce Brennfleck Shannon. 642 pages. 2000. 0-7808-0377-9. $78.

"Public libraries will find the book useful for reference and as a beginning research point for students, parents, and caregivers."
—*American Reference Books Annual, 2001*

"The strength of this work is that it compiles many basic fact sheets and addresses for further information in one volume. It is intended and suitable for the general public. This sourcebook is relevant to any collection providing health information to the general public."
—*E-Streams, Nov '00*

"From preventing retardation to parenting and family challenges, this covers health, social and legal issues and will prove an invaluable overview."
—*Reviewer's Bookwatch, Jul '00*

Obesity Sourcebook

Basic Consumer Health Information about Diseases and Other Problems Associated with Obesity, and Including Facts about Risk Factors, Prevention Issues, and Management Approaches

Along with Statistical and Demographic Data, Information about Special Populations, Research Updates, a Glossary, and Source Listings for Further Help and Information

Edited by Wilma Caldwell and Chad T. Kimball. 376 pages. 2001. 0-7808-0333-7. $78.

"The book synthesizes the reliable medical literature on obesity into one easy-to-read and useful resource for the general public."
— *American Reference Books Annual 2002*

"This is a very useful resource book for the lay public."
—*Doody's Review Service, Nov '01*

"Well suited for the health reference collection of a public library or an academic health science library that serves the general population." —*E-Streams, Sep '01*

"Recommended reference source."
—*Booklist, American Library Association, Apr '01*

" Recommended pick both for specialty health library collections and any general consumer health reference collection." — *The Bookwatch, Apr '01*

Ophthalmic Disorders Sourcebook

Basic Information about Glaucoma, Cataracts, Macular Degeneration, Strabismus, Refractive Disorders, and More

Along with Statistical and Demographic Data and Reports on Current Research Initiatives

Edited by Linda M. Ross. 631 pages. 1996. 0-7808-0081-8. $78.

Oral Health Sourcebook

Basic Information about Diseases and Conditions Affecting Oral Health, Including Cavities, Gum Disease, Dry Mouth, Oral Cancers, Fever Blisters, Canker Sores, Oral Thrush, Bad Breath, Temporomandibular Disorders, and other Craniofacial Syndromes

Along with Statistical Data on the Oral Health of Americans, Oral Hygiene, Emergency First Aid, Information on Treatment Procedures and Methods of Replacing Lost Teeth

Edited by Allan R. Cook. 558 pages. 1997. 0-7808-0082-6. $78.

"Unique source which will fill a gap in dental sources for patients and the lay public. A valuable reference tool even in a library with thousands of books on dentistry. Comprehensive, clear, inexpensive, and easy to read and use. It fills an enormous gap in the health care literature." — *Reference and User Services Quarterly, American Library Association, Summer '98*

"Recommended reference source."
— *Booklist, American Library Association, Dec '97*

Osteoporosis Sourcebook

Basic Consumer Health Information about Primary and Secondary Osteoporosis and Juvenile Osteoporosis and Related Conditions, Including Fibrous Dysplasia, Gaucher Disease, Hyperthyroidism, Hypophosphatasia, Myeloma, Osteopetrosis, Osteogenesis Imperfecta, and Paget's Disease

Along with Information about Risk Factors, Treatments, Traditional and Non-Traditional Pain Management, a Glossary of Related Terms, and a Directory of Resources

Edited by Allan R. Cook. 584 pages. 2001. 0-7808-0239-X. $78.

"This would be a book to be kept in a staff or patient library. The targeted audience is the layperson, but the therapist who needs a quick bit of information on a particular topic will also find the book useful."
—*Physical Therapy, Jan '02*

"This resource is recommended as a great reference source for public, health, and academic libraries, and is another triumph for the editors of Omnigraphics."
— *American Reference Books Annual 2002*

"Recommended for all public libraries and general health collections, especially those supporting patient education or consumer health programs."
—*E-Streams, Nov '01*

"Will prove valuable to any library seeking to maintain a current, comprehensive reference collection of health resources. . . . From prevention to treatment and associated conditions, this provides an excellent survey."
—*The Bookwatch, Aug '01*

"Recommended reference source."
—*Booklist, American Library Association, July '01*

SEE ALSO Women's Health Concerns Sourcebook

Pain Sourcebook, 1st Edition

Basic Information about Specific Forms of Acute and Chronic Pain, Including Headaches, Back Pain, Muscular Pain, Neuralgia, Surgical Pain, and Cancer Pain

Along with Pain Relief Options Such as Analgesics, Narcotics, Nerve Blocks, Transcutaneous Nerve Stimulation, and Alternative Forms of Pain Control, Including Biofeedback, Imaging, Behavior Modification, and Relaxation Techniques

Edited by Allan R. Cook. 667 pages. 1997. 0-7808-0213-6. $78.

"The text is readable, easily understood, and well indexed. This excellent volume belongs in all patient education libraries, consumer health sections of public libraries, and many personal collections."
— *American Reference Books Annual, 1999*

"A beneficial reference." — *Booklist Health Sciences Supplement, American Library Association, Oct '98*

"The information is basic in terms of scholarship and is appropriate for general readers. Written in journalistic style . . . intended for non-professionals. Quite thorough

664

in its coverage of different pain conditions and summarizes the latest clinical information regarding pain treatment." — *Choice, Association of College and Research Libraries, Jun '98*

"Recommended reference source."
— *Booklist, American Library Association, Mar '98*

■

Pain Sourcebook, 2nd Edition

Basic Consumer Health Information about Specific Forms of Acute and Chronic Pain, Including Muscle and Skeletal Pain, Nerve Pain, Cancer Pain, and Disorders Characterized by Pain, Such as Fibromyalgia, Shingles, Angina, Arthritis, and Headaches

Along with Information about Pain Medications and Management Techniques, Complementary and Alternative Pain Relief Options, Tips for People Living with Chronic Pain, a Glossary, and a Directory of Sources for Further Information

Edited by Karen Bellenir. 670 pages. 2002. 0-7808-0612-3. $78.

■

Pediatric Cancer Sourcebook

Basic Consumer Health Information about Leukemias, Brain Tumors, Sarcomas, Lymphomas, and Other Cancers in Infants, Children, and Adolescents, Including Descriptions of Cancers, Treatments, and Coping Strategies

Along with Suggestions for Parents, Caregivers, and Concerned Relatives, a Glossary of Cancer Terms, and Resource Listings

Edited by Edward J. Prucha. 587 pages. 1999. 0-7808-0245-4. $78.

"An excellent source of information. Recommended for public, hospital, and health science libraries with consumer health collections." — *E-Streams, Jun '00*

"Recommended reference source."
— *Booklist, American Library Association, Feb '00*

"A valuable addition to all libraries specializing in health services and many public libraries."
— *American Reference Books Annual, 2000*

■

Physical & Mental Issues in Aging Sourcebook

Basic Consumer Health Information on Physical and Mental Disorders Associated with the Aging Process, Including Concerns about Cardiovascular Disease, Pulmonary Disease, Oral Health, Digestive Disorders, Musculoskeletal and Skin Disorders, Metabolic Changes, Sexual and Reproductive Issues, and Changes in Vision, Hearing, and Other Senses

Along with Data about Longevity and Causes of Death, Information on Acute and Chronic Pain, Descriptions of Mental Concerns, a Glossary of Terms, and Resource Listings for Additional Help

Edited by Jenifer Swanson. 660 pages. 1999. 0-7808-0233-0. $78.

"This is a treasure of health information for the layperson." — *Choice Health Sciences Supplement, Association of College & Research Libraries, May 2000*

"Recommended for public libraries."
— *American Reference Books Annual, 2000*

"Recommended reference source."
— *Booklist, American Library Association, Oct '99*

SEE ALSO *Healthy Aging Sourcebook*

■

Podiatry Sourcebook

Basic Consumer Health Information about Foot Conditions, Diseases, and Injuries, Including Bunions, Corns, Calluses, Athlete's Foot, Plantar Warts, Hammertoes and Clawtoes, Clubfoot, Heel Pain, Gout, and More

Along with Facts about Foot Care, Disease Prevention, Foot Safety, Choosing a Foot Care Specialist, a Glossary of Terms, and Resource Listings for Additional Information

Edited by M. Lisa Weatherford. 380 pages. 2001. 0-7808-0215-2. $78.

"Recommended reference source."
— *Booklist, American Library Association, Feb '02*

"There is a lot of information presented here on a topic that is usually only covered sparingly in most larger comprehensive medical encyclopedias."
— *American Reference Books Annual 2002*

■

Pregnancy & Birth Sourcebook

Basic Information about Planning for Pregnancy, Maternal Health, Fetal Growth and Development, Labor and Delivery, Postpartum and Perinatal Care, Pregnancy in Mothers with Special Concerns, and Disorders of Pregnancy, Including Genetic Counseling, Nutrition and Exercise, Obstetrical Tests, Pregnancy Discomfort, Multiple Births, Cesarean Sections, Medical Testing of Newborns, Breastfeeding, Gestational Diabetes, and Ectopic Pregnancy

Edited by Heather E. Aldred. 737 pages. 1997. 0-7808-0216-0. $78.

"A well-organized handbook. Recommended."
— *Choice, Association of College and Research Libraries, Apr '98*

"Recommended reference source."
— *Booklist, American Library Association, Mar '98*

"Recommended for public libraries."
— *American Reference Books Annual, 1998*

SEE ALSO *Congenital Disorders Sourcebook, Family Planning Sourcebook*

Prostate Cancer Sourcebook

Basic Consumer Health Information about Prostate Cancer, Including Information about the Associated Risk Factors, Detection, Diagnosis, and Treatment of Prostate Cancer

Along with Information on Non-Malignant Prostate Conditions, and Featuring a Section Listing Support and Treatment Centers and a Glossary of Related Terms

Edited by Dawn D. Matthews. 358 pages. 2001. 0-7808-0324-8. $78.

"Recommended reference source."
—Booklist, American Library Association, Jan '02

"A valuable resource for health care consumers seeking information on the subject....All text is written in a clear, easy-to-understand language that avoids technical jargon. Any library that collects consumer health resources would strengthen their collection with the addition of the *Prostate Cancer Sourcebook*."
— American Reference Books Annual 2002

■

Public Health Sourcebook

Basic Information about Government Health Agencies, Including National Health Statistics and Trends, Healthy People 2000 Program Goals and Objectives, the Centers for Disease Control and Prevention, the Food and Drug Administration, and the National Institutes of Health

Along with Full Contact Information for Each Agency

Edited by Wendy Wilcox. 698 pages. 1998. 0-7808-0220-9. $78.

"Recommended reference source."
— Booklist, American Library Association, Sep '98

"This consumer guide provides welcome assistance in navigating the maze of federal health agencies and their data on public health concerns."
— SciTech Book News, Sep '98

■

Reconstructive & Cosmetic Surgery Sourcebook

Basic Consumer Health Information on Cosmetic and Reconstructive Plastic Surgery, Including Statistical Information about Different Surgical Procedures, Things to Consider Prior to Surgery, Plastic Surgery Techniques and Tools, Emotional and Psychological Considerations, and Procedure-Specific Information

Along with a Glossary of Terms and a Listing of Resources for Additional Help and Information

Edited by M. Lisa Weatherford. 374 pages. 2001. 0-7808-0214-4. $78.

"An excellent reference that addresses cosmetic and medically necessary reconstructive surgeries. . . . The style of the prose is calm and reassuring, discussing the many positive outcomes now available due to advances in surgical techniques."
— American Reference Books Annual 2002

"Recommended for health science libraries that are open to the public, as well as hospital libraries that are open to the patients. This book is a good resource for the consumer interested in plastic surgery."
—E-Streams, Dec '01

"Recommended reference source."
—Booklist, American Library Association, July '01

■

Rehabilitation Sourcebook

Basic Consumer Health Information about Rehabilitation for People Recovering from Heart Surgery, Spinal Cord Injury, Stroke, Orthopedic Impairments, Amputation, Pulmonary Impairments, Traumatic Injury, and More, Including Physical Therapy, Occupational Therapy, Speech/ Language Therapy, Massage Therapy, Dance Therapy, Art Therapy, and Recreational Therapy

Along with Information on Assistive and Adaptive Devices, a Glossary, and Resources for Additional Help and Information

Edited by Dawn D. Matthews. 531 pages. 1999. 0-7808-0236-5. $78.

"This is an excellent resource for public library reference and health collections."
—American Reference Books Annual, 2001

"Recommended reference source."
— Booklist, American Library Association, May '00

■

Respiratory Diseases & Disorders Sourcebook

Basic Information about Respiratory Diseases and Disorders, Including Asthma, Cystic Fibrosis, Pneumonia, the Common Cold, Influenza, and Others, Featuring Facts about the Respiratory System, Statistical and Demographic Data, Treatments, Self-Help Management Suggestions, and Current Research Initiatives

Edited by Allan R. Cook and Peter D. Dresser. 771 pages. 1995. 0-7808-0037-0. $78.

"Designed for the layperson and for patients and their families coping with respiratory illness. . . . an extensive array of information on diagnosis, treatment, management, and prevention of respiratory illnesses for the general reader."
— Choice, Association of College and Research Libraries, Jun '96

"A highly recommended text for all collections. It is a comforting reminder of the power of knowledge that good books carry between their covers."
— Academic Library Book Review, Spring '96

"A comprehensive collection of authoritative information presented in a nontechnical, humanitarian style for patients, families, and caregivers."
—Association of Operating Room Nurses, Sep/Oct '95

Sexually Transmitted Diseases Sourcebook, 1st Edition

Basic Information about Herpes, Chlamydia, Gonorrhea, Hepatitis, Nongonoccocal Urethritis, Pelvic Inflammatory Disease, Syphilis, AIDS, and More

Along with Current Data on Treatments and Preventions

Edited by Linda M. Ross. 550 pages. 1997. 0-7808-0217-9. $78.

■

Sexually Transmitted Diseases Sourcebook, 2nd Edition

Basic Consumer Health Information about Sexually Transmitted Diseases, Including Information on the Diagnosis and Treatment of Chlamydia, Gonorrhea, Hepatitis, Herpes, HIV, Mononucleosis, Syphilis, and Others

Along with Information on Prevention, Such as Condom Use, Vaccines, and STD Education; And Featuring a Section on Issues Related to Youth and Adolescents, a Glossary, and Resources for Additional Help and Information

Edited by Dawn D. Matthews. 538 pages. 2001. 0-7808-0249-7. $78.

"Recommended for consumer health collections in public libraries, and secondary school and community college libraries."
— *American Reference Books Annual 2002*

"Every school and public library should have a copy of this comprehensive and user-friendly reference book."
— *Choice, Association of College & Research Libraries, Sep '01*

"This is a highly recommended book. This is an especially important book for all school and public libraries." — *AIDS Book Review Journal, Jul-Aug '01*

"Recommended reference source."
— *Booklist, American Library Association, Apr '01*

"Recommended pick both for specialty health library collections and any general consumer health reference collection." — *The Bookwatch, Apr '01*

■

Skin Disorders Sourcebook

Basic Information about Common Skin and Scalp Conditions Caused by Aging, Allergies, Immune Reactions, Sun Exposure, Infectious Organisms, Parasites, Cosmetics, and Skin Traumas, Including Abrasions, Cuts, and Pressure Sores

Along with Information on Prevention and Treatment

Edited by Allan R. Cook. 647 pages. 1997. 0-7808-0080-X. $78.

"... comprehensive, easily read reference book."
— *Doody's Health Sciences Book Reviews, Oct '97*

SEE ALSO *Burns Sourcebook*

Sleep Disorders Sourcebook

Basic Consumer Health Information about Sleep and Its Disorders, Including Insomnia, Sleepwalking, Sleep Apnea, Restless Leg Syndrome, and Narcolepsy

Along with Data about Shiftwork and Its Effects, Information on the Societal Costs of Sleep Deprivation, Descriptions of Treatment Options, a Glossary of Terms, and Resource Listings for Additional Help

Edited by Jenifer Swanson. 439 pages. 1998. 0-7808-0234-9. $78.

"This text will complement any home or medical library. It is user-friendly and ideal for the adult reader."
— *American Reference Books Annual, 2000*

"A useful resource that provides accurate, relevant, and accessible information on sleep to the general public. Health care providers who deal with sleep disorders patients may also find it helpful in being prepared to answer some of the questions patients ask."
— *Respiratory Care, Jul '99*

"Recommended reference source."
— *Booklist, American Library Association, Feb '99*

■

Sports Injuries Sourcebook

Basic Consumer Health Information about Common Sports Injuries, Prevention of Injury in Specific Sports, Tips for Training, and Rehabilitation from Injury

Along with Information about Special Concerns for Children, Young Girls in Athletic Training Programs, Senior Athletes, and Women Athletes, and a Directory of Resources for Further Help and Information

Edited by Heather E. Aldred. 624 pages. 1999. 0-7808-0218-7. $78.

"While this easy-to-read book is recommended for all libraries, it should prove to be especially useful for public, high school, and academic libraries; certainly it should be on the bookshelf of every school gymnasium." — *E-Streams, Mar '00*

"Public libraries and undergraduate academic libraries will find this book useful for its nontechnical language." — *American Reference Books Annual, 2000*

■

Stress-Related Disorders Sourcebook

Basic Consumer Health Information about Stress and Stress-Related Disorders, Including Stress Origins and Signals, Environmental Stress at Work and Home, Mental and Emotional Stress Associated with Depression, Post-Traumatic Stress Disorder, Panic Disorder, Suicide, and the Physical Effects of Stress on the Cardiovascular, Immune, and Nervous Systems

Along with Stress Management Techniques, a Glossary, and a Listing of Additional Resources

Edited by Joyce Brennfleck Shannon. 600 pages. 2002. 0-7808-0560-7. $78.

Substance Abuse Sourcebook

Basic Health-Related Information about the Abuse of Legal and Illegal Substances Such as Alcohol, Tobacco, Prescription Drugs, Marijuana, Cocaine, and Heroin; and Including Facts about Substance Abuse Prevention Strategies, Intervention Methods, Treatment and Recovery Programs, and a Section Addressing the Special Problems Related to Substance Abuse during Pregnancy

Edited by Karen Bellenir. 573 pages. 1996. 0-7808-0038-9. $78.

"A valuable addition to any health reference section. Highly recommended."
— *The Book Report, Mar/Apr '97*

". . . a comprehensive collection of substance abuse information that's both highly readable and compact. Families and caregivers of substance abusers will find the information enlightening and helpful, while teachers, social workers and journalists should benefit from the concise format. Recommended."
— *Drug Abuse Update, Winter '96/'97*

SEE ALSO *Alcoholism Sourcebook, Drug Abuse Sourcebook*

■

Transplantation Sourcebook

Basic Consumer Health Information about Organ and Tissue Transplantation, Including Physical and Financial Preparations, Procedures and Issues Relating to Specific Solid Organ and Tissue Transplants, Rehabilitation, Pediatric Transplant Information, the Future of Transplantation, and Organ and Tissue Donation

Along with a Glossary and Listings of Additional Resources

Edited by Joyce Brennfleck Shannon. 628 pages. 2002. 0-7808-0322-1. $78.

■

Traveler's Health Sourcebook

Basic Consumer Health Information for Travelers, Including Physical and Medical Preparations, Transportation Health and Safety, Essential Information about Food and Water, Sun Exposure, Insect and Snake Bites, Camping and Wilderness Medicine, and Travel with Physical or Medical Disabilities

Along with International Travel Tips, Vaccination Recommendations, Geographical Health Issues, Disease Risks, a Glossary, and a Listing of Additional Resources

Edited by Joyce Brennfleck Shannon. 613 pages. 2000. 0-7808-0384-1. $78.

"Recommended reference source."
— *Booklist, American Library Association, Feb '01*

"This book is recommended for any public library, any travel collection, and especially any collection for the physically disabled."
— *American Reference Books Annual, 2001*

Women's Health Concerns Sourcebook

Basic Information about Health Issues That Affect Women, Featuring Facts about Menstruation and Other Gynecological Concerns, Including Endometriosis, Fibroids, Menopause, and Vaginitis; Reproductive Concerns, Including Birth Control, Infertility, and Abortion; and Facts about Additional Physical, Emotional, and Mental Health Concerns Prevalent among Women Such as Osteoporosis, Urinary Tract Disorders, Eating Disorders, and Depression

Along with Tips for Maintaining a Healthy Lifestyle

Edited by Heather E. Aldred. 567 pages. 1997. 0-7808-0219-5. $78.

"Handy compilation. There is an impressive range of diseases, devices, disorders, procedures, and other physical and emotional issues covered . . . well organized, illustrated, and indexed."
— *Choice, Association of College and Research Libraries, Jan '98*

SEE ALSO *Breast Cancer Sourcebook, Cancer Sourcebook for Women, 1st and 2nd Editions, Healthy Heart Sourcebook for Women, Osteoporosis Sourcebook*

■

Workplace Health & Safety Sourcebook

Basic Consumer Health Information about Workplace Health and Safety, Including the Effect of Workplace Hazards on the Lungs, Skin, Heart, Ears, Eyes, Brain, Reproductive Organs, Musculoskeletal System, and Other Organs and Body Parts

Along with Information about Occupational Cancer, Personal Protective Equipment, Toxic and Hazardous Chemicals, Child Labor, Stress, and Workplace Violence

Edited by Chad T. Kimball. 626 pages. 2000. 0-7808-0231-4. $78.

"As a reference for the general public, this would be useful in any library."
— *E-Streams, Jun '01*

"Provides helpful information for primary care physicians and other caregivers interested in occupational medicine. . . . General readers; professionals."
— *Choice, Association of College & Research Libraries, May '01*

"Recommended reference source."
— *Booklist, American Library Association, Feb '01*

"Highly recommended." — *The Bookwatch, Jan '01*

Worldwide Health Sourcebook

Basic Information about Global Health Issues, Including Malnutrition, Reproductive Health, Disease Dispersion and Prevention, Emerging Diseases, Risky Health Behaviors, and the Leading Causes of Death

Along with Global Health Concerns for Children, Women, and the Elderly, Mental Health Issues, Research and Technology Advancements, and Economic, Environmental, and Political Health Implications, a Glossary, and a Resource Listing for Additional Help and Information

Edited by Joyce Brennfleck Shannon. 614 pages. 2001. 0-7808-0330-2. $78.

"Named an Outstanding Academic Title."
> —*Choice, Association of College & Research Libraries, Jan '02*

"Yet another handy but also unique compilation in the extensive Health Reference Series, this is a useful work because many of the international publications reprinted or excerpted are not readily available. Highly recommended."
> —*Choice, Association of College & Research Libraries, Nov '01*

"Recommended reference source."
> —*Booklist, American Library Association, Oct '01*

Teen Health Series

*Helping Young Adults Understand, Manage,
and Avoid Serious Illness*

Diet Information for Teens
Health Tips about Diet and Nutrition

*Including Facts about Nutrients, Dietary Guidelines,
Breakfasts, School Lunches, Snacks, Party Food, Weight
Control, Eating Disorders, and More*

Edited by Karen Bellenir. 399 pages. 2001. 0-7808-0441-4. $58.

"Full of helpful insights and facts throughout the book.
. . . An excellent resource to be placed in public libraries
or even in personal collections."
—*American Reference Books Annual 2002*

"Recommended for middle and high school libraries
and media centers as well as academic libraries that
educate future teachers of teenagers. It is also a suitable
addition to health science libraries that serve patrons
who are interested in teen health promotion and education."
—*E-Streams, Oct '01*

"This comprehensive book would be beneficial to collections that need information about nutrition, dietary
guidelines, meal planning, and weight control. . . . This
reference is so easy to use that its purchase is recommended."
—*The Book Report, Sep-Oct '01*

"This book is written in an easy to understand format
describing issues that many teens face every day, and
then provides thoughtful explanations so that teens can
make informed decisions. This is an interesting book
that provides important facts and information for
today's teens."
—*Doody's Health Sciences
Book Review Journal, Jul-Aug '01*

"A comprehensive compendium of diet and nutrition.
The information is presented in a straightforward,
plain-spoken manner. This title will be useful to those
working on reports on a variety of topics, as well as to
general readers concerned about their dietary health."
—*School Library Journal, Jun '01*

Drug Information for Teens
Health Tips about the Physical and Mental Effects of Substance Abuse

*Including Facts about Alcohol, Anabolic Steroids, Club
Drugs, Cocaine, Depressants, Hallucinogens, Herbal
Products, Inhalants, Marijuana, Narcotics, Stimulants,
Tobacco, and More*

Edited by Karen Bellenir. 400 pages. 2002. 0-7808-0444-9. $58.

Mental Health Information for Teens
Health Tips about Mental Health and Mental Illness

*Including Facts about Anxiety, Depression, Suicide,
Eating Disorders, Obsessive-Compulsive Disorders,
Panic Attacks, Phobias, Schizophrenia, and More*

Edited by Karen Bellenir. 406 pages. 2001. 0-7808-0442-2. $58.

"In both language and approach, this user-friendly entry
in the *Teen Health Series* is on target for teens needing
information on mental health concerns." —*Booklist,
American Library Association, Jan '02*

"Readers will find the material accessible and informative, with the shaded notes, facts, and embedded glossary insets adding appropriately to the already interesting and succinct presentation."
—*School Library Journal, Jan '02*

"This title is highly recommended for any library that
serves adolescents and parents/caregivers of adolescents."
—*E-Streams, Jan '02*

"Recommended for high school libraries and young
adult collections in public libraries. Both health professionals and teenagers will find this book useful."
—*American Reference Books Annual 2002*

"This is a nice book written to enlighten the society,
primarily teenagers, about common teen mental health
issues. It is highly recommended to teachers and parents as well as adolescents."
—*Doody's Review Service, Dec '01*

Sexual Health Information for Teens
Health Tips about Sexual Development, Human Reproduction, and Sexually Transmitted Diseases

*Including Facts about Puberty, Reproductive Health,
Chlamydia, Human Papillomavirus, Pelvic Inflammatory Disease, Herpes, AIDS, Contraception, Pregnancy, and More*

Edited by Deborah A. Stanley. 400 pages. 2002. 0-7808-0445-7. $58.

Health Reference Series